Adolescent Rheumatology

Adolescent Rheumatology

Edited by
Janet E. McDonagh
University of Birmingham
Birmingham, UK

Patience H. White
George Washington University School of Medicine and Health Sciences
Washington, DC, USA

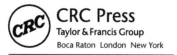

CRC Press
Taylor & Francis Group
Boca Raton   London   New York

CRC Press is an imprint of the
Taylor & Francis Group, an **informa** business

CRC Press
Taylor & Francis Group
6000 Broken Sound Parkway NW, Suite 300
Boca Raton, FL 33487-2742

First issued in paperback 2019

© 2008 by Taylor & Francis Group, LLC
CRC Press is an imprint of Taylor & Francis Group, an Informa business

No claim to original U.S. Government works

ISBN-13: 978-0-8493-9890-2 (hbk)
ISBN-13: 978-0-367-38767-9 (pbk)

Library of Congress Cataloging-in-Publication Data

Adolescent rheumatology/edited by Janet E. McDonagh, Patience H. White.
    p. ; cm.
Includes bibliographical references and index.
ISBN-13: 978-0-8493-9890-2 (hb : alk. paper)
    ISBN-10: 0-8493-9890-8 (hb : alk. paper) 1. Adolescent rheumatology. I. McDonagh,
Janet E. II. White, Patience H.
    [DNLM: 1. Rheumatic Diseases. 2. Adolescent. WE 544 A239 2008]
    RJ482.R48A33 2008
    618.92'723–dc22   2007033151

Visit the Taylor & Francis Web site at
http://www.taylorandfrancis.com

and the CRC Press Web site at
http://www.crcpress.com

To
Chris, DJ, Niall, Cara, and Nate,
and to all those young people who are, have been,
and will be in our care as rheumatologists.

Preface

The exemplars of childhood-onset chronic illnesses usually listed in the adolescent health literature rarely include rheumatic disease despite its having a similar or greater prevalence than other conditions, such as childhood diabetes or cystic fibrosis, and significant reported morbidities. Young people with rheumatic disease and their families therefore richly deserve a book dedicated solely to them and their health care.

Adolescent Rheumatology aims to provide a unique clinical approach that concentrates on the adolescent-specific aspects of health and rheumatic disease. We hope it will be useful and informative to the whole multidisciplinary rheumatology team, pediatric as well as adult, and to the other professionals who come into contact with young people with rheumatic disease. The international group of contributors was specifically selected to reflect the multidisciplinary nature of adolescent rheumatology and to include both pediatric and adult rheumatology professionals and young people themselves.

Adolescent Rheumatology starts with chapters that describe the context of being a young person in the twenty-first century, highlighting the impact of rheumatic disease on adolescent development. The interplay of the biological, psychological, and social elements of adolescent development and the interface with peers, family, and the wider community are fundamental to adolescent rheumatology. This importance is reflected in the attention developmental medicine receives throughout *Adolescent Rheumatology*. The next chapters address specific adolescent issues related to the main conditions in the adolescent rheumatology spectrum, namely juvenile idiopathic arthritis, systemic lupus erythematosus, chronic idiopathic pain syndromes, back pain, sports injuries, and osteoporosis. The following chapters remind us that young people with rheumatic disease are teenagers first and foremost. They explore the generic issues that characterize adolescence, including the "sex, drugs, and rock 'n' roll." Evidence suggests that young people with rheumatic disease are just as exploratory and risk-taking as their healthy peers but face a "double whammy" from both the potential dangers of such behaviors and the effect such behaviors can have on their condition and/or therapy. Chapters addressing parenting and peer issues in the context of rheumatic disease are also included, reflecting the importance of the dynamic nature of relationships with parents and friends throughout adolescence.

Envisioning futures is an important characteristic of adolescent rheumatology whether it be choosing the proactive rather than reactive approach to care or considering the prognosis of rheumatic disease into adulthood. The final chapters of *Adolescent Rheumatology* are therefore future-focused, addressing the coordination of the transition process as young people move from child- to adult-centered care and, in particular, how the vocational aspects of adolescent development are addressed in this process. The penultimate chapters of the book address two areas rarely included in standard pediatric rheumatology books that are of particular importance in the relatively new world of adolescent rheumatology—training in adolescent health and quality improvement. Although training programs are well established in Australia and North America, they are currently in their relative infancy in Europe. This has obvious implications for the quality of adolescent service provision such specialties as rheumatology. The consultation with and participation of young people is an important quality criteria of young person-friendly rheumatology services. The book's final chapter has been uniquely written by young people with rheumatic disease from several countries, enabling some of their voices to be heard. Young people truly have the last word!

Janet E. McDonagh
Patience H. White

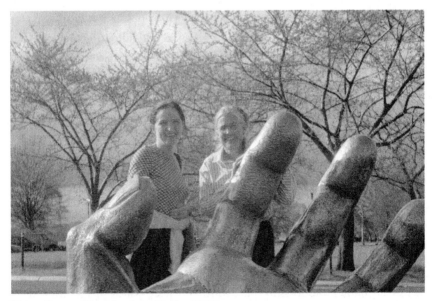

The editors, Washington, D.C., 2003!

Acknowledgments

As this book is published, I will celebrate 10 years of friendship with and mentorship from my co-editor, Professor Patience H. White. Our collaboration began with my award of a traveling fellowship from the Royal College of Physicians and Surgeons of Glasgow (Scotland) to spend time at the Adolescent Employment Readiness Center at the Children's National Medical Center in Washington, D.C. At the same time, I wrote up an audit project on behalf of the British Paediatric Rheumatology Group that revealed 82% of units seeing children with rheumatic disease in the United Kingdom had no specific service arrangements for adolescents. So, if you are a rheumatology trainee, beware where you travel during your training and carefully consider the nature of any audit question you ask as they can truly shape your future career!

However, the real experts in adolescent rheumatology are the young people themselves. It was therefore with extra delight that the publishers agreed to include a chapter written (Chapter 19) by young people with rheumatic disease. As one 15-year-old girl so eloquently writes:

Kids have changed over the years; they don't sit back and listen anymore. If there is a chance for their point to be heard, they will say it. Teenagers like to have fun and be childish at times but we do like to be treated as adults and given choices, not have choices made for us.

—Katie

And so it is for Katie and for all the other young people with rheumatic disease to whom this book is dedicated, who continue to be my most effective teachers of adolescent health and who deserve to be listened to *and* heard!

Contents

ix

Contributors

Amy Abrams Coventry, U.K.

Maria Luisa Bianchi Bone Metabolism Unit, Istituto Auxologico Italiano, IRCCS, Milano, Italy

Priscilla L. Campbell-Stokes Paediatric Department, Hutt Hospital, Lower Hutt, Wellington, New Zealand

Rolando Cimaz Department of Pediatrics, Meyer Children's Hospital, Firenze, Italy

Heather Clarke Department of Paediatric and Adolescent Rheumatology, Birmingham Children's Hospital, Birmingham, U.K.

Jacqui G. Clinch Adolescent Pain Management Service, Royal National Hospital for Rheumatic Diseases, Bath, U.K.

Rebecca A. Demorest Department of Orthopedics and Sports Medicine, Children's National Medical Center, and The George Washington University School of Medicine and Health Sciences, Washington D.C., U.S.A.

Marcelle de Sousa University College Hospital, University College London Hospitals NHS Foundation Trust, London, U.K.

Fabienne Dobbels Center for Health Services and Nursing Research, Katholieke Universiteit Leuven, Leuven, Belgium

Helena Fonseca Pediatric Division, Hospital de Santa Maria, Faculdade de Medicina de Lisboa, Lisboa, Portugal

Boel Andersson Gäre Futurum Academy of Health and Care, Jönköping County Council, Jönköping, and Department of Pediatrics, Linköping University, Linköping, Sweden

Marjorie M. Godfrey The Dartmouth Institute for Health Policy and Clinical Practice, Dartmouth Medical School, Lebanon, New Hampshire, U.S.A.

Donald E. Greydanus Michigan State University College of Human Medicine, Michigan State University/Kalamazoo Center for Medical Studies, Kalamazoo, Michigan, U.S.A.

Janine Hackett Department of Paediatric and Adolescent Rheumatology, Birmingham Children's Hospital, Birmingham, U.K.

Bernadette Johnson Department of Paediatric and Adolescent Rheumatology, Birmingham Children's Hospital, Birmingham, U.K.

Yukiko Kimura Section of Pediatric Rheumatology, Joseph M. Sanzari Children's Hospital, Hackensack University Medical Center, Hackensack, and University of Medicine and Dentistry of New Jersey (UMDNJ) Medical School, Newark, New Jersey, U.S.A.

David Lewis Birmingham, U.K.

Suzanne C. Li Section of Pediatric Rheumatology, Joseph M. Sanzari Children's Hospital, Hackensack University Medical Center, Hackensack, and University of Medicine and Dentistry of New Jersey (UMDNJ) Medical School, Newark, New Jersey, U.S.A.

Liza J. McCann Department of Paediatric Rheumatology, Royal Liverpool Children's Hospital, Alder Hey, Liverpool, U.K.

Janet E. McDonagh Division of Reproductive and Child Health, University of Birmingham, Birmingham, U.K.

Toni Neufille London, U.K.

Jon C. Packham Staffordshire Rheumatology Centre, Haywood Hospital, Stoke on Trent, and Primary Care Musculoskeletal Research Centre, Keele University, Staffordshire, U.K.

Dilip R. Patel Michigan State University College of Human Medicine, Michigan State University/Kalamazoo Center for Medical Studies, Kalamazoo, Michigan, U.S.A.

Akikur Rahman Birmingham, U.K.

Lindsay Robertson Department of Rheumatology, Derriford Hospital, Plymouth, U.K.

Debajit Sen University College London Hospital, Middlesex NHS Trust and Great Ormond Street NHS Trust, London, U.K.

Karen L. Shaw School of Health Sciences, University of Birmingham, Birmingham, U.K.

Nick J. Shaw Departments of Rheumatology and Endocrinology, Birmingham Children's Hospital, Birmingham, U.K.

Lori B. Tucker Division of Rheumatology, Centre for Community Child Health Research, BC Children's Hospital, Vancouver, British Columbia, Canada

Gerald Ullrich   Department of Pediatric Pulmonology and Neonatology, Children's Hospital, Hannover Medical School, Hannover, Germany

Patience H. White   Departments of Medicine and Pediatrics, The George Washington University School of Medicine and Health Sciences, and Arthritis Foundation, Washington, D.C., U.S.A.

1

Being a Teenager in the Twenty-First Century

Janet E. McDonagh

Division of Reproductive and Child Health, University of Birmingham, Birmingham, U.K.

INTRODUCTION

For readers of this book who are 30 years or older(!) the world we now live in is very different from the world when we were teenagers, and it is likely to continue to change at a rapid pace throughout this century. The social profile and adolescent trajectory is changing. As a result, adolescence is becoming a more complex life stage, longer in duration, and (potentially) more risky, with new rights and responsibilities for young people themselves. Adolescents constitute a significant percentage of the population, have a distinct pattern of health and illness, and are one subset of the general population that has experienced little or least improvement in overall health status over the past 40 years.

Chapter 19 encourages us to listen further to the voices of young people, but perhaps we can start with one of the best descriptions in the published literature, from a young participant with juvenile idiopathic arthritis (JIA) in the first controlled study of transitional care—"...it's not about arthritis—it's about living with it." (1).

DEFINING ADOLESCENCE

Adolescence is a biopsychosocial construct that, by definition, cannot be limited by an age criterion—it's "a stage, not an age"! Adolescence can be described as a variable period between childhood and adulthood characterized by rapid development and change in the psychological, social, and biological domains. In any professional meeting where adolescent matters are discussed, the topic of age criteria for adolescence is rarely absent. However, there are as many definitions as there are adolescents (Table 1). Although 19 years is frequently accepted as the upper age limit in the United Kingdom and the United States (3,4), other policy documents have considered this age group and found them wanting (6–8). A disproportionate prevalence of disadvantage is reported in the 16- to 25-year-old age group (7), the age band within which many of the transitions described above are likely to take place. Reassuringly, the definition of youth by both the European Union (5) and the World Health Organization (2) include the "invisible early twenties" (9). There have been recent calls from psychologists to recognize the early 20s as another stage of adolescent development—that of "emerging adulthood" —particularly in the light of the sociocultural shifts that serve to delay many of the normal adolescent transitions (8,9). This period of late adolescence and young adulthood is too often at risk of becoming a twilight zone, with young people falling out of pediatrics but not yet falling into adult medicine. When the impact of illness on adolescent development is then considered, age criteria become even more irrelevant, as developmental tasks are at risk, resulting in delay and/or limited achievement.

EPIDEMIOLOGY OF ADOLESCENTS AND ADOLESCENT RHEUMATOLOGY

In most developed countries, young people aged between 10 and 20 years account for 13% to 15% of the population, with increased representation among the ethnic minorities (10). The latter is of particular relevance in the multicultural populations of these countries and of major relevance in the sociocultural context of adolescent health.

The epidemiology of adolescent rheumatology has not been widely reported: other chronic illnesses are more frequently discussed in generic adolescent literature. However, musculoskeletal symptomatology is the third most common presentation among teenagers in primary care in the United Kingdom (11), and adolescent arthritis or rheumatism (lasting six months or

Table 1 Definitions of Adolescence

World Health Organization	10–19 years (2)
World Health Organization (Youth)	15–24 years (2)
American Academy of Pediatrics	14–19 years (3)
U.K. National Service Framework for Children, Young People, and Maternity Services	up to 19 years (4)
European Union (Youth)	15–25 years (5)

more) affects 7 per 1000 of adolescents (age 12–19 years), as reported in a nationally representative survey exploring the health status and behaviors of Canadians (12). In addition, 30 per 1000 adolescents unaffected by arthritis or rheumatism, reported chronic back problems (12). Furthermore, greater effects on measures of mental health, health services uses, school, work, and home activities of affected individuals (12- to 19-year-olds) compared with individuals without chronic disease or with other chronic disease have been reported (12). The burden of illness is not limited to adolescence either. Minden et al. reported considerable estimated 12-month costs into adulthood, although these differ among the various JIA subgroups (13).

The epidemiology of adolescent rheumatology cannot be considered in isolation. It is also important to reflect upon the predictors of adult disease identified during this developmental stage. In a study of 668 premenopausal women aged 18 to 35 years, menarche at age 15, physical inactivity as an adolescent, and low body weight were identified as independent predictors of low bone mass (14). Pain reports in childhood and early adolescence have been reported to be associated with the report of pain in early adulthood, supporting the need for effective pain management during adolescence (15). Of relevance to rheumatologists is the fact that the majority of childhood pain is musculoskeletal in origin (16). Of concern, a cost-of-illness to U.K. Society of Adolescent Chronic Pain discussed later in Chapter 9 has been estimated at approximately £3840 million in one year (17).

In addition to the reported associated morbidities of childhood-onset rheumatic disease into adulthood (18–27); (see also Chapters 6–12), health-risk behaviors adopted in adolescence track into adult life, with the antecedents of adult ill-health easily recognizable during adolescence (e.g., mental health, diet, exercise, cardiovascular risk, smoking, and injury). If such challenges are going to be effectively addressed, rheumatology professionals must learn to "think outside the health box," acknowledging that every health care encounter with an adolescent is a potential health-promotion opportunity, particularly in view of the pattern of health care utilization among adolescents (28). Adolescent behaviors have implications for health, many of which are directly relevant to the management of chronic rheumatic conditions, such as contraception for young people on teratogenic medication and alcohol use in young people on methotrexate (29).

Self-management patterns are also set down in adolescence, e.g., health care utilization, chronic disease self-management (see below), and therefore have potential implications for adult health. The importance of these adolescent antecedents to adult health and ill-health were echoed in a ground-breaking document about adolescent health from the professional colleges in the United Kingdom, which stated that "health services must pay greater attention to the special needs of young people if they wish to improve the emotional, psychological and physical health of the population" (6). There are no exemptions for rheumatology.

TASKS AND TRANSITIONS OF ADOLESCENCE

The key tasks of adolescence are listed in Table 2.

Alongside these tasks are several important life transitions, including moving from primary to secondary education and eventually from secondary education to either work or further education. There is also the transition from living in the family home to living independently, although the average age at which this happens is increasing in Western Europe (10). Finally there is the transition from pediatric to adult health care providers, a transition all young people are likely to make, although it is more pronounced for those with a chronic illness. Children and young people with chronic rheumatic conditions have been reported to be higher users of physicians compared to young people with other chronic illnesses (12,30). The tasks and transitions of adolescence are themselves interdependent and cannot be considered in isolation. Reciprocal influences should be acknowledged, in addition to the impact of illness on each.

KEY PRINCIPLES OF ADOLESCENT HEALTH CARE

Resilience Framework

One of the fundamental principles of adolescent health is that it is founded on the resilience framework (31,32) as opposed to the biomedical model of traditional health care. The latter is deficit and problem focused, with a paternalistic approach and delivery, whereas the resilience framework focuses on strengths, resilience, competencies, and successes and is egalitarian in approach and delivery.

Differences in Pediatric, Adolescent, and Adult Rheumatology Care Provision

There are major differences between pediatric, adolescent, and adult rheumatology care provision. These are summarized in Table 3, and many are discussed in other chapters of this book. Only when these differences are acknowledged by rheumatology professionals will adolescent rheumatology become truly established.

The key principles of adolescent health care in rheumatology are listed in Table 4.

Table 2 The Key Tasks of Adolescence

To consolidate personal identity (including sexual)
To establish relationships outside the family
To achieve interdependence with parents
To find a vocation

Table 3 Differences in Pediatric, Adolescent, and Adult Rheumatology Care

Age range
Growth and development
Consultation dynamics
Communication skills
Role of parents/family
Role of peers
Generic health issues, e.g., sexual health, substance use
Educational issues
Vocational issues
Consent and confidentiality issues
Different disease spectrum and manifestations
Impact of disease
Tolerance of immaturity
Procedural pain management
Legislation

Adolescents as New Users of Health Services

It is useful to further consider the idea that adolescents are "new users" of health services. In infancy and childhood, health services are accessed by parents on behalf of their sons/daughters. During adolescence, however, young people increasingly access health services independently. A potential predictor of the effectiveness of such utilization is the young person's acquisition of the necessary skills for doing so. In the context of chronic rheumatic disease, such skills training may be negatively affected by overprotective parenting, as is exemplified by the fact that a minority of adolescents are seen in adolescent clinics independently of their parents (33–35). Young people want to be assured privacy and confidentiality before choosing to be seen alone (1,36). Confidentiality has been reported as the main attribute of an adolescent-friendly service by young people (37,38); some young people will actually forgo health care if they think their parents

Table 4 Key Principles of Adolescent Health Care

Age and developmentally appropriate
Acknowledges the reciprocal influences of health and disease
   on adolescent development (physical, psychosocial, cognitive)
Promotes health and prevents disease
Transitional care
Views adolescents as "new users" of health services
Multidisciplinary and interagency

will find out (39). Commencement of such skills training starts early, as doctors involve children more in the consultation. In an interesting study of 302 consecutive outpatient pediatric encounters, children's contributions were limited to 4%, and pediatricians directed only one in every four statements to the child (40). Although pediatricians asked children a lot of medical questions (26%), only a small amount of the medical information (13%) was directed at the children (40). Other key skills young people need include self-medication and other forms of self-management, to know how to contact health care providers directly, get prescriptions and so on; these are integral components of transitional care (41). They are further discussed in Chapter 16. It remains important to acknowledge the differences between self-management for adolescents with chronic illness from that of adults (42) and to involve young people directly in service development in this area.

The Multidisciplinary Nature of Adolescent Health

Adolescent health care is, by definition, multidisciplinary and interagency. It involves professionals in primary and secondary health care, education and vocational services, social services, and the voluntary sector. Key players in adolescent rheumatology are listed in Table 5.

Provider characteristics have been reported to be the main predictor of satisfaction with health care by adolescents with and without chronic illness (38,43). Several behavioral factors amenable to training have been reported by young people with a range of chronic illnesses including JIA (38). The limited opportunities for formal adolescent health training in some countries remain a concern. (6). Significant unmet educational, and training needs among rheumatology professionals in the United Kingdom has been reported, reflecting this lack of training (44). Of concern, although professionals knowledgeable in transitional care—an important component of adolescent rheumatology management—was considered best practice by users and providers alike, but is considered feasible in only a few hospitals in the United Kingdom (45). It is reassuring that training, when available, makes a difference. In a randomized controlled trial of adolescent health training in primary care, large sustainable improvements in knowledge, skill, and self-perceived competency were reported in the short term (46). At 5-year follow-up, scores were all significantly higher than at baseline, with improvements sustained between 12 months and five years, with 54% of doctors receiving further training in the interim (47,48) Other reported positive outcomes of training include higher rates of desired clinical practices, for example, confidentiality, screening (46,49–51), greater number of adolescents seen, and a greater tendency to engage in continuing education in adolescent health (52).

The coordination of all these individuals is demanding and challenging but vital for quality care provision at this important stage of development In pediatric care, such coordination has been reported to increase parent

Table 5   Key Players in Adolescent Rheumatology
Health Care Provision

The adolescent
The young person him- or herself
Parents/caregivers
Siblings
Friends and peers
Health-care providers
Primary health-care provider/general practitioner
School nurse
Community pediatrician
Adult rheumatologist (in late adolescence)
Endocrinologist
Ophthalmologist
Orthopedic surgeons
Other specialties, e.g., renal, dermatology (SLE)
Occupational therapist
Physiotherapist
Psychologist
Social services
Social worker
Youth services
Youth worker
Local youth groups
Education/vocation
School teachers
School counselors
Careers advisors

Abbreviation: SLE, systemic lupus erythematosus.

satisfaction, as reported by the Pediatric Alliance for Coordinated Care (53). Other studies have supported a role for a key worker in chronic illness management (3,4,54–56). The size of the adolescent health team, even if virtual, creates very real demands on interprofessional communication. The challenges of translating policy into clinical practice has been highlighted in various audits, including limited documentation of adolescent health issues in rheumatology case notes (57), limited transition plans for both out-patients (57,58) and inpatients (59), and the lack of development of a written transition policy in centers participating in a controlled trial of a transitional care program (57).

SUMMARY

Adolescent rheumatology, as the rest of adolescent health, is gradually coming into its own and is being recognized as having specific age and developmental issues that must be addressed by appropriately trained professionals on the rheumatology team. Perhaps adolescent rheumatology should consider plagiarizing the publicity campaign of the teacher training agency in the United Kingdom and call for professionals who want to work with people who will teach them new words, who are potentially the most exciting people in the country, and who have not yet made up their minds on many things.

REFERENCES

1. Shaw KL, Southwood TR, McDonagh JE. Users' perspectives of transitional care for adolescents with juvenile idiopathic arthritis. Rheumatology 2004; 43: 770–8.
2. World Health Organisation. The Health of Young People. Geneva: WHO, 1993
3. Society for Adolescent Medicine. A position statement of the Society for Adolescent Medicine. J Adolesc Health 1995; 16:413.
4. Department of Health. National Service Framework for Children, Young People and Maternity Services. September 2004. www.dh.gov.uk
5. European Commission. *Europe and Youth: A New Impetus* 2001 (http://www. europa.eu.int/comm/youth/doc/publ/fl_youth_en.pdf last accessed 170206).
6. Royal College of Paediatrics and Child Health. Bridging the Gap: Health Care for Adolescents. June 2003 (www.rcpch.ac.uk).
7. Office of the Deputy Prime Minister. *Transitions: Young Adults with Complex Needs* 2005. ODPM Publications. Wetherby, UK www.socialexclusion.gov.uk
8. Dovey-Pearce G, Hurrell R, May C, et al. Young adults' (16–25 years) suggestions for providing developmentally appropriate diabetes services: a qualitative study. Health Soc Care Community 2005; 13:409–19.
9. Arnett JJ. Emerging adulthood: A theory of development from the late teens through the twenties. Am Psychologist 2000; 55:469–80.
10. Coleman J, Schofield J. Key data on Adolescence 2005. Brighton, UK: Trust for the Study of Adolescence, 2005.
11. Churchill R, Allen J, Denman S, et al. Do the attitudes and beliefs of young teenagers towards general practice influence actual consultation behaviour? Br J Gen Pract 2000; 50:953–7.
12. Adam V, St-Pierre Y, Fautrel B, et al. What is the impact of adolescent arthritis and rheumatism? Evidence from a national sample of Canadians. J Rheumatol 2005; 32:354–61.
13. Minden K, Niewerth M, Listing J, et al. Burden and cost of illness in patients with juvenile idiopathic arthritis. Ann Rheum Dis 2004; 63:836–42.
14. Hawker GA, Jamal SA, Ridout R, Chase C. A clinical prediction rule to identify pre-menopausal women with low bone mass. Osteoporos Int 2002; 13(5):400–6.
15. Brattberg G. Do pain problems in young school children persist into early adulthood? A 13-year follow-up. Eur J Pain 2004; 8:187–99.
16. Roth-Isigkeit A, Thyen U, Stoven H, Schwarzenberger J, Schmucker P. Pain among children and adolescents: restrictions in daily living and triggering factors. Pediatrics 2005; 115(2):e152–62.

17. Sleed M, Eccelston C, Beecham J, Knapp M, Jordan A. The economic impact of chronic pain in adolescence: methodological considerations and a preliminary costs-of-illness study. Pain 2005; 119(1–3):183–90.

18. Oen K, Malleson PN, Cabral DA, et al. Disease course and outcome of juvenile rheumatoid arthritis in a multicentre cohort. J Rheumatol 2002; 29:1989–99.

19. Packham JC, Hall MA. Long-term follow-up of 246 adults with juvenile idiopathic arthritis: education and employment. Rheumatology (Oxford) 2002; 41:1436–9.

20. Packham JC, Hall MA. Long-term follow-up of 246 adults with juvenile idiopathic arthritis:social function, relationships and sexual activity. Rheumatology (Oxford) 2002; 41:1440–3.

21. Packham JC, Hall MA. Long-term follow-up of 246 adults with juvenile idiopathic arthritis: functional outcome. Rheumatology (Oxford) 2002; 41: 1428–35.

22. Packham JC, Hall MA, Pimm TJ. Long-term follow-up of 246 adults with juvenile idiopathic arthritis: predictive factors for mood and pain. Rheumatology (Oxford) 2002; 41:1444–9.

23. Packham JC, Hall MA. Premature ovarian failure in women with juvenile idiopathic arthritis (JIA). Clin Exp Rheumatol 2003; 21:347–50.

24. Petersen LS, Mason T, Nelson AM, et al. Psychosocial outcomes and health studies in adults who have had juvenile arthritis: a controlled population based study. Arthritis Rheum 1997; 40:2235–40.

25. Foster HE, Marshall N, Myers A, et al. Outcome in adults with juvenile idiopathic arthritis. Arthritis Rheum 2003; 48:767–75.

26. Zak M, Hassager C, Lovell DJ, et al. Assessment of bone mineral density in adults with a history of juvenile chronic arthritis: a cross sectional long-term follow-up study. Arthritis Rheum 1999; 42:790–8.

27. Ostensen M, Almberg K, Koksvik HS. Sex, reproduction and gynecological disease in young adults with a history of juvenile chronic arthritis. J Rheumatol 2000; 27:1783–7.

28. Oppong-Odiseng ACK, Heycock EG. Adolescent health services – through their eyes. Arch Dis Child 1997; 77:115–9.

29. Nash AA, Britto MT, Lovell DJ, et al. Substance use among adolescents with JRA. Arthritis Care Res 1998; 11:391–6.

30. Palmero TM. Impact of recurrent and chronic pain on child and family daily functioning: a critical review of the literature. J Dev Behav Pediatr 2000;21: 58–69.

31. Olsson CA, Bond L, Burns JM, Vella-Brodrick DA, Sawyer SM. Adolescence resilience: a concept analysis. J Adolesc 2002; 26:1–11.

32. Patterson J, Blum RJ. Risk and resilience among children and youth with disabilities. Arch Pediat Adolesc Med 1996; 150:692–8.

33. Britto MT, Rosenthal SL, Taylor J, et al. Improving rheumatologists screening for alcohol use and sexual activity. Arch Pediatr Adolesc Med 2000; 154:478–83

34. Robertson LP. Hickling P, Davis PJC, et al. A comparison of paediatric vs adult rheumatology clinics. (1) The doctor perspective. Rheumatology 2003; 42:51.

35. Shaw KL, Southwood TR, McDonagh JE. Growing up and moving on in Rheumatology: a multicentre cohort of adolescents with Juvenile Idiopathic Arthritis. Rheumatology 2005; 44:806–12.

36. Beresford B, Sloper P. Chronically ill adolescents' experiences of communicating with doctors: a qualitative study. J Adolesc Health 2003; 33:172–9.
37. McPherson A. Primary health care and adolescence. In: MacFarlane A, ed. Adolescent Medicine. London: Royal College of Physicians, 1996:33–41.
38. Klostermann BK, Slap G, Nebrig DM, et al. Earning trust and losing it: adolescents' views on trusting physicians. J Family Pract 2005; 54(8):679–87.
39. Cheng TL, Savageau JA, Sattler AL, et al. Confidentiality in health care. A survey of knowledge, perceptions and attitudes among high school students. J Am Med Assoc 1993; 269:1404–7.
40. Van Dulmen AM. Children's contributions to pediatric outpatient encounters. Pediatrics 1998; 102:563–8.
41. McDonagh JE. Growing up and Moving on. Transition from pediatric to adult care. Pediatric Transplant 2005; 9:364–72.
42. Sawyer SM, Aroni RA. Self-management in adolescents with chronic illness. What does it mean and how can it be achieved? Med J Aust 2005; 183(8):405–9.
43. Freed LH, Ellen JM, Irwin CE, Millstein SG. Determinants of adolescents' satisfaction with health care providers and intentions to keep follow-up appointments. J Adolesc Health 1998; 22:475–9.
44. McDonagh JE, Southwood TR, Shaw KL. Unmet education and training needs of rheumatology health professionals in adolescent health and transitional care. Rheumatology (Oxford) 2004; 43(6):737–43.
45. Shaw KL, Southwood TR, McDonagh JE. Transitional Care for Adolescents with Juvenile Idiopathic Arthritis: Results of a Delphi Study. Rheumatology 2004; 43:1000–6.
46. Sanci LA, Coffey CM, Veit FC, et al. Evaluation of the effectiveness of an educational intervention for general practitioners in adolescent health care: randomised controlled trial. Br Med J 2000; 320(7229):224–30.
47. Sanci L, Coffey C, Patton G, et al. Sustainability of change with quality general practitioner education in adolescent health: a 5 year follow-up. Med Educ 2005; 39(6):557–60.
48. Evans T, Bearinger L, Ireland M, et al. Self-reported competencies of adolescent health professionals: changes in the last decade. J Adolesc Health 1998; 22:149.
49. Middleman AB, Binns HJ, Durant RH. Factors affecting pediatric residents' intentions to screen for high risk behaviours. J Adolesc Health 1995; 17:106–12.
50. Lustig JL, Ozer EM, Adams SH, et al. Improving the delivery of adolescent clinical preventive services through skills-based training. Pediatrics 2001; 107:1100–7.
51. Marks A, Fisher M, Lasker S. Adolescent medicine in pediatric practice. J Adolesc Health Care 1990; 11:149–53.
52. Key JD, Marsh LD, Darden PM. Adolescent medicine in paediatric practice: a survey of practice and training. Am J Med Sci 1986; 7:18–21.
53. Palfrey JS, Sofis LA, Davidson EJ, et al. The Pediatric Alliance for Coordinated Care: Evaluation of a medical home model. Pediatrics 2004; 113:1507–16.
54. McDonagh JE, Southwood TR, Shaw KL. Growing up and moving on in rheumatology: development and preliminary evaluation of a transitional care

programme for a multicentre cohort of adolescents with juvenile idiopathic arthritis. J Child Health Care 2006; 10(1):22–42.

55. Garwick AW, Kohrman C, Wolman C, et al. Families' recommendations for Improving Services with chronic conditions. Arch Pediatr Adolesc Med 1998; 152:440–8.

56. Joseph Rowntree Foundation. Implementing Key Worker Services: A Case Study of Promoting Evidence-Based Practice. York: Joseph Rowntree Foundation, 1999. (www.jrf.org.uk)

57. Robertson LP, McDonagh JE, Southwood TR, et al. Growing up and moving on. A multicentre UK audit of the transfer of adolescents with Juvenile Idiopathic Arthritis JIA from paediatric to adult centred care. Ann Rheum Dis 2006; 65:74–80.

58. Lotstein DS, McPherson M, Strickland B, Newacheck PW. Transition planning for youth with special health care needs: results from the national survey of children with special health care needs. Pediatrics 2005; 115:1562–8.

59. Lam PY, Fitzgerald BB, Sawyer SM. Young adults in children's hospitals: why are they there? Med J Aust 2005; 182(8):381–4.

2

The Teenage Brain

Gerald Ullrich

Department of Pediatric Pulmonology and Neonatology, Children's Hospital, Hannover Medical School, Hannover, Germany

"People who have something better to do don't suffer as much."
(1)

INTRODUCTION

The field of adolescent medicine began in 1952 when internist J.R. Gallagher established the first adolescent unit to ensure a physician's tendency to consider his or her patient and not just focus upon disease alone (3). Unlike with children, the developmental characteristics of adolescents have long been neglected—misleadingly, since adolescence differs in many ways from adulthood, too. The most prominent characteristic of adolescence is the occurrence of multiple transitions (2) ranging from biological to psychological and social processes, all of which are strongly interrelated. Starting with activities of the hormonal regulatory systems, puberty is characterized by rapid growth in height and weight, changes in body composition and tissues, and the acquisition of primary and secondary sex characteristics (see Chapter 3) (4). In addition to these very profound biological transformations, the young person also has to face a multitude of additional psychosocial adaptations and transformations (see "Developmental Issues and Chronic Illness"). These are labeled normative stresses since everybody has to cope with them more or less at the same time (5, 6). Not surprisingly, coping with normative stresses may severely be affected by non-normative stresses, such as a chronic illness: "an adolescent without any significant health problems can have a difficult enough time coping with all these changes, which are occurring more or less concurrently. Consider the impact of a chronic health disorder on one or more of these components of development: the effect can be devastating" (3).

13

DEVELOPMENTAL ISSUES AND CHRONIC ILLNESS

Most discussions of developmental aspects during adolescence refer to the widely accepted concept of "developmental tasks" (7), which has a focus on the psychosocial dimension (8). However, there are also profound transformations on a more basic level, that is, the adolescent's information processing. The following section summarizes typical ways in which adolescents perceive their world differently from children. This is then followed by a discussion on divergent conceptualizations of adolescence, and an exploration of problems created by the emergence of chronic illness during adolescence. Finally, the specific issues of rheumatic disease during adolescence are discussed.

Adolescence and Information Processing

As with adolescence in general, the cognitive transformations are psycho-somatic in a literal sense: changes in the brain (including synaptogenesis, electroencephalographic patterns, and metabolic function) at the start of puberty closely match the emergence of major discontinuation in behavior and cognition (9). As regards the cognitive transformations, Piaget's model of cognitive stages has received utmost attention (10). It implies that the child processes information from the environment in very different ways, depending on the respective developmental stage. Piaget differentiated the pre-logic stage (first years of life), the concrete logic stage (elementary school age), and the logical thinking stage, the latter usually beginning in early adolescence and characterized by cognitive abilities that increasingly correspond to the adult's way of information processing. Although not without critiques (8,10) there is general agreement that development pro-ceeds "from simple to complex, from concrete to abstract, and from ego-centric to decentered" (8). "Egocentric" in cognitive terminology is quite different from being selfish. It means that the reasoning is still fixed to the subject's perspective, that the child is not yet able to imagine the world from another person's point of view. Unlike the child, the young adolescent is increasingly able to perceive the world from different perspectives and becomes even able to abstract from the world as it is and to imagine how it could be (Table 1). This ability of hypothetical reasoning brings about profound irritation as for the credibility and reliability of the adult world which now may be questioned. Hypothetical reasoning together with an enhanced concept of time also provides a more thorough understanding of terms like chronic illness or long-term impact of disease activity. And as youngsters are increasingly able to refer to their own cognitive processing (introspection), a discrepancy between real and ideal self emerges which constitutes their typical psychological vulnerability and irritability during adolescence.

Table 1 Developmental Gains in Cognitive Functioning During Adolescence

■ Ability to reflect on hypothetical problems
■ Ability to systematically explore solutions
■ Abstract thinking
■ Ability to reflect on one's own thinking
■ Advanced concept of future

Source: Adapted from Ref. 10.

Other characteristic modes of perception, although not purely cognitive in nature, are the strong desire to compare oneself with peers and to be alike. This is heavily influenced by the divergence in physical growth and development, especially at the start of puberty. Not surprisingly, then, "the worst fear of young adolescents is to be excluded by the crowd"(8). As a consequence of being able to reflect on oneself (discover the self), adolescents also tend to overestimate their uniqueness ("personal fable") and to disregard that statistical rules (like risk ratios) may also apply to themselves, leaving the characteristic feeling of invulnerability (6,11). This may trigger risk taking behavior, although the latter is often determined by motives belonging to the developmental process of identity formation, rather than merely resulting from cognitive misinterpretations (6). However, these may at least exaggerate respective tendencies.

Finally, adolescents are often said to be erratic, including their convictions and preferences, at least that they "typically struggle with some uncertainty while they are deciding on their future commitments" (12,13). Although several studies have reported that turmoil is the exception rather than the rule, adolescents are perceived to be somewhat more changeable and unpredictable at least by adult standards (8). However, we should keep in mind that this "lack" of stability and accountability is functional with respect to the ongoing process of identity formation (12).

Adolescence—A Stage or a Passage?

There are numerous theories of adolescence, which mostly refer to one of two paradigms: at one end of the continuum, adolescence is perceived as a passage, characterized by certain transitions, leading to pre-fixed developmental endpoints. This is concisely exemplified in the concept of developmental tasks (7). At the other end, the characteristics of adolescence are rather described as a stage or developmental "moratorium," a period characterized by experimentation and defining one's own identity and self. While the transitions approach focuses on pre-fixed developmental tasks and is directed to the future, the "moratorium" approach (most prominently purported by Erickson) focuses on the individual's autonomy and identity formation and is centered on the present (14,10). As outlined by Reinders (14), both theoretical concepts differ with respect to the underlying dimensions: time (future vs. present) and generation (adulthood vs. peers). They should not, however, be perceived as exclusive. On the contrary, adolescent development may be described within these coordinates (Table 2).

As Reinders (14) further exemplifies, internal (personality and personal resources) as well as external influences (family, society) may determine the course of the developmental pathways: there is either potential and appeal to speed up transition in order to fulfill adult roles or to remain in the adolescent orientation stage and to protract the "moratorium." This typology may serve as a useful tool to describe developmental pathways beyond the well known but exaggerated lament of adolescence as a turmoil or as a notoriously rebellious phase (which wrongly equates adolescence with the "segregation" pathway; Table 2). As Ingersoll rightly states, "an

Table 2   Typology of Adolescent Pathways

+

Assimilation	Integration
High identification with	Socio-cultural autonomy
standards of the adult world,	of the adolescent stage
low intergenerational	equally important as
conflict; strongly future	the transition to the
oriented	adult world

Passage orientation

Stage orientation

−   +

Marginalization	Segregation
Undetermined as to whether to relate to peers or to adults,	Demarcation from adults and focus on peer-related
low future orientation and	culture and values, ("sub-
low engagement in peer	culture"-type); strongly
activities	oriented to the present

−

Source: Adapted from Ref. 14.

image of adolescents as generally stressed, tumultuous, and anxiety-ridden is misleading and potentially harmful" (8). Weiner even goes one step further, highlighting the fact that psychosocial adaptation is the rule and if there are overt signs of conflict, these must not be played down as a transient adolescent unrest, "symptom formation is pathologic" (12). According to the same author, findings from comparative studies on healthy adolescents with minor symptoms versus disturbed adolescents provide guidelines for differentiating normal from abnormal development: the more symptoms are displayed, the longer these persist, and the more the symptom picture is marked not only by feelings of anxiety and depression but also disturbed thinking or antisocial behavior, the more likely it is that the young person has a definite psychopathologic condition.

Adolescence and Chronic Illness

Given the tasks imposed by the emergence of a chronic disease, and bearing in mind the characteristics of the normal (healthy) adolescent, adolescence is probably the most untimely period for disease manifestation (Table 3). Blum and Geber particularly stress the adverse effects when chronic illness influences the pubertal development itself: "Whether delayed or precocious, pubertal changes have profound social and emotional consequences for all youth" (15). Strasburger and Brown say that the emergence of a chronic illness may even have a "devastating effect" since the disease and or the therapeutic regime may impact on several components of development, concurrently (3). Similarly, Fritz (16) describes a negative impact of chronic illness on nearly each of the four main domains: attainment of physical maturity; development of autonomy and separation from parents; sexual identity and the formation of mature relationships with both sexes; and preparing for a productive place in society. Successful adaptation, therefore, may not to be taken for granted (15). Not surprisingly, then, young people with chronic illnesses were the target of countless studies. As will be seen in

Table 3 Why Chronic Illness Is Particularly Untimely During Adolescence

- Interference of disease with pubertal/physical development at a time when normal variation may already lead to turmoil
- Illness- or drug-dependent alterations of appearance at a time of increased fear of rejection
- Being different from peers at a time of maximum desire for conformity
- Increased dependence on parents at a time of expected stepwise separation
- Being obliged to follow a rigid therapeutic discipline at a time of impulsiveness and volatility
- Being dependent on adult counselors at a time of heightened skepticism towards the adult world (values and credibility)

more detail with respect to studies on young people with rheumatic disease, there is a trend towards reporting less noticeable problems, as study designs are increasingly sophisticated and methodologically sound. However, longitudinal data are mostly lacking. Data from a German longitudinal study on coping in adolescents with insulin-dependent diabetes mellitus is therefore of major interest (17,18), particularly in view of its explicit developmental orientation. The authors referred to the focal theory of adolescence, developed by Coleman (19), who discovered that interest in and concerns about different topics peaked at different points in adolescence. Different issues come "into focus" at different times, according to this theory. The question under study was, what would happen to the common developmental process and topics if the youngsters had to cope with major non-normative stresses, demanding their immediate attention? Interestingly, the authors found developmental delay only during the first interviews, but not in the long-term (17). Age appropriate developmental tasks were initially postponed except for educational issues, where the youngsters even displayed better results than healthy controls (18). Referring to the typology of adolescence discussed in the previous section, these adolescents fast-tracked the "vertical" development (14). As Figure 1 further shows, the majority of adolescents in the German study successfully integrated developmental and disease related tasks. A third of adolescents primarily focused on illness management to the detriment of developmental tasks, especially regarding the peer-related dimensions [less "horizontal" development (14)]. A minority resolved the conflict of developmental and illness related tasks to the detriment of the latter. They appeared to even speed up their normal development in so far as they often displayed premature and socially deviant (acting out) behavior and largely neglected alarming HbA_{1c}-scores. That is, they purely

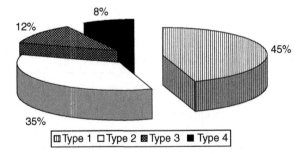

Figure 1   Types of coping in adolescents with insulin-dependent diabetes mellitus: Type 1: successful integration of developmental and illness-related tasks; no long-term developmental leeway. Type 2: focusing on illness adjustment to the detriment of developmental tasks. Type 3: focusing on developmental tasks to the detriment of illness adjustment. Type 4: maladjustment and failure. *Source*: Adapted from Ref. 18.

focused on "horizontal" development according to the typology outlined in Table 2. A residual category of adolescents came from families, who seemed overwhelmed altogether. Developmental as well as illness related targets were largely missed.

The emergence of a chronic disease may therefore indeed be overwhelming and may lead to respective symptoms either with regard to insufficient psychosocial development or with regard to insufficient disease control (or both). However, as the public perception of normal adolescence constantly exaggerates turmoil, there may also be a bias towards an overly skeptical view of adolescents with a chronic illness. Furthermore, their likely short term problems may not be good predictors against successful long-term adaptation. Since short term problems may frequently be present, it may be particularly difficult to define good adaptation, at all. Fritz (16) cites an early definition of Mattson (20) which still appears to be appropriate, today (Table 4).

ADOLESCENCE AND RHEUMATIC DISEASES

We will adopt a distinction made by Harrington et al. (21) and discuss recent empirical studies according to (a) the impact of adolescence on the disease and (b) the impact of the disease on development. However, we would like to highlight on the spectrum of the disease, first.

Disease Spectrum and Diversity

Unlike other chronic illnesses like diabetes, rheumatic diseases may vary considerably with respect to symptoms, course of the disease, prognosis, and therapy, all of which contribute to the psychosocial impact. Table 5 gives a list of important disease-related symptoms and factors. Drug-induced symptoms as well as severe functional impairment are associated with a more severe course of the disease. This occurs more often in patients with systemic or polyarticular onset juvenile idiopathic arthritis (JIA) (22,23) as well as in SLE patients (24). Functional impairment not only has implications for daily activities with peers, but may cause problems at school (absenteeism, transportation), too (25,26). Siegel and Baum (27), in an excellent paper on JIA and sexuality, also describe the impact of functional

Table 4 How to Identify Good Adaptation in the Chronically Ill

- Age-appropriate dependence on family
- Minimal need for secondary gains from the illness
- Acceptance of the limits and responsibilities imposed by the disease
- Development of compensatory sources of satisfaction

Source: Adapted from Ref. 20; cited from Ref. 16.

Table 5 Disease-Related Symptoms and Factors That May Impair Functioning and Psychosocial Maturation and Health

Body image[a]
  Growth failure
  Pubertal delay
  Localized growth anomalies (e.g., a short digit, micrognathia)
  Joint deformities (including leg-length discrepancies)
  Drug-induced altered distribution of fat stores
  Change in skin appearance and body shape (either pathognomonic: rash,
    Raynaud's syndrome; or drug-induced: acne, hirsutism, striae, cushingoid
    appearance)
  Scars from previous surgery
Self-esteem and social maturation
  Inability to perform household tasks
  Physical dependence from parents
  Limited mobility
  Functional limitations (due to stiffness, joint deformity, pain, or impaired vision)
  Reduced fitness
Mental health
  Impaired body image, self-esteem, and social maturation
  Pain
  Loss of control/sense of helplessness
  Parental overprotection ("vulnerable child syndrome")
  Lack of sympathetic peers and significant others

[a]*Source*: Adapted from Ref. (53).

impairment on sexual activities. As regards the sense of helplessness and/or low sense of self-efficacy, patients with rheumatic disease may be more vulnerable than other chronic patients given the fact that—unlike for diabetes and other well-controllable diseases—there is only limited promise that adherence with therapy will prevent future symptoms and flares. Furthermore, there is also a greater risk of unsympathetic reactions from peers and significant others (including teachers): being a young person and suffering from a "disease of elderly people" may provoke insulting reactions from peers. Furthermore, rheumatic symptoms may vary extremely during the course of one day, which may falsely undermine credibility (regarding sick role).

On the other hand, among adolescents with rheumatic diseases, there are also some with minimal or no limitations at all, or whose disease is in remission. This occurs more often in JIA patients with an oligoarticular onset (22,23).

Age at disease manifestation may further act as an important modulating factor (28). Pelkonen (29), for instance, mentioned that disease onset in adolescence may eventually end up as a "disaster" [similarly (30)]. Late disease manifestation characteristically occurs in patients with rheumatoid factor positive JIA, enthesitis related JIA, and SLE.

In other words, there is a tremendous diversity both within and among the JIA groups, as well as among the broader spectrum of rheumatic diseases. This should be kept in mind if studies report on results of "rheumatic" patients.

Developmental Influences on Disease Perception and Management

Harrington et al. (21) outlined three important developmental differences between adolescents and children: (1) the conception of their illness becomes more complex and realistic (even though misperceptions and gaps may eventually remain undetected), (2) growing independence and responsibility for therapy (with nonadherence occurring frequently), (3) more pronounced, adult-like pain perception (possibly due to the broader knowledge of the disease and symptoms, which are increasingly being perceived as signs of later impairment).

To date, studies have primarily focused on adherence and pain, rather than the beliefs about illness. Nevertheless, the early studies on disease conception proved to be influential inasmuch as recent research approaches adolescents as "consumers" and "experts" (31–35). This reflects a developmental understanding of adolescents who are now being perceived as individuals with specific needs—and that these needs have to be addressed if interventions and services are to be effective.

Nonadherence

Studies on nonadherence usually focus on medication taking (36) and disregard avoidance of risk taking behavior as a further dimension of compliance (37). Given the fact, that experimentation is typically associated with adolescence and early adulthood (11), the paucity of literature on experimentation/risk taking and chronic illness is somewhat puzzling. Frequently, for JIA patients risk taking behavior even includes involvement in common activities like skiing (36). Certainly, there are more obvious risk taking behaviors (38,39), such as smoking, alcohol and drug misuse, unsafe sex and early pregnancy, which remain important considerations in JIA patients, too. Depending upon the medication prescribed there may even be specific adverse effects of risk taking behavior in young people with rheumatic disease. A study of 55 mostly female American adolescents with JIA (mean age 14 years) reported alcohol use in 31% and this was slightly less frequent (24%) in patients currently treated with methotrexate (40). The authors also asked whether or not adolescents, during their regular contacts with the rheumatologist, would occasionally be interviewed alone. Only one in four patients consented! Given that adolescents often limit self-disclosure if their parents are present (30,41) this figure should prompt concerns and emphasizes the importance of providing adolescents opportunities to be seen separately from their parents with assurances of confidentiality (see Chapters 4 and 14).

Adolescent Pain Perception

Pain perception of adolescents has been described as comparable to that of adults rather than children (21). As in adulthood, pain becomes more of a problem for the adolescent with rheumatic disease. A Swedish study (42) on 125 patients with JIA (mean age 14 years) showed that pain was even the most powerful predictor of their well-being (explaining 55% of variance)!

Other recent studies try to elucidate moderating factors of pain perception, particularly the role of pain coping strategies. Two studies (43,44) identified "catastrophizing" as a powerful factor of intensified pain perception whereas "pain control thinking" seemed to be the beneficial counterpart (45). "Catastrophizing" also appeared to be the mediating factor between a positive parental history of pain and the child's own pain perception and poor health (43). The authors of this study suggest that by gathering information from parents about their own pain histories, health care providers may be able to identify children at risk for developing maladaptive pain coping strategies and higher levels of disease-related pain and disability. Another pattern of health related interactions was identified in a recent study on 215 children (mean age 12.4 year) with either headaches, JIA ($n = 63$) or sickle cell disease and their parents (46). The authors analyzed the children's pain intensity and frequency, their level of anxiety and depression and the parental response style to children's pain behavior as well as functional disability (child and parent rating). Interestingly, they found an interaction of child distress and solicitousness of the parent in response to their child's pain, in that for those children who reported greater depressive and anxiety symptoms, child report of parental solicitousness was associated with greater child-reported functional disability.

Impact of Illness on Development and Psychosocial Functioning

A review of studies on the psychosocial impact of rheumatic disease suggests that the outlook appears to be less grim than early studies suggested (21). However, there certainly remains a vulnerability towards internalizing symptoms (anxiety, depression, adjustment disorder) during adolescence in the context of chronic rheumatic disease and considerable restrictions in the social domain. Similarly, a meta-analysis (47) showed a low to moderate effect (0.30) of the disease on rate of psychological disturbance. This was more pronounced for internalizing symptoms (0.47) and negligible with respect to externalizing behavior and self-concept (<0.15, respectively). However, since most of the studies solely relied on parental accounts "it is unclear to what extent inclusion of child report of adjustment problems would change the nature of the results of the meta-analysis" (47).

If child reports of adjustment problems are included, results appear to be even more favorable: compared to schoolmates, young people with JIA (23 children and 24 adolescents from the Netherlands) did not display more psychopathology nor differ with respect to internalizing symptoms (48). The only difference of adolescents was in the social competence domain but was at least partly related to the disease itself (participation in sports, number of subjects at school). However, playing with or seeing friends was similar. This fits to the overall result of a recent American study which used a longitudinal, case-controlled study design to assess the social functioning of young people with JIA (49). As in the first part of the longitudinal study (50), although 74 young people with JIA were found to be similar to their case-control classmates on all measures of social functioning and behavior, the follow-up study on 57 adolescents (mean age 13 years) did not show differences on any of the measures of social reputation or social acceptance. In addition, children with JIA were not different from controls with respect to non-social attributes, "suggesting that peers did not perceive these children as chronically ill" (49) With respect to the obvious psychological hardiness of these young people, the authors conclude " that the social development of children is highly protected, with maladjustment occurring only with exposure to severe adversity" (49). Since patients with more severe or active disease showed subtle decrements over time, these results would best fit a dose response model of disease effects.

Finally, results of studies on young adults with JIA may also contribute important details to our understanding of the disease impact during the transition from childhood to adulthood. A British study assessed 246 adults (mean age 28 years) individually by interview, various questionnaires, and physical examination. The physical outcome showed a remarkably high percentage of patients with clinically active arthritis (43%) and severe functional limitations (37–43%). However, the sample was biased towards patients with the worst long-term prognosis [i.e. systemic and rheumatoid factor positive polyarthritis constitute 14% of common pediatric rheumatology populations but constituted 36% of the study group (51)]. The educational level of the study group was higher than national average, as well as compared to patients' siblings (52). However, unemployment was higher than in the national population (137%). With respect to social maturation the study group revealed a moderate delay: age of onset of sexual activity was higher than in the general population, the percentage of single patients was 12% higher than for their siblings and the percentage of married or cohabitating persons 11% lower than that for their siblings (53). Of 83% sexually active adults, 58% experienced difficulties related to their disease which is in agreement with Siegel and Baum (27) who stressed the importance of the disease impact in this respect. Even more disturbing was that 30% of those who were not sexually active felt that this was due to their illness. Most of these ($n = 10$) individuals "felt they were not perceived as sexual beings" (53)!

Psychopathology—assessed by the Hospital Anxiety and Depression Scale (54)—showed low rates of depression (5% above threshold) but elevated rates of anxiety (32% above threshold) (55). Multiple regression analysis of psychopathology and several other scales identified self-efficacy as the most important predictor. Self-efficacy explained 31% variance of anxiety scores, and 18% variance of depression scores (with 74%/54% total explained variance, respectively). Regarding differences between diagnostic subsets patients with oligoarthritis were significantly less anxious than other subsets and experienced less pain, too. Adults with systemic onset JIA had elevated levels of both anxiety and depression.

Compared to the previously mentioned results of adolescents with JIA, this long-term follow-up study reveals a more distressing picture of the disease impact and highlights on the importance of transitional care (see Chapter 16).

BEYOND DISTURBANCE: RESILIENCE

Although rheumatic diseases may certainly impact on the psychosocial health of the afflicted, the lack of differences between young people with JIA and healthy controls is "more impressive than the differences" (56). Successful coping under bad conditions (such as chronic disease) is at the core of studies belonging to the resilience paradigm.

Terminology

Unfortunately, earlier terms like "stress-resistance" or "invulnerability" were misleading inasmuch as they insinuate that some children and young people were so constitutionally tough that they would not succumb to the pressure of stress and adversity (57). Nowadays, resilience is considered as "an ability to recover from negative events" (58). This does not presuppose absence of any kind of impact following exposure to adversity. Rather, it means absence of lasting disturbance. Similarly, Fonagy et al. (59) described resilience as "normal development under difficult conditions."

Studies on Resilience

Research on resilience usually focuses on social competence despite bad conditions. The latter are most often described as major negative life events. Apart from methodological limitations in assessing life events (60) it should be kept in mind, that there may also be a profound (cumulative or even exponential) interactive effect if more than one bad condition is present (58,57). Also, life stress not only results from major life events; the chronic influence of so-called "daily hassles" may represent bad, stressful conditions, too. Daily hassles are irritating, frustrating experiences that occur in everyday transactions with the environment. The idea that daily hassles can be stressors seems particularly important with respect to JIA since the presence of the disease often leads to lots of small, daily reminders of

Table 6 Key Elements of Resilience

Dispositional attributes of the child
Constitution (positive temperament, robust neurobiology)
Sociability (responsiveness to others, pro-social attitude to others)
Intelligence (academic achievement, planning and decision making)
Communication skills (developed language)
Personal attributes (tolerance for negative affect, self-efficacy, self-esteem, internal locus of control)
Family level
Atmosphere and support (parental warmth, cohesion and care, belief in the child, non-blaming)
Income and status (material resourced)
Community level
School experiences (supportive peers, positive teacher influence)
Supportive communities (provisions and resources to assist, nonpunitive)

Source: Adapted from Ref. 58.

misery that may well be categorized as daily hassles and sources of stress. Surprisingly, most studies on stress in children and young people with JIA did not assess stressors specific to the lives of children with arthritis (61).

What are the "ingredients" of resilience? Garmezy's distinction is still valid which identifies three categories of resilience enabling factors: (1) dispositional attributes of the child, (2) family cohesion and warmth, (3) the availability and use of external support systems by parents and children [(62), according to (60)]. Olsson et al. (58) further differentiate the most influential processes and factors, all of which are empirically substantiated (Table 6).

Even though dispositional attributes of the child are certainly of great importance, it must be kept in mind that resilience is not an attribute born into the child (59). As Rutter noted, resilience is the concerted effect of a certain way of responding to external stressors (active coping instead of mere reacting), feelings of self-efficacy and of self-esteem (both of which are prerequisites of active coping), and a secure attachment to family members and significant others [(63), according to (64)].

CONCLUSION

Earlier reports on the psychosocial disease impact in children and young people with rheumatic disease tended to be negatively biased due to weak study designs (56) and due to the prevailing focus on disturbance instead of resilience in the pediatric psychology literature. In the meantime, more sophisticated studies have substantially corrected this picture. However, at least some authors suspect that we might overemphasize normalcy, today. Some even argued that the ostensible normalcy of JIA patients might be their problem in that it showed a kind of hyperadaptation (48,65). Two editorials on studies with overwhelmingly "positive" results did not go that far but explicitly questioned the positive overall impressions (66,67). They claim that future research should focus more on the severely ill young people who—by virtue of the low frequency of the underlying diseases—mostly represent small subsets in previous studies. It may well be that psychosocial consequences emerge only at or above certain levels of disease severity, functional impairment, and treatment intensity. The reciprocal influences of adolescent psychosocial development and the diversity of the rheumatic diseases have not yet been adequately addressed, especially regarding rheumatic diseases beyond the JIA spectrum (SLE, vasculitis, etc.). On the other hand, disease characteristics have not demonstrated a consistent relationship with psychosocial adjustment, so that identifying those at greatest risk for problems will not be a simple task. As the most recent study shows, negative attitude towards illness may well be one important stress processing factor (61). Therefore, future research should rely more on homogeneous samples (regarding diversity) and should focus more on mediating factors than on the general issue of a disease related, increased risk of disturbances. Finally, we should keep in mind the "power of positive thinking" (68): these young people as well as their healthy peers (should) focus on real-life targets, and having meaningful goals to pursue will help them overcome some of the inescapable strains of illness.

REFERENCES

1. Fordyce WE. Pain and suffering: a reappraisal. Am Psychol 1988; 43:276–83.
2. Pattan GC, Viner R. Pubertal transitions in health. The Lancet 2007; 369: 1130–9.
3. Strasburger VC, Brown RT. Adolescent Medicine. A Practical Guide. 1st ed. Boston, Toronto, London: Little, Brown and Company 1991.
4. Kreipe RE. Normal somatic adolescent growth and development. In: McAnarney ER, Kreipe RE, Orr DP, et al., eds. Textbook of Adolescent Medicine. Philadelphia, London: WB Saunders, 1992:44–67.
5. Hauser ST, Bolds MK. Stress, coping and adaptation within adolescence: diversity into resilience. In: Feldman S, Elliot G, eds. At the Threshold: for the Developing Adolescent. Cambridge: University Press, 1990:388–413.
6. Seiffge-Krenke I. Gesundheitspsychologie des Jugendalters [Health psychology of adolescence]. Göttingen, Bern, Toronto, Seattle, Hogrefe Verlag für Psychologie, 1994.
7. Havighurst RJ. Developmental Tasks and Education. 3rd edn. New York: McKay, 1972.
8. Ingersoll GM. Psychological and social development. In: McAnarney ER, Kreipe RE, Orr DP, et al., eds. Textbook of Adolescent Medicine. Philadelphia, London: WB Saunders, 1992:91–8.

9. Watkins JM, Williams ME. Cognitive neuroscience and adolescent development. In: McAnarney ER, Kreipe RE, Orr DP, et al., eds. Textbook of Adolescent Medicine. Philadelphia, London: WB Saunders, 1992:99–106.

10. Mussen PH, Conger JJ, Kagan J, et al. Child Development and Personality. New York: Harper Collins Publications, 1990.

11. Hurrelmann K, Lösel F, eds. Health Hazards in Adolescence. Berlin: De Gruyter, 1990.

12. Weiner IB. Normality during adolescence. In: McAnarney ER, Kreipe RE, Orr DP, et al., eds. Textbook of Adolescent Medicine. Philadelphia, London: WB Saunders, 1992:86–90.

13. Kimmel DC, Weiner IB. Adolescence: A Developmental Transition. New York; Wiley, 1985: Chap. 8.

14. Reinders H. Jugendtypen. Ansätze zu einer differentiellen Theorie der Adoleszenz [Types of youth. Steps to a differential theory of adolescence]. Opladen: Leske & Budrich, 2003.

15. Blum RW, Geber G. Chronically ill youth. In: McAnarney ER, Kreipe RE, Orr DP, et al., eds. Textbook of Adolescent Medicine. Philadelphia, London: WB Saunders, 1992:222–8.

16. Fritz GK. Chronic illness and psychological health. In: McAnarney ER, Kreipe RE, Orr DP, et al., eds. Textbook of Adolescent Medicine. Philadelphia, London: WB Saunders, 1992:1133–7.

17. Boeger A, Seiffge-Krenke I, Roth M. Symptombelastung, Selbstkonzept und Entwicklungsverzögerung bei gesunden und chronisch kranken Jugendlichen: Ergebnisse einer 4 1/2jährigen Längsschnittsudie. [Psychopathology, self concept and developmental delays in healthy and chronically ill adolescents: results of a 4–5-year follow-up study] Z Kinder Jugendpsychiatr 1996; 24: 231–9.

18. Seiffge-Krenke I. Chronisch kranke Jugendliche und ihre Familien: Das Dilemma zwischen altersgemäßer Entwicklung und Krankheitsanpassung. [Chronically ill adolescents and their families: The dilemma of age-apropriate development and adjustment to illness]. In: Oerter R, Hagen VV, Röper G, et al., eds. Klinische Entwicklungspsychologie. Ein Lehrbuch [Clinical Developmental Psychology. A Textbook]. Weinheim: Psychologie Verlags Union, 1999:691–710.

19. Coleman JC. Current contradictions in adolescent theory. J Youth Adolesc 1978; 7:1–11.

20. Mattson A. Long-term physical illness in childhood: A challenge to psychosocial adaptation. Pediatrics 1972; 52:801–11.

21. Harrington J, Kirk A, Newman ST. Developmental issues in adolescents and the impact of rheumatic disease. In: Isenberg DA, Miller III JJ, eds. Adolescent Rheumatology. London: Martin Dunitz, 1999:21–33.

22. Oen K, Malleson, PN, Cabral DA, et al. Disease course and outcome of juvenile rheumatoid arthritis in a multicenter cohort. J Rheumatol 2002; 29(9): 1989–99.

23. Minden K, Kiessling U, Listing J, et al. Prognosis of patients with juvenile chronic arthritis and juvenile spondyloarthropathy. J Rheumatol 2000; 27(9): 2256–63.

24. Sandborg CI. Childhood systemic lupus erythematosus and neonatal lupus syndrome. Curr Opin Rheumatol 1998; 10(5):481–7.

25. Spencer CH, Fife RZ, Rabinovich CE. The school experience of children with arthritis. Coping in the 1990s and transition into adulthood. Pediat Clinics N Am 1995; 42(5):1285–98.

26. Taylor J, Passo MH, Champion V. School problems and teacher responsibilities in juvenile rheumatoid arthritis. J School Health 1987; 57:186–90.

27. Siegel DM, Baum J. Adolescent rheumatic disease and sexuality. In: Isenberg DA, Miller III JJ, eds. Adolescent Rheumatology. London: Martin Dunitz, 1999:291–9.

28. Singsen BH, Johnson MA, Bernstein BA. Psychodynamics of juvenile rheumatoid arthritis. In: Miller JJ, ed. Juvenile Rheumatoid Arthritis. Littleton, MA, PSG, 1979; 249–65.

29. Pelkonen PM. Impact of arthritis and its consequences on the psychosocial development of adolescents. Rev Rhum (Engl. Edition) 1997; 64(10):191S–3S.

30. Leak AM. The management of arthritis in adolescence. Br J Rheumatol 1994; 33:882–8.

31. Barlow JH, Shaw KL, Harrison K. Consulting the 'experts': children's and parents' perceptions of psycho-educational interventions in the context of juvenile chronic arthritis. Health Educ Res 1999; 14(5):597–610.

32. Shaw KL, Southwood TR, McDonagh JE. User perspectives of transitional care for adolescents with juvenile idiopathic arthritis. Rheumatology 2004;43 (6):770–8.

33. Ullrich G, Mattussek S, Dressler F, et al. How do adolescents with juvenile chronic arthritis consider their disease related knowledge, their unmet service needs, and the attractiveness of various services? Eur J Med Res 2002; 7(1): 8–18.

34. Wright C, Russo K, Karp M, et al. Listening to adolescents with JIA—A user involvement initiative for relationship and sexuality education. Clin Exp Rheumatol 2003; 21(4):538.

35. Aasland, Flato B, Vandvik IH. Patient and parent experiences with health care services in pediatric rheumatology. Scand J Rheumatol 1998; 27(4):265–72.

36. Kroll I, Barlow JH, Shaw K. Treatment adherence in juvenile rheumatoid arthritis—a review. Scand J Rheumatol 1999; 28(1):10–8.

37. Meichenbaum D, Turk DC. Facilitating Treatment Adherence. A Practitioner's Guidebook. New York, London: Plenum Press, 1987.

38. Ginsburg KR, Slap GB. Unique needs of the teen in the health care setting. Curr Opin Pediatr 1996; 8(4):333–7.

39. Malus M. Towards a separate adolescent medicine [editorial]. Br Med J 1992; 305:789–90.

40. Nash AA, Britto MT, Lovell DJ, et al. Substance abuse among adolescents with juvenile rheumatoid arthritis. Arthritis Care Res 1998; 11(5):391–6.

41. Society for Adolescent Medicine. Confidential health care for adolescents: Position paper of the Society for Adolescent Medicine. J Adoles Health 1997; 21:408–15.

42. Sallfors C, Hallberg LR, Fasth A. Well-being in children with juvenile chronic arthritis. Clin Exp Rheumatol 2004; 22(1):125–30.

43. Schanberg LE, Anthony KK, Gil KM, et al. Family pain history predicts child health status in children with chronic rheumatic disease. Pediatrics 2001; 108(3):E47.
44. Thastum M, Zachariae R, Herlin T. Pain experience and pain coping strategies in children with juvenile idiopathic arthritis. J Rheumatol 2001; 28:1091–8.
45. Schanberg LE, Lefebvre JC, Keefe FJ, et al. Pain coping and the pain experience in children with juvenile chronic arthritis. Pain 1997; 73(2):181–9.
46. Peterson CC, Palermo TM. Parental reinforcement of recurrent pain: the moderating impact of child depression and anxiety on functional disability. J Pediatr Psychol 2004; 29(5):331–41.
47. LeBovidge JS, Lavigne JV, Donenberg GR, et al. Psychological adjustment of children and adolescents with chronic arthritis: a meta-analytic review. J Pediatr Psychol 2003; 28(1):29–39.
48. Huygen AC, Kuis W, Sinnema G. Psychological, behavioural, and social adjustment in children and adolescents with juvenile chronic arthritis. Ann Rheum Dis 2000; 59(4):276–82.
49. Reiter-Purtill J, Gerhardt CA, Vannatta K, et al. A controlled longitudinal study of the social functioning of children with juvenile rheumatoid arthritis. J Pediatr Psychol 2003; 28(1):17–28.
50. Noll RB, Kozlowski K, Gerhardt C, et al. Social, emotional, and behavioral functioning of children with juvenile rheumatoid arthritis. Arthritis Rheum 2000; 43(6):1387–96.
51. Packham JC, Hall MA. Long-term follow-up of 246 adults with juvenile idiopathic arthritis: functional outcome. Rheumatology (Oxford) 2002; 41(12):1428–35.
52. Packham JC, Hall MA. Long-term follow-up of 246 adults with juvenile idiopathic arthritis: education and employment. Rheumatology (Oxford) 2002; 41(12):1436–9.
53. Packham JC, Hall MA. Long-term follow-up of 246 adults with juvenile idiopathic arthritis: social function, relationships and sexual activity. Rheumatology (Oxford) 2002; 41(12):1440–3.
54. Snaith RP, Zigmond AS. HADS—Hospital Anxiety and Depression Scale. Windsor, UK: NFER Nelson, 1994.
55. Packham JC, Hall MA, Pimm TJ. Long-term follow-up of 246 adults with juvenile idiopathic arthritis: predictive factors for mood and pain. Rheumatology (Oxford) 2002; 41(12):1444–9.
56. Miller III JJ. Psychosocial factors related to rheumatic diseases in childhood. J Rheumatol 1993; 20(Suppl. 38):1–11.
57. Woodgate RL. Conceptual understanding of resilience in the adolescents with cancer: Part I. J Pediat Oncol Nursing 1999; 16(1):35–43.
58. Olsson CA, Bond L, Burns JM, et al. Adolescent resilience: a concept analysis. J Adolesc 2003; 26(1):1–11.
59. Fonagy P, Steele M, Steele H, et al. The Emanuel Miller Memorial Lecture 1992. The theory and practice of resilience. J Child Psychol Psychiat 1994; 35:231–57.
60. Luthar SS, Zigler E. Vulnerability and competence: a review of research on resilience in childhood. Am J Orthopsychiat 1991; 61(1):6–22.

61. LeBovidge JS, Lavigne JV, Miller ML. Adjustment to chronic arthritis of childhood: The roles of illness-related stress and attitude toward illness. J Pediatr Psychol 2005; 30(3):273–86.

62. Garmezy N. Stress-resistant children: the search for protective factors. In: Stevenson JE, ed. Recent Research in Developmental Psychopathology. Oxford: Pergamon Press, 1985:213–33.

63. Rutter M. Resilience in the face of adversity. Protective factors and resistance to psychiatric disorder. Br J Psychiat 1985; 147:598–611.

64. Lösel F, Bliesener T, Köferl P. Psychische Gesundheit trotz Risikobelastung in der Kindheit: Untersuchungen zur "Invulnerabilität." In: Seiffge-Krenke I, eds. Jahrbuch der medizinischen Psychologie (Band 4): Krankheitsverarbeitung bei Kindern und Jugendlichen. [Mental Health in Spite of Negative Life Events During Childhood: Studies on "Invulnerability." In: Yearbook of Medical Psychology (vol. 4)] Berlin, Heidelberg: Springer-Verlag, 1990:103–23.

65. Vandvik IH, Hoyeraal HM. Juvenile chronic arthritis: a biobehavioral disease. Some unsolved questions. Clin Exp Rheumatol 1993; 11:669–80.

66. Dahlquist LM. Commentary: Are children with JRA and their families at risk or resilient? J Pediatr Psychol 2003; 28(1):45–6.

67. Routh DK. Commentary: juvenile rheumatic disease as a psychosocial stressor. J Pediatr Psychol 2003; 28(1):41–3.

68. Jacobs JC. Pediatric rheumatology for the practitioner. 3rd edn. New York, Berlin, Heidelberg: Springer-Verlag, 1993.

3

Growing Pains: Growth and Puberty

Priscilla L. Campbell-Stokes

Paediatric Department, Hutt Hospital, Lower Hutt, Wellington, New Zealand

Nick J. Shaw

Departments of Rheumatology and Endocrinology, Birmingham Children's Hospital, Birmingham, U.K.

INTRODUCTION

Growth and development are unique to children and young people. Statural growth and pubertal development, just like any other aspect of growth and development, are complex processes requiring a healthy balance of both internal (metabolic) and external (psychosocial) factors in order to proceed normally. Disruption of such development may consequently occur due to a multitude of factors, many of which can be exemplified in chronic rheumatic disease.

In order to recognize and subsequently address potential issues related to statural growth and pubertal development in young people with chronic rheumatic diseases, one needs to be familiar with the factors and processes that are required for normal growth and development. This chapter first reviews normal statural growth and pubertal development. How these may be adversely impacted by chronic rheumatic disease is then discussed. This is followed by an outline to guide initial assessment of young people with chronic rheumatic disease with associated short stature and/or delayed puberty. Finally, general principles for managing these complications are discussed.

NORMAL GROWTH AND DEVELOPMENT

Stature

Although the process of physical maturation that occurs during adolescence, puberty, incorporates the final growth spurt and attainment of final adult height, we first need to consider the aspects of growth prior to this period. As in any aspect of development throughout life, there is normal variation in the development of stature. On top of this normal variation, chronic rheumatic illness can variably impact growth in the prepubertal years and can subsequently impact growth further during the pubertal process.

Growth data, provided in the form of growth reference charts, forms the basis for assessing the "normality" of stature. There are various growth reference charts available for this purpose derived from different populations at different times. Growth reference charts derived from longitudinal data, repeated measurements of the same children over time, more accurately reflect an individual's growth compared to those derived from cross-sectional data, measurements of different children at different ages (1). The normal range is often between the 3rd and 97th percentiles, but varies a little, for example, between the 2nd and 98th percentiles using U.K. 1990 standards (Figs. 1 and 2). Children and young people growing outside these limits may still be growing normally, however, and other factors need to be taken into consideration.

During the first one to two years of life most infant's length adjusts either upwards or downwards, reflecting a transition from intrauterine growth determinants (including maternal size and fetal nutrition) to their genetic (familial and ethnic) growth potential (1). During the childhood years (age 2–9 years) a child is expected to grow along the same percentile, as determined by their genetic growth potential. This is simply estimated (provided no parental growth pathology) by calculating the mid parental height range (MPHR) (2) as follows:

For a male child, MPHR

$$= \frac{\text{Father's height} + \text{Mother's height} + 12.5 \text{ cm}}{2} +/-10 \text{ cm}$$

For a female child, MPHR

$$= \frac{\text{Father's height} + \text{Mother's height} - 12.5 \text{ cm}}{2} +/-8.5 \text{ cm}$$

The MPHR is the 95% confidence interval for that family, indicating that 95% of the couple's sons/daughters are expected to attain final adult heights within the range (in the absence of pathology).

Changing percentiles during puberty reflects the wide normal variation in timing and rate of the pubertal growth spurt. Some growth charts provide percentiles for early and late developers, in addition to average developers (Figs. 1 and 2).

The early stages of growth failure are more readily apparent when height velocity (growth rate) is compared to recognized standards (2) (Figs. 3 and 4). The normal range is between the 25th and 75th percentiles. Height velocity is slowest just prior to the pubertal growth spurt.

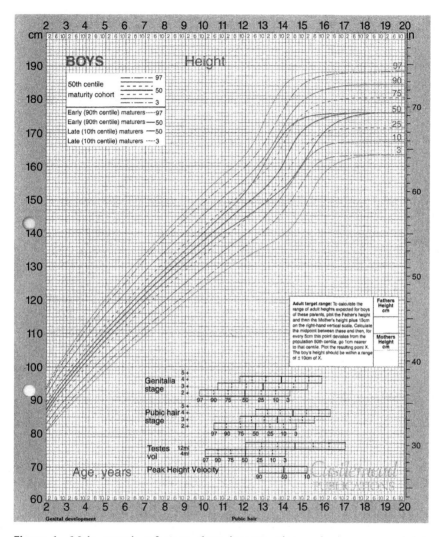

Figure 1 Male growth reference chart incorporating early, average, and late puberty-onset growth percentiles.

Puberty

Hormonal Regulation of Puberty

The pubertal process of physical maturation results in the attainment of final adult height, sex-specific changes in body fat and lean body mass, and the development of the secondary sex characteristics. There is wide individual variation in the timing of both the onset and duration of this process.

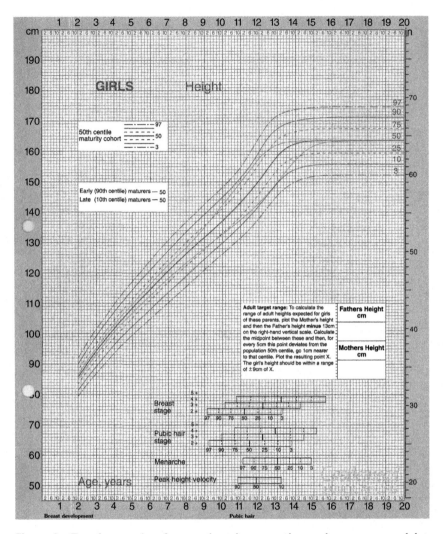

Figure 2 Female growth reference chart incorporating early, average, and late puberty-onset growth percentiles.

However, knowing the average age-of-onset and duration of each phase, the predictable sequential progression through the stages, and an understanding of the overall process will help identify young people not progressing through the process as anticipated.

The exact factor(s) initiating the pubertal process remains unknown, although current thinking proposes a body clock concept (housed in the hypothalamus) under the control of yet to be found "master genes" (3). The

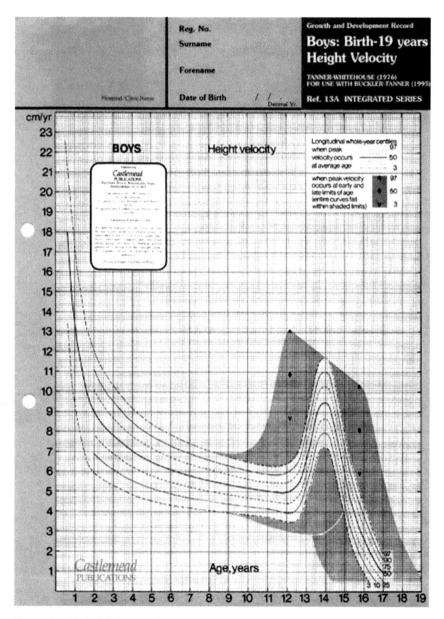

Figure 3 Male height-velocity chart.

control of subsequent physiologic events via the hypothalamic-pituitary-gonadal (HPG) axis is better defined.

The gonadotrophin releasing hormone (GnRH)-producing hypothalamic cells release GnRH in a pulsatile manner throughout life, leading to

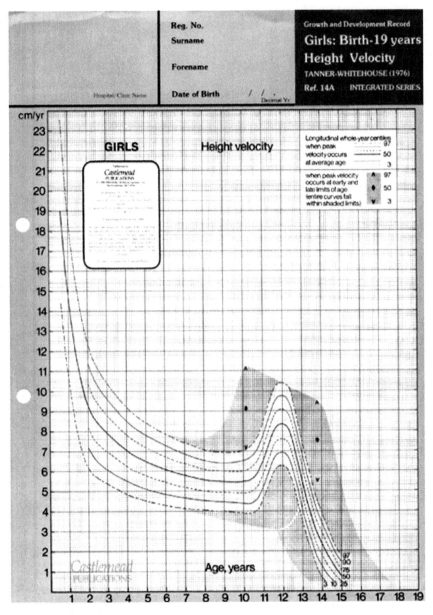

Figure 4   Female height-velocity chart.

pulsatile secretions of the pituitary luteinizing and follicle stimulating hormones (LH and FSH). The axis is relatively dormant during childhood as a
consequence of central inhibitory mechanisms. With the onset of puberty
this inhibition is released and there is a progressive reduction in the

sensitivity of the GnRH-producing hypothalamic cells to the negative feedback of circulating gonadal steroids (estrogen and testosterone). As a consequence there is an increase in both the amplitude and frequency of LH and FSH release, during sleep initially, with FSH increasing more than LH as puberty approaches. LH primarily regulates the subsequent increases in estrogen and testosterone levels in females and males, respectively (4).

Estrogen and testosterone initiate and maintain the process of development of secondary sexual characteristics as well as contribute to the growth spurt, other physical changes, and the development of fertility. Although breast development is the first overt sign of puberty onset in females, estrogen levels are known to increase well in advance of this, commencing enlargement of internal genital organs two years before breast budding. Estrogen levels in females rise more steadily and less dramatically than testosterone levels in males, with pubertal testosterone levels reaching more than 20 times adult levels (4).

The development of a positive feedback loop between the ovary (estrogen), hypothalamus (GnRH) and pituitary (LH) occurs late in the pubertal process and results in menstrual cycles. This process of positive feedback may take some time to fully mature, hence the irregularity of cycles in the first few years following menarche.

The onset and progress of puberty is also influenced by genetic factors (family history of puberty onset), under- and overnutrition, chronic illness, psychosocial factors, and possibly undefined growth factors. The relationship between body weight and the onset of puberty is illustrated by the steady decrease in age of menarche during the last century (which has recently plateaued) due to a steady increase in body size resulting from improved general health and nutrition (3). Pubertal onset requires an increase in leptin levels from adipose tissue, perhaps signaling the attainment of an appropriate nutritional and metabolic milieu in which puberty can proceed, although this is not the primary initiating mechanism as once thought (3).

While the hormones of the HPG axis have the primary role in the pubertal process, other hormones are still important. Growth hormone (GH), and hence insulin-like growth factor 1 (IGF-1), are increased by the gonadal hormones. Without GH, full height potential will not be attained. Likewise, full height attainment is dependent on the presence of thyroid hormone, although thyroid hormone levels do not alter during puberty. In contrast, the increase in adrenal hormones [dehydroepiandrosterone (DHEA) and DHEA-sulphate] via the hypothalamic-pituitary-adrenal (HPA) axis is not necessary for pubertal height acceleration. Instead increased adrenal hormones, a consequence of the adrenarche, influence development of axillary and pubic hair, especially in females (4).

In terms of the pubertal growth spurt, estrogen and testosterone are the main promoters in females and males, respectively, with GH and IGF-1 the important secondary effectors. The latter affect the rate of growth while estrogens and/or androgens control bone maturation (closure of the epi-physes) and hence duration of the pubertal growth spurt (4).

Physical Changes During Puberty

Around 15% of final adult height is attained during the pubertal spurt (on average 25 cm in females and 30 cm in males). Following the prepubertal deceleration in height velocity, the female accelerates soon after the onset of breast development to a peak velocity in mid puberty, 6 to 12 months prior to the menarche. The remaining attainable height averages 5 cm following the menarche, more in those with earlier menarche and vice versa. Males, on the other hand, start their height spurt later into puberty, usually when the testes are of 8 ml volume, getting on average two extra years of prepubertal growth than females. They have a higher growth rate, reaching an average peak height velocity of 9 cm per year, and continue to grow for longer, leading to an average difference between adult males and females of 12.5 cm (3, 4).

Despite asynchrony between the HPG axis (breast and genital develop-ment) and the HPA axis (pubic hair development) and the different stages varying at different rates (Fig. 5), as a general rule, most pubertal events are approximately normally distributed with a standard deviation (SD) of one year. An approximate estimation of the normal range for a particular pubertal event can be calculated by adding and subtracting two years from the average age of the event (3) (Table 1). However, young people found to be outside these ranges need more careful clinical evaluation to differentiate those whose pubertal progress may still be normally variable, from those whose progress is pathological.

Tanner and Marshall devised a five-stage pubertal progression of the secondary sexual characteristics, from the prepubertal Stage 1 through to the adult stage 5 (5,6). These are illustrated and described in Figures 6 and 7. Estimation of testicular volume is commonly undertaken with the Prader orchidometer (Fig. 8). Progression from 3 to 4 mL testes with thinning of scrotum indicates the onset of puberty in the male. Up to two-thirds of males may develop breast enlargement (gynecomastia), and this is most prominent in late puberty (G4), and as in the female may be non-pathologically asymmetrical. In the female, estrogen also promotes devel-opment of the internal genitalia (vagina, uterus, and ovaries) concurrently with the above external changes.

The other physiologic changes that occur during puberty include:

- Change in body composition. Females start to lay down more body fat from 7 years of age, developing twice as much as males by age 16 years. Meanwhile males undergo an acceleration of lean body mass growth from around 9 years, doubling their muscle and skeletal mass by 16 to 17 years. This lean body mass increase starts more peripherally in the hands and feet, and progresses centrally, with truncal growth occurring last (4).

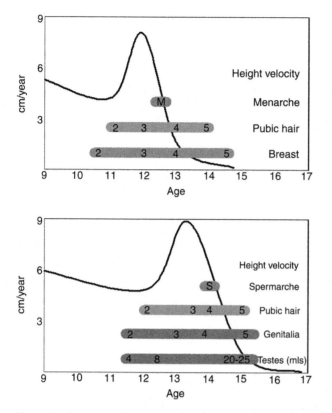

Figure 5 Progress of male and female pubertal development.

- Bone accretion. Estrogen and testosterone primarily regulate bone accretion which peaks in the second decade of life, and is complete by 16 to 17 years in females, but not until the early twenties in males. General nutrition, calcium intake, vitamin D levels, exercise, and menstrual history are also contributing factors.
- Development of facial hair and a deepening of the voice occur in late male development, stage G3–4.
- Increase in bone-derived alkaline phosphatase levels during the growth spurt.
- Increase in hematocrit, hemoglobin, and cholesterol with increased levels of testosterone.

IMPACT OF CHRONIC RHEUMATIC DISEASE ON GROWTH AND DEVELOPMENT

The two main disturbances of growth and pubertal development seen in young people with chronic rheumatic disease are growth failure and

Table 1   Average Age of Pubertal Development

Pubertal event	Females Average age	Stage	Bone age	Males Average age	Stage	Bone age
Puberty onset						
Breasts	10.5	B2	11			
Genitalia/ testes				11.5	G2 O4	12
Pubic hair	11	P2		12–12.5	P2	
Menarche/ spermarche	12–13	B3–4		14	G3–4	
Start of height spurt	11	B2	11	12.5	G2–3 O6–8	13
Peak of height spurt	12	B2–3	14	13.5	G3–4	14
Puberty end	14–15	B5 P5	15	16–17	G5 O20– 25 P5	17

Abbreviations: B, breasts; G, penis and scrotum; O, testes volume as per orchidometer; P, pubic hair.

pubertal delay. Young people with such conditions may experience either condition or both. Together they can result in short stature, reduced bone density (see Chapter 12), low self-esteem, poor body image, and delayed development of the psychosocial tasks of adolescence (see Chapter 1).

Outcome studies in juvenile idiopathic arthritis (JIA) from as early as the 1950s and up to the present day describe significant generalized and localized growth disturbances, short stature, and shortened bones respectively. Conclusions from these studies have changed little from the earlier descriptions by Ansell and Bywaters in 1956 (7). They found from a survey of 119 children less than 14 years of age with Still's disease (now known as JIA systemic onset) that disease activity retarded growth resulting in infantile proportions and that this was exacerbated by systemic steroid treatment. In addition, they saw catch-up growth during disease remission, especially in the younger children, but not in those with longstanding and severe disease activity.

Subsequent studies have found that growth failure is most severe in the systemic onset and polyarticular subtypes of JIA and particularly those with a more severe course and/or treated with systemic steroids. The individual contribution from each of these two factors is difficult to establish. Zak et al. found the mean final height of 65 adults with all subtypes of JIA to be −0.25 standard deviation score (SDS), not significantly different from the general population (8). However, their heights were not normally distributed, and 10.7% had a final height more than two SD below the general population mean. Just over a quarter also had significantly reduced arm span, a

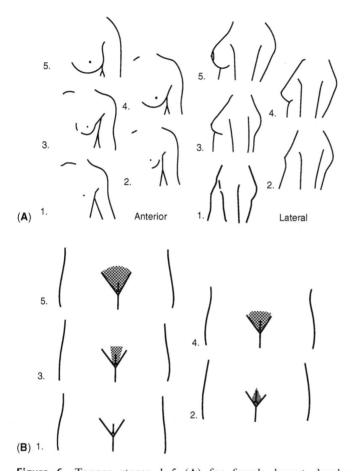

Figure 6 Tanner stages 1–5 (**A**) for female breast development. *Stage 1*: Preadolescent: elevation of papilla only. *Stage 2*: Breast bud stage: elevation of breast and papilla as small mound. Enlargement of areola diameter. *Stage 3*: Further enlargement and elevation of breast and areola, with no separation of their contours. *Stage 4*: Projection of areola and papilla to form a secondary mound above the level of the breast. *Stage 5*: Mature stage: projection of papilla only due to recession of the areola and general contour of the breast. Tanner stages 1–5 (**B**) for female pubic hair development. *Stage 1*: Preadolescent: The vellus over the pubes is not further developed than that over the abdominal wall, i.e., no pubic hair. *Stage 2*: Sparse growth of long, slightly pigmented downy hair, straight or slightly curled, chiefly along labia. *Stage 3*: Considerably darker, coarser, and more curled. The hair spreads sparsely over the junction of the pubes. *Stage 4*: Hair now adult type, but the area covered is still considerably smaller than in the adult. No spread to medial surface of thighs. *Stage 5*: Adult in quantity and type with distribution of the horizontal (or classical "feminine") pattern. Spread to the medial surface of the thighs but not up the linea alba or elsewhere above the base of the inverse triangle (spread up linea alba occurs late and rated stage 6).

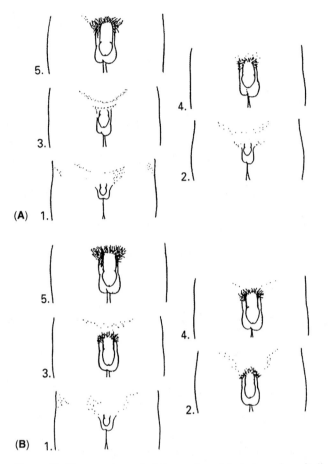

Figure 7   Tanner stages 1–5 for male pubic hair and genitalia development. Pubic
hair stages (**A**) as per females (see page 41). Tanner stages 1–5 (**B**) for male genitalia
development. *Stage 1*: Preadolescent: testes, penis and scrotum are of about the same
size and proportion as in early childhood. *Stage 2*: Enlargement of scrotum and
testes. Skin of scrotum reddens and changes in texture. Little or no enlargement of
the penis at this stage. *Stage 3*: Enlargement of penis, which occurs at first mainly in
length. Further growth of testes and scrotum. *Stage 4*: Increased size of penis with
growth in breadth and development of glans. Testes and scrotum larger; scrotal skin
darkened. *Stage 5*: Genitalia adult in size and shape.

consequence of both generalized and localized growth disturbance. Twenty-
five to 30% of the variation in these growth disturbances was related to JIA
subtype (systemic onset and polyarticular versus oligoarticular), systemic
steroid treatment, and Steinbrocker functional class (II–IV vs. I).

   More recently, a larger study of 246 adults with JIA found males and
females to be on average 4.2 and 3.8 cm shorter respectively than the male

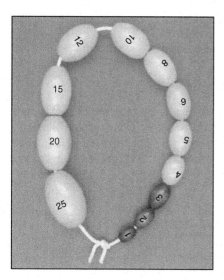

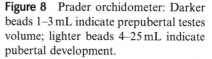

Figure 8 Prader orchidometer: Darker beads 1–3 mL indicate prepubertal testes volume; lighter beads 4–25 mL indicate pubertal development.

and female general populations (9). Reduced final height was significantly associated with duration of systemic steroid treatment, again implicating both systemic steroid treatment and disease severity.

A smaller study of 24 patients with JIA systemic onset receiving oral steroids for at least two years, retrospectively, described growth from diagnosis, through childhood disease activity to final height (10). At diagnosis mean height SDS for age was −0.03 and not significantly different from height expected for genetic potential. After 4 years of disease activity they experienced a significant loss of height with a mean height −2.7 SDS. The reduction in height velocity correlated with duration of systemic steroid. Following discontinuation of oral steroids 70% had a partial catch up in height (mean of 1 SDS) with mean final height −1.5 SDS, while 30% had persistent poor height velocity and mean final height of −3.6 SDS. The mean final height was strongly correlated with height SDS at discontinuation of oral steroids. In addition, greater catch-up growth was seen in those growing above their genetic potential at diagnosis. Overall 41% had final heights more than two SD below the general population mean, and 87% failed to attain heights within their genetic potential. This study highlighted two critical periods impacting final height, which become important when considering intervention and prevention: the active disease phase and the period following systemic steroid discontinuation.

The impact of disease activity on growth in the absence of steroid use is illustrated by Chedeville et al. (11) who showed improved height and height velocity in 21 prepubertal children with JIA who responded to Methotrexate compared to 6 prepubertal children with JIA who did not respond to Methotrexate by one year. The improved growth was still significant after three years.

There is no published research describing growth during puberty in young people with JIA, and little describing their pubertal course. In a cohort of 13 young people with JIA (systemic onset or polyarticular requiring oral steroids) and receiving GH, 9 had entered puberty at a mean age of 12.8 years (9.6–15.4) and 15.5 (12.5–16.3) in females and males respectively (12). Rusconi et al. (13) found that menarche occurred later in 83 females with JIA compared to their mothers and healthy Italian controls, and more so in those on oral steroids or with systemic onset. Other studies have found no difference in age of menarche compared to the general population (14,15). However, clinical experience indicates that pubertal delay is common in young people with JIA systemic onset. Glucocorticoids, particularly in high doses may cause menstrual irregularities, including primary or secondary amenorrhea.

Few final height data are available from other chronic rheumatic disease groups such as the connective tissue disorders, presumably due to their lower prevalence and greater heterogeneity. Short stature in addition to asymmetric growth abnormalities have been reported in the connective tissue disorders of SLE, JDMS, and scleroderma (16). It has been shown, however, that for the same systemic steroid doses, those with JIA experience greater reductions in height than those with SLE, highlighting the disease specific contributions to growth failure (17).

The main contributing factors to growth failure are the following:

- Chronic active systemic inflammation
- Chronic localized inflammation (hyperemia, local growth and inflammatory factors) damaging the growth plate and accelerating epiphyseal maturation
- Glucocorticoid treatment
- Osteoporosis with vertebral collapse
- Undernutrition (anorexia, increased caloric requirements—inflammation/infection)
- Adverse impact of chronic illness on emotional state
- Pubertal delay

In addition, there are issues associated with adolescent development that can impact on the course of the illness and its management, which in turn may further affect physical growth and development (18). These include:

- Increased caloric need for the pubertal growth spurt
- Changing hepatic and renal metabolism, necessitating medication dose adjustment

- Reduced adherence to management, which may be a consequence of delayed cognitive development, competing priorities, and exploration of health risk behaviors

Figure 9 depicts the GH–IGF-1 axis regulating growth along with some of the factors leading to growth failure. The most important determinant appears to be the net circulating level of IGF-1 activity (19).

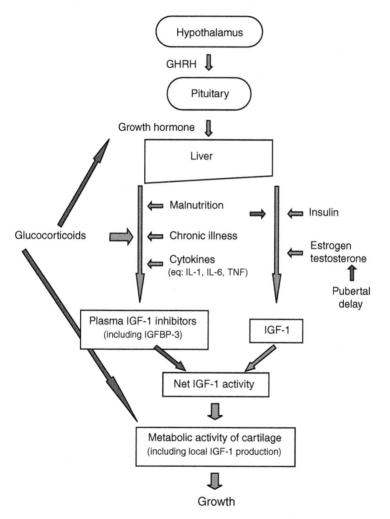

Figure 9 Mechanisms of growth failure in chronic rheumatic disease involving the GH–IGF-1 axis. *Abbreviations*: GHRH, growth hormone releasing hormone; IGF-1, insulin-like growth factor-1; IGFBP-3, insulin-like growth factor binding protein-3; IL-1, interleukin-1; IL-6, interleukin-6; TNF, tumor necrosis factor. *Source*: Adapted from Ref. 19.

Glucocorticoids have a normal physiologic function in mediating catabolic processes such as proteolysis. As a consequence, in supra-physiologic amounts, such as treatment with oral steroids, growth is inhibited and height velocity slows. The mechanism for this is thought to be a combination of suppression of GH secretion, stimulation of IGF-1 inhibitors, and direct effects on the growth plate (20–22). It has been established that this occurs in doses equivalent to at least 0.25 mg per kg per day of prednisolone (23,24). Following oral or intravenous administration of prednisolone, IGF-1 activity levels fall over the first 4–6 hours respectively, with recovery by 24 hours (19). The use of alternate day oral steroids allows a period of normal IGF-1 activity, and therefore the potential for normal height velocity and growth to be maintained (19). However, disease control is not often able to be maintained with alternate day regimes and potentially may lead to protracted steroid therapy.

There have been several small studies in children with JIA assessing GH secretion as well as IGF-1 levels, with variable results. Touati et al. (25) treated 14 children with severe systemic onset or polyarticular JIA and growth failure receiving oral steroids with GH for one year. Baseline measurements revealed spontaneous nocturnal GH levels more than two SD below the mean in half the children, normal stimulated GH levels in all but one, low-normal IGF-1 levels in 12 and normal IGFBP-3 levels in all children. With GH treatment (0.46 mg/kg/wk) IGF-1 and IGFBP-3 levels rose, as did the IGF-1/IGFBP-3 ratio, indicating an overall increase in IGF-1 activity. Davies et al. (26) found baseline 24-hour GH profiles in 12 prepubertal children with JIA and growth retardation to be the same as those seen in "short normal" children. Levels of IGF-1 and IGF BP-3 however were lower than controls. Following treatment with GH, levels of IGF-1 increased within four days and correlated with height velocity.

CLINICAL ASSESSMENT

Stature

Assessment of stature starts with regular height measurement (Box 1). This requires consistent and correct technique for reliable data. It is helpful, if

---

Box 1   Assessment of Stature

- Accurate height measurement
- Calculation of height velocity
- Comparison with appropriate growth charts and standards
- Calculation of mid-parental height range
- Correct interpretation of data

possible, for young people to be measured by the same person at each visit, especially when the young person has significant joint deformities or treatment decisions are being considered, to minimize interobserver error.

Measuring Technique

A correctly installed stadiometer should be used, which is checked regularly for accuracy. The young person should be positioned in bare feet, with their heels, buttocks, and shoulder blades against the back wall/plate. The head should be held so that the Frankfurt plane (the imaginary line from the center of the ear hole to the lower border of the eye socket) is horizontal. The head board should exert a gentle downward pressure to allow good contact with the head. The height should be read at maximum stretch, but without having caused lifting or overextension (2).

When there are significant joint deformities, particularly of the spine and lower limbs, an accurate description of this should be noted, as changing joint deformity (with changing disease activity) can affect the ability to position a young person correctly for measurement and can therefore affect the measurement obtained.

Height measurements should be plotted on an appropriate growth reference chart for sex and age. By definition, short stature is when a person's height is below the 2nd percentile (more than two SD below the mean). Despite this, the person's height may be normal for their genetic potential (compare height percentile to that of the mid-parental height range) or pubertal stage. Pathological short stature is indicated by a poor growth velocity.

Calculation of Height Velocity

Height velocity should be calculated with a minimum of six months between height measurements, as growth does not occur in a smooth linear fashion and often has a seasonal influence. A 1-year interval overcomes the seasonal effect on growth, but may not allow timely recognition of growth slowing.

Height velocity (cm per year)

$$= \frac{\text{Current height} - \text{Previous height}}{\text{Months between measures}} \times 12$$

These calculations can then be plotted against recognized standards for sex, age, and pubertal stage (Figs. 3 and 4). Early growth failure can be recognized when height velocities are consistently below the 25th percentile.

The differential diagnosis of short stature and an approach to clinical evaluation and investigation (1) is outlined in Table 2. First an assessment is made between normal variant short stature and pathologic short stature. If pathologic, body proportions are measured to distinguish proportionate from disproportionate. Thirdly, for those with proportionate short stature, timing of onset (pre- or postnatal) is determined to further narrow the likely

Table 2 Differential Diagnosis of Short Stature

Condition	Features/investigations
Normal variants	
Familial short stature	Predicted final height within MPHR (albeit short)
	Bone age normal for chronological age
	Normal history and examination
	Normal height velocity (growth parallel to 3rd percentile for average pubertal development)
Constitutional delay of growth and development	Bone age delayed by more than 2 SD
	Delayed puberty and growth spurt (otherwise normal history and examination)
	Height velocity normal for bone age (growth parallel to 3rd percentile for late pubertal development)
	Family history delayed puberty
	Normal final height
Pathologic	
Proportionate	Normal US:LS ratio for age (mean 1.0 after 7 yrs)
	Normal arm span–height for age (0 cm 8–12 yrs; + 1 cm for females and + 4 cm for males at 14 yrs)
Postnatal: Birth growth parameters appropriate for gestational age	
Chronic illness and/or malnutrition	History/examination/screening and confirmatory tests
Endocrine disorders	History/examination/
Hypopituitarism	Respective hormone profiles
Growth hormone deficiency	
Hypothyroidism	
Cushing syndrome	
Psychosocial deprivation	Social and dietary history/developmental examination
Prenatal: Small at birth for gestational age	
IUGR	Antenatal/maternal history/examination/ TORCH screen
Chromosomal disorders (including Turner syndrome)	Dysmorphic/congenital anomalies/karyotype
Dysmorphic syndromes	Dysmorphic/congenital anomalies/radiology

(Continued)

Table 2 Differential Diagnosis of Short Stature (*Continued*)

Condition	Features/investigations
Disproportionate	Abnormal US:LS ratio for age
	Abnormal arm span–height for age
Skeletal dysplasias	Skeletal radiology
Rickets	History/examination/calcium/phosphate/
	alkaline phosphatase/radiology

Abbreviations: MPHR, mid-parental height range; TORCH, toxoplasmosis, other, rubella, cytomegalovirus, herpes; US:LS, upper body segment height:lower body segment height.

diagnosis. It should also be noted that these diagnoses are not necessarily mutually exclusive, with some young people having a combination of factors contributing to their short stature. For example, a young person may have familial short stature exacerbated by chronic rheumatic disease and delayed puberty.

Puberty

Adolescence is a time when young people become particularly sensitive to their appearance and differences from their peers (see Chapter 2). They also are anxious about puberty onset and progress, although they may not overtly express these anxieties. For example, males more commonly present for assessment of delayed puberty, although there is little indication that the incidence varies much between the sexes (4). Common working definitions

---

Box 2 Assessment of Pubertal Delay

Trigger questions:

■ How do you compare yourself to peers in your class? Are you small? Do they appear more or less developed than you?
■ How do you like your body? What about it would you like to be different?
■ Have your periods started?

Bear-in-mind factors influencing pubertal development:

■ Ethnicity—black females enter puberty around one year earlier than white females and proceed through menarche around 6 months earlier
■ Family history—there is some concordance with parental age of puberty onset
■ Nutrition—chronic malnutrition can delay, while overnutrition can advance, puberty onset
■ Bone age—a young person's bone age, rather than chronological age, best concurs with pubertal development

of delayed puberty requiring assessment are: no breast development by 13 years or no menses by 15 years in females and prepubertal testes volume (<4 mL) at 14 years in males. While the majority will have constitutional delay, assessment is required to identify those requiring intervention, whether for psychological reasons or for pathologic delay. It is also important to try and ascertain which is more distressing to the young person: lack of pubertal changes or the associated short stature.

Just as height is assessed at each visit, an assessment of pubertal stage should also be made (Box 2). This allows for early identification of abnormalities, as well as allowing reassurance to be given. Historical information in addition to the chronic rheumatic disorder and its management should include: parental ages of puberty onset; symptoms suggestive of other hormonal disorders; past illnesses, their treatment and any surgery. Physical assessment should include: current and previous height and weight; pubertal staging according to Tanner and Marshall (Figs. 6 and 7) including determination of any significant discrepancy between gonadal (breast or testes) and adrenal (pubic hair) development; body proportions; and dysmorphic features. Assessment following referral to a pediatric endocrinologist will also involve neurological examination, visual fields, fundoscopy, and sense of smell.

Young people often find pubertal assessment embarrassing. Pictorial and written aids for self-assessment have been developed for use by adolescents. Studies assessing the reliability and validity of such assessments in different adolescent populations have shown inconsistent results (27–32). Concordance with physician examination ranged from fair to good with both over- and underestimation, varied by aspect of development (genital vs. pubic hair), ethnicity, and sex, with female self-assessments generally more reliable. If used in a clinical setting, they should not be relied upon for treatment decisions, but rather as a screening tool.

One of the most useful initial investigations is an X-ray of the left hand and wrist to assess bone age. However, this is unlikely to be useful in a proportion of young people with chronic rheumatic conditions with delayed growth and development. Those with JIA systemic onset or polyarthritis and associated growth abnormalities are more likely to have growth-plate damage in the hand and wrist secondary to their arthritis, making a bone age assessment difficult.

Delayed puberty in those with chronic rheumatic conditions is most commonly reversible, whether from a constitutional delay (family history of delayed puberty) or active inflammation and its treatment, particularly systemic steroids. If a bone age can be obtained, a delayed bone age is usually found, indicating potential for further height growth.

Table 3 outlines the differential diagnosis of delayed puberty (4,33–36). While not exhaustive it provides an approach to clinical evaluation and investigation. Two broad categories can be established by baseline

Table 3 Differential Diagnosis of Delayed Puberty

Condition	Features/investigations
Hypogonadotrophic hypogonadism: Low LH and FSH	
Reversible deficiency	
Constitutional delay of growth and pubertal development	Bone age delayed by more than 2 SD
	Delayed puberty and growth spurt (otherwise normal history and examination)
	Height velocity normal for bone age (growth parallel to 3rd percentile for late pubertal development)
	Family history delayed puberty
	Normal final height
Chronic illness and/or malnutrition	History/examination/screening and confirmatory test
Psychogenic disorders	History/examination
Excessive exercise	History/examination
Endocrine disorders	History/examination/respective hormone profiles
Cushing syndrome	
Hyperprolactinemia	
Hypothyroidism	
Permanent deficiency	
Hypothalamic-pituitary defects	
Acquired	
Chemotherapy/irradiation/ surgery	History/examination Neurological examination/MRI head
Tumors	
Congenital	
Panhypopituitarism	
Isolated gonadotrophin deficiency	LHRH test with other pituitary hormones
Kallman syndrome	Normal childhood growth, LHRH test with other pituitary hormones
Congenital midline defects	Normal childhood growth /sense of smell, LHRH test
	History/examination/MRI head
Hypergonadotrophic hypogonadism: High LH and FSH	
Chromosomal disorders	Dysmorphic features/body proportions/ karyotype
Klinefelter syndrome (47 XXY)	
Turner syndrome (45 X0) and variants	
Other variants of ovarian and testicular gonadal dysgenesis	

(Continued)

Table 3   Differential Diagnosis of Delayed Puberty (*Continued*)

Condition	Features/investigations
Testicular abnormalities	
Anorchism/cryptorchism/ testicular torsion	History/examination
Chemotherapy/irradiation/surgery to gonads	History
Viral infections, e.g., mumps orchitis	History
Some types of congenital adrenal hyperplasia e.g., 17α-hydroxylase deficiency	Biochemical evaluation
Autoimmune disorders, e.g., oophoritis	Serum autoantibodies

Abbreviations: LHRH, luteinizing hormone-releasing hormone; SD, standard deviation.

LH and FSH levels. In addition, there is a group of miscellaneous disorders, for example, Prader-Willi syndrome, Noonan syndrome, and testicular feminization.

It can often be difficult distinguishing between constitutional delay and other causes of hypogonadotrophic hypogonadism, and referral to a pediatric endocrinologist is recommended. Those with constitutional delay tend to also have delayed adrenarche (low DHEA-sulphate levels), while those with permanent causes of hypogonadotrophic hypogonadism tend to have normal onset of adrenarche, and therefore appropriately increasing DHEA-sulphate levels (37). There is however considerable overlap between the two groups. Recently, further attempts to help this distinction have included measurement of 8am testosterone levels: for those with levels greater than 0.7 nmol/L, 77% will have an increase in testicular volume to 4 ml or more within 12 months, and 100% within 15 months; while only 12% and 25% will do so within 12 and 15 months respectively with levels below 0.7 nmol/L (37). More definitive measures are still awaited while we continue to mostly rely on the passage of time to give the ultimate answer.

In addition, females may enter puberty normally and progress without establishing menstruation, while others may progress through menarche but then develop secondary amenorrhea. The differential diagnoses for primary amenorrhea in a pubertal female and secondary amenorrhea (36) are presented in Table 4.

MANAGEMENT

Short Stature

Despite the availability of GH, the primary consideration in the management of growth failure in chronic rheumatic disorders remains aiming for

Table 4 Differential Diagnosis of Amenorrhea Postpubertal Onset

Condition	Features/investigations
Primary amenorrhea with puberty onset	
Polycystic ovary syndrome	History/examination/pelvic ultrasound/androgens
Müllerian duct anomalies (adysplasia of vagina/cervix/uterus)	Pelvic ultrasound
Gonadal dysgenesis	Elevated LH/FSH, Karyotype
Hyperprolactinaemia	Prolactin levels
Testicular feminization	Minimal adrenarche, karyotpye
Secondary amenorrhea	
Elevated FSH	
Milder and partial forms of disorders causing hypergonadotrophic hypogonadism in Table 3	
Onset of acquired disorders in Table 3 during puberty for example, SLE treated with systemic steroids	
FSH not elevated	
Low estrogen	
Milder and partial forms of disorders causing hypogonadotrophic hypogonadism in Table 3	Karyotype
Variants of Turner syndrome	Very high androgen levels/adrenal
Virilization	suppression tests/ultrasound
Normal estrogen	
Extraovarian endocrine conditions Pregnancy, hypothyroidism, under-/overnutrition	History/examination/relevant hormones
Disturbance of cyclic LH release Psychogenic stress, hyperprolactinaemia	History/examination/relevant hormones
Hyperandrogenism (polycystic ovary syndrome)	History/examination/pelvic ultrasound/androgens

optimal control of inflammatory activity, minimizing the use of systemic steroids, and maintaining adequate nutrition (see Box 3). It must be emphasized that while systemic steroids reduce height growth, they do not reduce skeletal maturation to the same extent, therefore complete catch-up growth may not be achievable, and every effort must be made to limit the use of systemic steroids to maximize final height potential.

Unfortunately there are some prepubertal young people with chronic rheumatic conditions in whom remission cannot be adequately achieved, or

---

Box 3   Treatment of Short Stature

- Primary objective is disease control
- Catch-up growth potential reduced but greater the earlier disease is controlled before epiphyseal closure
- Use systemic steroid alternatives where possible
- If systemic steroids are required, aim for $<0.25\,mg/kg/day$ prednisolone equivalent
- Ensure adequate caloric intake and nutrition
- Use of growth hormone can prevent further loss

---

in whom disease control only comes at the expense of using growth suppressing doses of systemic steroids. In such situations, height velocities are reduced and loss of height SD scores ensues. Previously it was hoped that the impact on systemic steroids on growth retardation could be minimized with the use of alternate-day steroids or derivatives of Prednisolone such as Deflazacort (38). Unfortunately in practice these alternative regimes usually do not maintain disease control, and are therefore not now commonly used.

The short-term response to GH treatment is generally positive as indicated by the response in the studies discussed earlier. All 14 children treated by Touati et al. (25) with GH (0.46 mg/kg/week) had improved height velocities, increasing from a mean height velocity of 1.9 to 5.4 cm per year. This had the net result of preventing further loss of height SDS with no overall catch-up growth. A moderate ($r = 0.56$) negative correlation was found between baseline IGF-1 levels and height velocity with GH, and is potentially of predictive value for assessing likely response to treatment.

Thirteen of these children went on to have 3 years of GH treatment, following a year without (12). Growth velocity and IGF-1 and IGFBP-3 levels returned to baseline off treatment. Again, even after 3 years of treatment, the net result was prevention of further loss of height SDS with no overall catch-up growth, with height velocities slowing after the first year of treatment. Marked individual variation was seen however, with those with more severe disease (higher inflammatory markers and systemic steroid doses) losing height SDS while those with less disease activity improved their height SDS.

The children treated by Davies et al. (26) also had significant increases in height velocity following a year of GH. Greater height velocities were seen in those with polyarticular rather than systemic disease, mild to moderate disease and in those treated with a higher dose of GH (24 vs. 12 IU/m^2). They also found that height velocity correlated negatively with CRP levels. Very similar findings have more recently been reported by Bechtold et al. (39,40) following 2 and 4 years of growth hormone treatment using two dose regimes (determined by growth hormone status) and a control group.

Box 4 Growth Hormone Use in JIA

- Mostly short-term studies (up to 3 years)
- No studies through to final height
- Dose of 0.3–0.5 mg/kg/week required
- Improved height velocity has been seen for up to 3 years
- Maintains but does not improve height SDS
- Highly variable response
- Best response in those with low disease activity and prednisolone dose < 0.25 mg/kg/day
- Potential role for prophylactic GH needs further study

Studies have not yet been completed looking at final height outcome in those with JIA treated with GH.

Another more recent initiative has been the use of GH prophylactically. Simon et al. (41) randomly assigned 30 children early in the course of their JIA, having been on Prednisolone for only 12–15 months, to either GH treatment (0.46 mg/kg/week) for 2 years or no GH. Those treated had higher height velocity SD scores with a small (0.2 ± 1.1) overall gain in height SDS at 2 years, while those untreated lost height (height SDS –1.2 ± 0.8) at 2 years. In addition, those treated gained lean body mass and lost fat mass, with the opposite occurring in those untreated.

These studies do indicate a role for GH in JIA associated growth failure (Box 4). It must be remembered that the response is highly variable, being particularly dependent on disease activity and systemic steroid dose. Young people in whom this treatment is being considered must be appropriately informed and counseled so as not to give false expectations regarding intended benefit and final height outcome. Its use is only appropriate for those young people who are still prepubertal or in early to mid puberty where there is still potential for growth. Potential for further growth may however be difficult to gauge, independent of pubertal status, as damaged growth plates may render bone age interpretation impossible and they may have prematurely fused. For the same reasons it is also difficult to determine how long to continue GH treatment for, especially when there is no final outcome data.

The other prerequisite to treatment is that the young person must be in agreement and prepared to have daily subcutaneous injections, which may be in addition to other injectable treatments such as methotrexate or etanercept.

While there may not be clear, long-term height advantages yet from GH use in those with chronic rheumatic-disease-associated growth failure, the potential for psychological benefits should not be discounted (12,39). GH counteracts the anti-lipolytic effect of glucocorticoids and can improve body composition and reduce cushingnoid appearances. On the other hand, there are potential side effects, including the development of glucose intolerance, which usually reverses on cessation of GH and rarely results in overt diabetes mellitus (12,39).

Delayed Puberty

Management should begin with counseling and reassurance. If possible, underlying causes of pubertal delay should be treated. If this is not possible, management is either directed towards puberty induction with short courses of low dose sex steroids in those with reversible delayed puberty, or to long-term sex hormone replacement therapy (Box 5).

Short courses of sex steroids induce puberty which then continues spontaneously, albeit sometimes at a slower rate. This is usually enough to result in the pubertal height spurt, development of secondary sex characteristics, and accretion of bone mass.

Issues to consider around the timing of treatment are: prepubertal growth and any concomitant GH therapy; psychological impact including delayed development of adolescent tasks; and the potential long-term effect of a prolonged delay till puberty induction on bone mass accretion.

The decision to treat or not to treat, and if so when, should be made in conjunction with the young person. Treatment is therefore individualized, taking into account all aspects of the young person's life, including health status and psychological effects, along with intended benefits.

The main error to avoid with treatment is accelerating the bone age faster than the chronological age, and thereby reducing final height. This error can be avoided with short, low-dose courses of sex steroids.

For males older than 14 years, a short course (3–6 months) of low-dose testosterone or androgens will often be enough to induce puberty, initiating changes of the external genitalia (penis and scrotum). Any increase in testicular size during treatment indicates the onset of normal puberty. Occasionally a second course may be required if puberty does not commence following the first course and a period of observation. The common regimes include:

- testosterone enanthate, 50 mg IM monthly for 4–6 months;
- oxandrolone, 2.5 mg orally daily for 3–6 months.

Box 5   Treatment of Delayed Puberty

- Primary objective is disease control
- Ensure adequate caloric intake and nutrition
- Counsel and reassure
- Use short courses of low-dose sex steroids to induce puberty (in consultation with the young person), avoiding acceleration of bone maturation

---

Those with permanent gonadotrophin deficiency will require long-term hormone replacement therapy starting usually around the average age of puberty. Testosterone enanthate is given IM every four weeks, starting at 50 mg and increasing by 50 mg every six months to a maintenance dose of 200–300 mg 3–4 weekly.

Short courses of treatment for pubertal induction are less commonly given to females, with reassurance and padded bras often being satisfactory unless puberty is markedly delayed. When treatment is considered low-dose androgens, such as oxandrolone orally daily for six months, may initially be used in the presence of short stature and a bone age of less than 11 years (35). Puberty (and feminization) can then be induced with ethinyl oestradiol 2 μg daily orally (or with a depot estradiol preparation) for six months.

If ongoing hormone replacement is required, the dose of ethinyl oestradiol is doubled every 6 to 12 months to 20 μg, simulating normal pubertal progression. Menarche usually occurs after two to three years of treatment, at which time a progestin, such as medroxyprogesterone acetate (MPA) can be added to cyclical estrogen. For example, give 5–10 mg of MPA daily for the last 5–7 days of a 21–25 day estrogen cycle per month. On attainment of final height, a low-dose estrogen combined oral contraceptive pill is then usually preferred (35).

SUMMARY

With recent and ongoing advances in new therapies for chronic rheumatic diseases, there is hope that in the future children and young people with these conditions will more readily establish disease control with minimal need for systemic steroids. Unfortunately, this is not yet the case and we still have children and young people with difficult-to-suppress inflammation and/or dependent on systemic steroids. Addressing the growth and puberty delaying consequences is an important ongoing part of the clinical assessment process. These issues need to be addressed early and in consultation with the young person in order to maximize both physical and psychological outcomes.

CLINICAL EXAMPLES

Short Stature

Case 1 was 2½ years old when she was diagnosed with JIA systemic onset. She was initially very unwell with associated bone marrow suppression, and she developed pericarditis during the first year of her illness. Her management included nonsteroidal anti-inflammatories, intermittent pulses of intravenous methylprednisolone, oral prednisolone in varying doses for 13 years, intra-articular steroids on six occasions, and methotrexate for 11 years.

Her statural growth during her disease course is shown in Figure 10. In addition to growth failure, her course was complicated by reduced bone

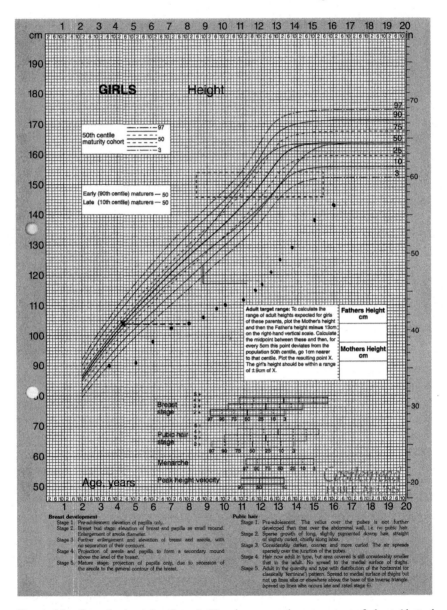

Figure 10 Growth chart for Case 1. X = bone age; bar near top of chart (dotted lines) indicates period of growth hormone treatment.

density and consequent vertebral crush fractures at 10 years of age. She was treated with three monthly cycles of pamidronate for a year and then oral alendronate for a year.

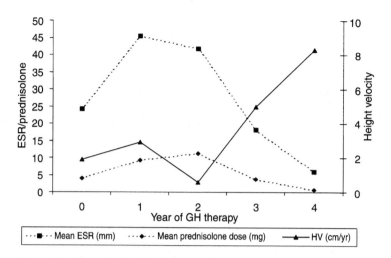

Figure 11 Interrelationship between disease activity (ESR and prednisolone dose) and height velocity as illustrated by Case 1.

Assessment of her growth failure included GH stimulation testing, which was normal, and her IGF-1 level, which was low-normal. GH treatment was commenced when she was nearly nine years old when her height SDS was –4.3. This was continued for 6½ years. Figure 11 shows her height velocity response to GH during the first four years of treatment, and also nicely demonstrates the influence of ongoing disease activity (as indicated by ESR and Prednisolone dose) on this response. The first two years of treatment coincided with disease flares and vertebral crush fractures. As has been described in many of the GH treatment studies in JIA, GH treatment maintained her height SDS between –4.4 and –4.7. It wasn't until she reached puberty late at 14 years and then had her pubertal growth spurt that her height SDS increased. This reached –3.2 SDS just following menarche in stage 4 puberty.

Delayed Puberty

Case 2 was diagnosed with enthesitis-related arthritis, particularly involving his hips and lumbosacral spine, when he was 11 years old. At diagnosis his height was on the 10th percentile. In the first year of his disease activity he had elevated ESR levels (up to 60 mm/hr) with subsequent levels all less than 25 mm/hr. He has been managed with regular nonsteroidal anti-inflammatories, Sulphasalzine and the occasional intra-articular triamcinolone hexacetonide injection. He has only once had low-dose (15 mg daily) oral prednisolone for two weeks following disease flare related to intercurrent infection.

At 14 years of age he was becoming more concerned with his height. Clinical assessment revealed delayed puberty with 4 ml testes at 14½ years.

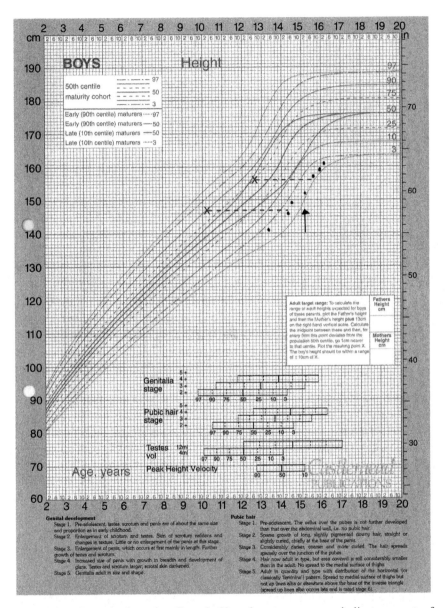

Figure 12 Growth chart for Case 2. X = bone age; arrow indicates onset of oxandrolone treatment.

His bone age at 14.25 years was accordingly significantly delayed at 10.2 years. After discussion he initially opted to allow nature to take its course. However, due to increasing self-consciousness regarding his short stature, he later opted for a 3-month course of oxandrolone (2.5 mg daily), which promoted further pubertal development and his pubertal growth spurt (Fig. 12). Catch-up growth into the normal range is anticipated as he continues through his pubertal growth spurt, with his bone age at 15.6 years still delayed at 12.8 years.

USEFUL RESOURCES

- www.thehormonefactory.com
  A website designed for young people addressing puberty and sexual health issues in early adolescence. The Hormone Factory was funded by the Bertarelli Foundation (Geneva) and developed by researchers and educators for the Australian Research Centre in Sex, Health & Society, Faculty of Health Sciences, La Trobe University, Australia. The Centre has a long-established record in research, policy and practice into sexual & reproductive health with a focus on young people, & in working with the school sector in sensitive issues.
- www.lifebytes.gov.uk/sex/sex_puberty.html
- www.mindbodysoul.gov.uk/sexual/puberty.html
- www.doctorann.org/body/stages/
- Rosen DS. Physiologic growth and development during adolescence. Pediatr Rev 2004; 25(6):194–9.
- Kulin HE, Muller J. The biological aspects of puberty. Pediatr Rev 1996; 3:75–86.
- Mehta A, Hindmarsh P. Guide to the assessment and treatment of delayed puberty. Prescriber 2004; 5(May):57–64.

REFERENCES

1. Mahoney CP. Evaluating the child with short stature. Pediatr Clin N Am 1987; 34(4):825–49.
2. Cox LA. A Guide to Measurement and Assessment of Growth in Children. Welwyn Garden City, UK: Castlemead Publications, 1992.
3. Rosen DS. Physiologic growth and development during adolescence. Pediatr Rev 2004; 25(6):194–9.
4. Kulin HE, Muller J. The biological aspects of puberty. Pediatr Rev 1996; 3: 75–86.
5. Marshall WA, Tanner JM. Variations in pattern of pubertal changes in boys. Arch Dis Child 1970; 45:13–23.
6. Marshall WA, Tanner JM. Variations in pattern of pubertal changes in girls. Arch Dis Child 1969; 44:291–303.
7. Ansell BM, Bywaters EGL. Growth in Still's disease. Ann Rheum Dis 1956; 15: 295–319.
8. Zak M, Muller J, Pedersen FK. Final height, armspan, subischial leg length and body proportions in Juvenile Chronic Arthritis. Horm Res 1999; 52:80–5.

9. Packham, J.C.; Hall, M.A. Long-term follow-up of 246 adults with juvenile idiopathic arthritis: functional outcome. Rheumatology 2002; 41, 1428–35.

10. Simon D, Fernando C, Czernichow P, et al. Linear growth and final height in patients with systemic juvenile idiopathic arthritis treated with longterm glucocorticoids. J Rheumatol 2002; 29:1296–300.

11. Chedeville G, Quartier P, Miranda M, et al. Improvements in growth parameters in children with juvenile idiopathic arthritis associated with the effect of methotrexate on disease activity. Joint Bone Spine 2005; 72:392–6 (Epub 2005).

12. Simon D, Lucidarme N, Prieur A-M, et al. Effects on growth and body composition of growth hormone treatment in children with juvenile idiopathic arthritis requiring steroid therapy. J Rheumatol 2003; 30:2492–9.

13. Rusconi R, Corona F, Grassi A, Carnelli V. Age at menarche in juvenile idiopathic arthritis. J Pediatr Endocrinol Metal 2003; 16 (Suppl. 2):285–8.

14. Ostensen M, Almberg K, Koksvik HS. Sex, reproduction and gynaecological disease in young adults with a history of juvenile chronic arthritis (JCA). J Rheumatol 2000; 27:783–7.

15. Laaksonen A. A prognostic study of juvenile rheumatoid arthritis. Acta Paed Scand 1966; 163 (Suppl.):49–55.

16. Ostrov BE, Levine RL. Interactions of puberty with rheumatic diseases, contraception and gynaecological issues. In Isenberg DA, Miller III LJ, eds. Adolescent Rheumatology. London: Martin Dunitz, 1999; 301–24.

17. Bernstein BH, Stobie D, Singsen BH, et al. Growth retardation in juvenile rheumatoid arthritis (JRA). Arthritis Rheum 1977; (Suppl. 20):212–6.

18. Suris J-C, Michaud P-A, Viner R. The adolescent with a chronic condition. Part 1: Developmental issues. Arch Dis Child 2004; 89:938–42.

19. Kappy MS. Regulation of growth in children with chronic illness. Am J Dis Child 1987; 141:489–93.

20. Morris HG. Growth and skeletal maturation in asthmatic children: Effect of corticosteroid treatment. Pediatr Res 1975; 9:579–83.

21. Baxter JD. Mechanism of glucocorticoid inhibition of growth. Kidney Int 1978; 14:330–3.

22. Allen RC, Jimenez M, Cowell CT. Insulin-like growth factor and growth hormone secretion in juvenile chronic arthritis. Ann Rheum Dis 1991, 50, 602–6.

23. McEnery P, Gonzalez L, Martin L, et al. Growth and development of children with renal transplants. J Pediatr 1973; 83:806–14.

24. Potter D, Holliday M, Wilson C, et al. Alternate day steroids in children after renal transplantation. Transplant Proc 1975; 7:79–82.

25. Touati G, Prieur A-M, Ruiz C, et al. Beneficial effects of one year growth hormone administration to children with juvenile chronic arthritis on chronic steroid therapy. I. Effects on growth velocity and body composition. J Clin Endocrinol Metab 1998; 832(2):403–9.

26. Davies UM, Jones J, Reeve J, et al. Juvenile rheumatoid arthritis. Effects of disease activity and recombinant human growth hormone on insulin-like growth factor 1, insulin-like growth factor binding proteins 1 and 3 and osteocalcin. Arthritis Rheum 1997; 40(2):332–40.

27. Schall JI, Edisio JS, Stallings VA, et al. Self-assessment of sexual maturity status in children with Crohn's disease. J Pediatr 2002; 141(2):223–9.
28. Wacharasindhu S, Pri-Ngam P, Kongchonrak T. Self-assessment of sexual maturation in Thai children by Tanner photograph. J Med Assoc Thai 2002; 85(3):308–19.
29. Taylor SJ, Whincup PH, Hindmarsh PC, et al. Performance of a new pubertal self-assessment questionnaire: a preliminary study. Paediatr Perinat Epidemiol 2002; 15(1):88–94.
30. Wu Y, Schreiber GB, Klementowicz V, et al. Racial differences in accuracy of self-assessment of sexual maturation among young black and white girls. J Adolesc Health 2001; 28(3):197–203.
31. Neinstein LS. Adolescent self-assessment of sexual maturation: reassessment and evaluation in a mixed ethnic urban population. Clin Pediatr (Phila) 1982; 21(8):482–4.
32. Duke PM, Litt IF, Gross RT. Adolescents' self-assessment of sexual maturation. Pediatrics 1980; 66(6):918–20.
33. Mehta A, Hindmarsh P. Guide to the assessment and treatment of delayed puberty. Prescriber 2004; 5(May):57–64.
34. Styne DM. Puberty and its disorders in boys. Endocrinol Metab Clin N Am 1991; 20(1):43–69.
35. Rosenfield RL. Puberty and its disorders in girls. Endocrinol Metab Clin N Am 1991; 20(1):15–42.
36. Crouch N, Creighton S. Amenorrhea in adolescents: Diagnosis and management. Prescriber 2004; 19(January):40–15.
37. Styne DM. New aspects in the diagnosis and treatment of pubertal disorders. Pediatr Clin N Am 1997; 44(2):505–29.
38. Markham A, Bryson HM. Deflazacort. A review of its pharmacological properties and therapeutic efficacy. Drugs 1995; 50(2):317–33.
39. Bechtold S, Ripperger P, Mühlbayer D, et al. GH therapy in juvenile chronic arthritis: Results of a two-year controlled study on growth and bone. J Clin Endocrinol Metab 2001; 86(12):5737–44.
40. Bechtold S, Ripperger P, Hafner R, et al. Growth hormone improves height in patients with juvenile idiopathic arthritis: 4-year data of a controlled study. J Pediatr 2003; 143:512–9.
41. Simon D, Bubuteishvili L, Ruiz JC, et al. Prevention of growth retardation with early rGH treatment in children, suffering from juvenile idiopathic arthritis, receiving glucocorticoid therapy: Results of a 2-year randomised controlled study. Horm Res 2004; 62 (Suppl. 2):28.

4

Creating a Listening Culture: Communicating with Young People

Janet E. McDonagh

Division of Reproductive and Child Health, University of Birmingham, Birmingham, U.K.

INTRODUCTION

Adolescence constitutes a time when health care professionals do not deal directly with adults, the latter whom share relatively similar describe views of social values and norms, acknowledging cultural differences. Furthermore, communication styles between serial visits with the same adolescent may vary considerably as the young person moves through the various stages of adolescent development. Communication strategies appropriate to pediatric or adult settings may not be effective in adolescent settings, and a different range of skills is required to create the listening culture so vital for this age group, who are the adults of the future. This chapter considers the characteristics of adolescent-friendly rheumatology services, discusses the principles of interviewing, and outlines useful communication strategies in clinical practice. Specific issues with respect to communication with parents are further discussed in Chapter 14.

ADOLESCENT-FRIENDLY RHEUMATOLOGY SERVICES

Adolescents, as all age groups, have the right to be looked after by appropriately trained professionals, to receive information in a form and at a pace they can assimilate in an environment that respects their privacy and dignity and spares them embarrassment. Current evidence suggests that there remains room for improvement in these aspects of adolescent rheumatology health-service delivery. National surveys in the United Kingdom have reported limited adolescent rheumatology service provision in the United Kingdom (1) and significant unmet education and training needs among rheumatology professionals in both the pediatric and adult sectors (2). A Delphi study of adolescents with juvenile idiopathic arthritis (JIA), their parents, and a range of professionals involved in their care agreed on a set of aspects for what constituted best practice (and that were also highly feasible) in a key aspect of adolescent transitional care (Table 1) (3). In addition, they identified three attributes of best practice that were considered feasible in only a few hospitals. The availability of professionals knowledgeable in transitional care was one of these attributes (3).

In a large cohort of adolescents with JIA, the perceived quality of care received by adolescents and their parents was lower than what they would like (4). Dissatisfaction is not just a feature of secondary care. In a U.K. study of 4000 adolescents (15–16 years) in primary care, 53% reported problems with consultations (5). In another U.K. study of school students, 27% of females aged 12 to 15 years felt quite/very uneasy talking to their general practitioner (6). It is not only the young people who perceive problems. Parents of adolescents reported that doctors lacked communication skills with their teenage children and appeared uncomfortable when discussing sensitive topics such as sexual behavior (7). Several authors have explored the barriers to effective communication between adolescents and health professionals and examples of these are detailed in Table 2 (8–10). Some of these areas will now be discussed in detail.

Table 1   Best Practice in Adolescent Transitional Care

Aspects of care strongly agreed to be best practice and deemed highly feasible:
  Address young people's psychosocial and educational/vocational needs
  Use an individualized approach
  Provide honest explanations of the adolescent's condition and associated
    health care
  Provide opportunities for adolescents to express opinions and make
    informed decisions
  Maintain continuity in health personnel
  Give adolescents the option of being seen by professionals without their
    parents present
Aspects of care agreed to be best practice, but deemed as having limited feasibility:
  Multidisciplinary teams (consultants only)
  Professionals who are knowledgeable about adolescent development
  Age-appropriate physical environment
  Dedicated adolescent environments (e.g., adolescent waiting areas)
  Providing opportunities to meet similar others

Source: Adapted from Ref. 3.

Table 2 Barriers to Effective Communication Between
Young People and Health Professionals

Practical
  Presence of parents
  Presence of students/trainees
  Gender of professional
  Time constraints
  Limited contact (duration and/or frequency)
  Not routinely seeing the adolescent alone
  Lack of assurance of confidentiality
Attitudinal
  Perceived attitudes towards adolescents
  Type of information needed
  Perceived lack of interest in wider impact of chronic illness
  Lack of perceived applicability
  Ambivalence about the role of the specialist
  Trust
  Honesty
  Fidelity
Behavioral
  Communication skills of the adolescent
  Communication skills of the health professional
  Lack of training of the professional
  Lack of comfort with adolescent issues
  Competency
  Honesty

FACTORS AFFECTING COMMUNICATION BETWEEN YOUNG PEOPLE AND HEALTH PROFESSIONALS

Confidentiality

When adolescents are asked to name the important attributes of an adolescent friendly service, confidentiality appears at the top of their list (11). Confidentiality underpins both the development of a therapeutic alliance and the development of future relationships with health professionals and is, by definition, based on mutual trust. If confidentiality is not assured, health-seeking behaviors during adolescence may be negatively influenced (12). In a U.S.-based study, over half of young people reported health concerns they wished to keep private from their parents, and a quarter said they would forgo health care in some situations if their parents found out (12). Unfortunately, pediatric practices appear less likely than family medicine to offer confidential services to adolescents (13). Furthermore, adolescents may be unaware of their right to confidentiality. It is important to stress that the right to confidentiality exists independently of competence to consent to treatment. Consent, competence, and confidentiality for young people are fundamentals of adolescent health and core knowledge for health professionals involved in the care of young people (14–16). Confidentiality should ideally be assured in every consultation with individual young people and their right to confidentiality should be explained to their parent/caregivers (16). Professionals must ensure that the services they work in have policies and practices that foster confidentiality and competence among adolescents attending their services (Fig. 1).

A practical aspect of confidentiality is the opportunity for the young person to choose to be seen independently of their parents (Fig. 2). Adolescents with JIA report appreciation of the opportunity to be seen alone but find it difficult to deal with their parents when the latter want to be present during the consultation (17). In the context of a chronic illness, independent visits should be viewed as a matter of choice—is the young person choosing to have their parent with them or is the parent choosing? If adolescents do choose to have someone with them, is it because they do not have the skills or confidence to be seen alone? Preparation and skills training for independent visits are an integral part of adolescent and transitional care as young people learn how to become "new users" of health services previously accessed by their parents on their behalf (see Chapter 1). In the United Kingdom 40% to 50% of 15- to 16-year-olds see their GP on their

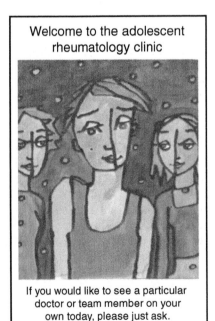

Welcome to the adolescent rheumatology clinic

If you would like to see a particular doctor or team member on your own today, please just ask. It's your health. Have your say.

Figure 1 Waiting room poster advocating that young people be seen independently of their parents when they so choose. *Source*: Courtesy of London Adolescent Network Group.

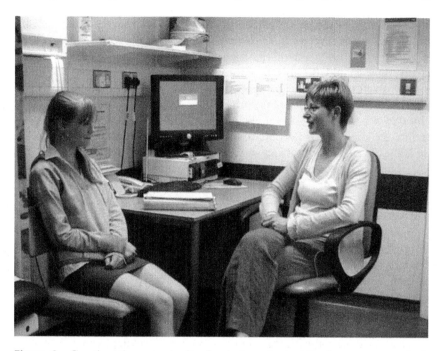

Figure 2 Creating the opportunity for independent visits for young people in adolescent rheumatology clinics.

own (18) in contrast to only 16% to 27% of adolescents in rheumatology clinics (19–21). Furthermore, only 12% of adolescents (14- and 17-year-olds) with JIA were seeing their GP alone (20). Young people with another chronic illness—cystic fibrosis—feel that 13 to 16 years is the best time for them to be seen independently (22). Independent visits were reported to be one of the five main methods of "demonstrating transition" by providers of health care for adolescents with sickle cell disease in the United States (23) along with encouraging patients to accept more responsibility, providing literature, making the patient more financially responsible, and having family conferences to discuss transition. Independent visits have also been identified as a baseline predictor of health related quality-of-life in a large U. K. cohort of adolescents with JIA (24) and a predictor of successful transfer in a cardiology population (25).

The presence of a parent(s) has also been reported to impact on the quality of communication between adolescents and professionals (9,26). In a study of 313 adolescents (aged 11–21 years), discussion of sexual issues was related to the absence of a parent and the positive attitudes and/or apparent comfort of the professional (26). Of note, few adolescents *initiated* discussion of sexual issues, requiring a proactive approach by the professional (26).

The right of the young person to choose a chaperone must also not be forgotten, as for any patient, particularly for the psychologically and/or physically sensitive parts of the interview and/or examination. However, ideally they should be able to choose whether it be a parent, friend or another professional. The components of the physical examination to be performed should be explained to the young person at the outset (including why they are necessary) and a chaperone offered. If the patient chooses to decline the use of a chaperone, it should be documented. There are useful guidelines available addressing such issues for the interested reader (27,28).

The impact of the presence of other strangers during the consultation, whether students or other professionals, has similarly been reported to impair communication between young people with chronic illnesse and professionals (9,17). This, however, has major implications to potential training opportunities in adolescent rheumatology. Adolescents with JIA reported perceived erosion of trust in the presence of such strangers (e.g., students, trainees), although they acknowledged that professionals needed to learn. Furthermore, they were willing to be involved in such training, but suggested that it not take place during their appointments (17).

If there is another team member in the room for some reason, it can be useful to consider using him or her in either a chaperoning or de-briefing role, e.g., walking out with the young person and checking to see if he or she is happy with everything before leaving the clinic.

Provider Characteristics

Provider behavior is another major determinant of adolescent's satisfaction with health care (12,29–34). A professional interested in adolescent problems was perceived by adolescents as another major attribute of an adolescent-friendly practice, second only to confidentiality (11). Freed et al. have found that adolescents' satisfaction with their visits may be more influenced by the *interpersonal style* of the health care provider than with the *content* of their actual discussions (31). However, young people (including those with JIA) have reported that health professionals should also be highly knowledgeable about their condition and highly rated the knowledge of their current staff (10,17,30,34).

Of all the interpersonal characteristics, honesty and trust are rated as key attributes of quality health care, regardless of the population under study (10,17,30,34). Adolescents have suggested that honesty includes "straight talk" which does not include condescension and false reassurance (30). Young people's requests for complete explanations of prognosis and treatment options have been documented previously (11,12,17,35–37). Unfortunately, both health professionals and parents may act, deliberately or inadvertently, as "gate-keepers" in the transmission of information (9,17,35,27). While this is often motivated by a desire to protect young people from emotional distress, it can impede effective communication of information. Other factors influencing communication between young people and professionals are detailed in Table 2 (9,21,38).

Adolescent health care provision is by definition multidisciplinary and potentially involves a wide range of professionals Table 3.

Effective communication by and among members of the virtual adolescent rheumatology team is a key principle of quality adolescent health care provision, acknowledging the recognition of confidentiality. These professionals should also be appropriately trained in adolescent health, a criterion not without its challenges considering the lack of formal training opportunities outside the mental health area currently available in the United Kingdom at the time of writing (39). Training issues with respect to adolescent rheumatology are discussed further in Chapter 17.

Environment

Young people with JIA in the United Kingdom have reported that pediatric environments were patronizing, adult environments distressing, and both isolating (17). They called for age-appropriate dedicated areas in hospitals where they would feel normal and valued (17). Unfortunately, although adolescent-focused environments were determined to be best practice by young people with JIA, their parents, and health professionals alike, they also considered them to be feasible in only a few U.K. hospitals in a Delphi study (3). In a U.K. study of secondary school students, 30% had been admitted to hospital after age of 13 years, 53% to a pediatric ward, 81% to an adult ward (40). Irrespective of where there were admitted, the majority felt out of place (40).

In the ambulatory-care setting, the need for longer clinic appointments for adolescents compared to both pediatric and adult clinics has been highlighted at a national level in the United Kingdom (39), and this has obvious implications for resource allocation in a financially constrained

Table 3   The Virtual Adolescent Rheumatology Team

Young person
Their family
Their friends
Primary health-care providers, including school nurses and counselors
Secondary health-care providers (medical workers, nurses, occupational
    therapists, physiotherapists, psychologists)
School teachers
Vocational services
Social services
Youth services
Voluntary sector

---

system of care. Time is vital to allow an unhurried approach, particularly for the anxious, quiet teenager or for young people with complex problems. Furthermore, during the transition from triadic consultations typical of pediatric practice to the more adult dyadic consultations, an individual clinic visit may start with the family interview, then the young person is seen independently, and then ending with a family briefing in other words, three separate consultations. In the context of multidisciplinary team, a hospital visit to an adolescent rheumatology department may involve consultations with various team members. Robertson et al. reported a significant difference in rheumatology-consultation duration between pediatric and adult clinics (34 vs. 15 minutes, respectively, $p < 0.001$) (19). In primary care, consultations involving 11- to 19-year-olds were the shortest of any age group by 23% (41)!

Difficulty getting a quick appointment has also been reported by young people as a major difficulty in accessing health services (5) which may impact their communication when eventually they are seen! It is important to realize that a lengthy wait is not only interpreted by users as a sign of inefficiency, but also as a lack of respect, in that it implies that the time of health professionals is more important than that of service users (30). Providing timely explanations for delays and making better use of waiting time (e.g., facilitating social networking among patients, completing transitional assessment forms) may help to minimize such feelings.

Examples of simple development strategies for adolescent-friendly rheumatology services are detailed in Table 4. Perhaps the most important strategy of all, however, is to involve young people themselves in any service developments (42)! The U.K. Department of Health have developed a useful summary document, highlighting the range of factors to address when developing adolescent-friendly health services (43)—and rheumatology services should be no exception!

INTERVIEWING AND ASSESSMENT SKILLS

The fundamental skill necessary for effective assessment of adolescents is empathy and a nonjudgmental approach. Praise of the young person is another, frequently forgotten aspect of communication with this age group, and is key to success. As in pediatrics, acknowledging the reciprocal influences of growth and development during adolescence on health and illness is imperative (44) (see Chapters 2,3). Using this development as a lens through which effective communication takes place is useful in practice.

Assessment of cognitive development is important when considering communication with young people, particularly the development of new cognitive skills, including abstract thinking capacities in mid adolescence. The "bullet proof" idea of personal invulnerability characteristic during mid adolescence has challenging implications for disease education and

Table 4 "You're Welcome": The 4 Ps of Young-Person-Friendly Rheumatology Service Delivery

---

People

Offer a professional of preferred gender when feasible. Acknowledge that this may vary between visits, depending on the needs of the young person at the time.

Involve all team members. For example, another team member can see the parent(s) when the young person is being seen alone. If another team member is in the clinic room, he or she could have debriefing role at the end of the visit, spending some time with the young person and going over what has been discussed.

Identify the key person for each young person who will help to coordinate the transition process.

Ensure professional sensitivity towards apparently routine clinic tasks, e.g., weighing, urine testing, ascertaining the date of the last menses for X-rays.

Provide training for all new staff members.

Involve the whole team, e.g., secretaries/receptionists should be trained to take messages from young people.

Use peers in disease-education programs.

Use role models, e.g., young adults with JIA who successfully made the transition to adult care, into work, etc.

Create an advisory panel of young people for service developments, etc.

Foster multidisciplinary and interagency involvement—among the health, social services, youth service, education, and voluntary sectors.

Place

Provide an emotionally and physically safe environment. A gender balance among staff is important, particularly where physical examinations are undertaken.

Hide toys if the area usually used by a pediatric service.

Dedicated clinic and waiting area

    May be within a larger general waiting area

    May be the later appointment slots of a general pediatric/adult clinic

Consider consultation room set up—position chairs to ensure maximum eye contact between professional and young person.

Consider need for additional rooms to facilitate independent visits and to meet needs of parents.

Access—ensure convenient timing of clinic appointments (e.g., after school) access for advice, text messaging, e-mail, helpline.

Process

Encourage all team members to encourage independent behavior, e.g, receptionists can give the young person the appointment slip; secretaries can encourage young people to phone with questions.

Aspire to continuity of care personnel between visits when possible.

Schedule appointments so friends can attend, to facilitate peer support.

(Continued)

Table 4 "You're Welcome": The 4 Ps of Young-Person-Friendly Rheumatology Service Delivery (*Continued*)

Paper

Provide age and developmentally appropriate information resources in a range of formats—paper-based, internet, text messaging.

Consider credit card–size information handouts, particularly for sensitive issues (e.g., sexual health advice), which the young person can to keep private in a wallet.

Make information available in a relatively private place to encourage use (e.g., toilets!) and avoid gatekeeping.

Hang posters describing confidentiality practices, generic health issues etc. In multiuser areas, consider use of projector and PowerPoint slide show for adolescent-friendly informational material.

Create computer access with reasonable privacy to encourage information-seeking behavior facilitate to anonymity when accessing sensitive information.

Keep notes. Document the patient's progress and preparation for independent visits, especially if personnel continuity cannot be guaranteed.

Send clinic letters routinely to young person, bearing in mind confidentiality issues in case letters are intercepted by parents. Consider asking the young person to bring a list of questions. ("Think of three questions for me for your next visit!") and remember to ask for them.

Send a follow-up letter to patient recapping the information exchanged during the clinic visit and suggesting issues that need further discussion or review at the next visit.

Provide up-to-date teenage magazines—for boys and girls! Ask your patients which ones to buy.

Place a suggestion box/book in waiting area to encourage feedback from patients.

---

prevention. The use of immediate motivators ("here and now") rather than future motivators ("if and then") to improve adherence is usually more fruitful at this stage (see Chapter 15). Chronic illnesses may impact cognitive development through the effect of certain therapies, pain, depression, fatigue, or school absence. Conversely, cognitive development will influence communication, health education, decision-making and self-care. Adolescence is also characterized by rapid change: as they get older, their developmental capacities change, and information provided earlier may need to be repeated. Reassessment of developmental needs is an important aspect of adolescent rheumatology care. This is shown in studies that report significant misunderstandings and lack of disease knowledge in established attendees of rheumatology clinics (45,46).

In practice, health professionals also need to assess and facilitate transfer of responsibility, communication, and "ownership" of disease from parents to the young person—key tasks of transitional care (see Chapter 16). In practical terms, it is useful to redefine relationships in early adolescence (e.g., at 11–12 years). This might be take the form of a discussion about the philosophy of transition and the transfer to an adolescent service. Using the comparison of changing schools (primary to secondary) at this time is useful— "After all, you wouldn't stay in primary/junior school for ever, would you?" Such discussions can usefully facilitate opportunities for young people to be seen alone for part or all of their consultation, assuring their parents some time to address their needs as well.

An interactive, rather than a traditional adult medicine interrogative approach, is preferable in adolescent rheumatology. Interview strategies can be divided into two types—unidirectional and bidirectional (47). The unidirectional approach is characterized by the provision of facts, opinions/ advice, closed questions, and suggestions of alternatives. This strategy requires the young person to have the confidence to interrupt the conversation and assert themselves. The bidirectional approach is more interactive and involves the professional asking for understanding, the use of problem solving, open questions, and posing hypothetical situations. The latter is the preferred strategy in adolescent health, as it conveys the real message that the young person has options and is expected to respond and/ or participate. In a study of health education, doctors were found to use bidrectional strategies only 22% of the time with an adolescent: doctor ratio for talking of 0.14 in the unidirectional discussions compared to the healthier 1.06 in the bidirectional discussions ($p = 0.004$) (47).

Taking a psychosocial history is a useful strategy for engaging young people, in addition to identifying risk factors and eventually formulating interventions. A useful interview tool described in the literature is HEADSS (Home, education, activities, drugs, sexual, health, suicide) (48,49). Unfortunately, the evidence suggests that general adolescent health issues are not always addressed in specialty clinics (21,50,51), but screening for such issues can be improved by participation in a coordinated transitional-care program (21). Adolescents have been reported to have more diverse and serious health concerns than expected by health care providers (52). Carroll et al. reported that adolescents with chronic illness report more age-related concerns, e.g., acne, menstrual periods, sexual health, worries about height and weight, substance use, etc., than their healthy peers (53). What is less well known is how such issues are addressed in specialty clinics. Since adult health behaviors become established during adolescence, every health-related encounter, irrespective of setting, should be considered a potential health-promotion opportunity. Barriers to such health promotion have been reported (21,38) and are reflected in Table 2.

A proactive approach to adolescent health facilitates the addressing of such issues in the rheumatology clinic, "if you have a problem about ———, know that you can come and talk to me; I'm willing to help." Including psychosocial issues in individualized transition plans (54) is a useful way to raise awareness among adolescents attending the clinic that such issues matter to the rheumatology team, and, even if they are not relevant immediately, when they do become so, adolescents will know that they can ask related questions when they come to clinic.

Useful interviewing strategies in the specific context of the triadic consultation involving parent(s) and the adolescent include circular questioning and turn-taking, which are detailed in Chapter 14. One of the most important skills for triadic consultations is to take care how the opinion of the parents is obtained, and to ensure it is not perceived as a lack of belief in the young person.

USEFUL COMMUNICATION STRATEGIES

Importance of the First Question

When seeing a new referral it is very important to clarify the perception (both adolescent and parental) of why the adolescent has been referred to you. Adolescent-parent discrepancies may be readily revealed, even at this early stage in the consultation! In several studies, the professional's lack of interest in the wider impact of the condition is reported by young people to impede effective communication (9,10,17). This is readily addressed by always starting the consultation with a non-disease-related question, for example, "What have you been up to since we last met?" rather than "How is your arthritis?" A useful aide-memoire is to draw a text box in the corner of the notes page with a reminder of an important event to ask about at the next visit, e.g., joined new football team, took part in a play, etc. The mere fact that you have remembered will convey the message that the young person has being listened to and that the rest of their life is important. Adolescent health professionals need to understand that the social context of health behaviors for adolescents can be very different from those of children and adults. Asking their opinion rather than making statements like, "When I was your age ..." is obviously the preferred strategy during this stage of development.

Providing a Verbal Plan for the Consultation

A useful strategy to use at with an adolescent is to explain at the beginning what is going to happen during the consultation. This is particularly pertinent for both the adolescent and their parent when young people are ready to be seen independently. Asking permission to ask sensitive questions as well as explaining why such questions are being asked is also useful, for example, "I want to ask you some personal questions now. This is standard practice with all the young people I see, and it helps to give me a picture of your overall health and who you are. Is that OK?" Intrinsic to these introductory strategies is the inclusion of an explanation and assurance of confidentiality, as discussed earlier.

Importance of Time and Listening

Young people are new users of health services; they may not have been given many opportunities to make decisions for themselves when they were younger or, indeed, even asked for their opinion. It is therefore important to give them both time to find the words they want to answer with and time to make their own decisions. In adolescent health, listening skills are more important than talking skills! Young people have reported that their own communication skills impact on their ability to communicate with doctors (9). It is therefore important to allow them time to find the words—a useful tip is: after asking a question which is met with initial silence, just to fiddle with your pen for a moment, giving them enough time to find the words to at least make a start at a response. Similarly with decision-making, "You don't need to decide which treatment to start today. I will write to you with the list of options, give you time to think about it, and I will phone you next week, and we can discuss it again."

Importance of Respect

Respect is also important. Health professionals should attempt to lessen inequality in status by respecting the young person as an expert in their disease (10). They after all are the ones with the condition! The reported discrepancies between adolescent and parental ratings of pain, disability, and health-related quality-of-life (55,56) highlights the importance in listening to both equally valid perspectives,. Parents will vary in their awareness, sensitivity, and tolerance of adolescent health concerns. In the clinical setting it remains imperative to consider, acknowledge, and actively believe in both perspectives, particularly as discordance may be associated with depressive symptoms in the adolescent (55).

Paraphrasing to Check Understanding

In view of adolescents' developing communication skills, it is important to make sure that you, the professional, understands that what they have just said matches what they meant to say! Summarizing what they have said and saying it back to them using different words is a useful strategy to help avoid misinterpretation on the part of the health professional.

Similarly, it is important to assess their understanding of what you have said! "What do you understand by 'barrier contraception'?" "Now that I have told you about arthritis, how would you explain it to your best friend?" "What does a unit of alcohol actually mean in terms of drinks?"

Trigger Questions

Finally, the use of "trigger questions" is particularly useful for exploring the more sensitive areas of enquiry. Several have been already used as examples in the preceding text. Table 5 lists some further examples of these useful

Table 5   Trigger Questions in Adolescent Rheumatology

Disease-related questions

Can you explain your condition in your own words? How would you tell someone about your condition?

What information have you found on your disease in books, the internet, on TV, and from experts?

Do you know other people who have the same condition?

Who knows that you have this illness?

What do other people think of you having this illness (peers, teachers, neighbors, etc.)?

Why do you think you have this condition?

What does this illness prevent you from doing (be very specific!) now and later in your life?

If your condition disappeared overnight, what would you spend tomorrow doing? (A useful question for parents as well!)

Therapy-related questions

Can you tell me why you need your particular treatments?

Who does what in your treatment? (What is your role? What is your parent's role?)

How do you approach the prescriptions, tasks?

How much time does managing the condition take you and/or your parents?

How does the schedule of the tasks fit into your schedule/social life/average day?

When was the last time you forgot to take your medicine/do your therapy?

Can you estimate what percentage of the prescribed treatment you took/performed in the last two weeks?

General health and well-being questions

Describe a typical day at home/school/on a weekend to me.

How do you compare yourself to peers in your class/grade? Are you small? Do they have more or less breast development compared to you? Have they started their periods yet?

What do you like about your body? What would about it you like to be different?

Have your periods started already?

Some young people experiment with cigarettes and alcohol. In your grade at school, do people smoke/drink/use illicit drugs? What about your friends? And you?

If you needed advice, for example, regarding alcohol/drug use or sexual health, where would you go?

What do you enjoy in life?

Tell me about your friends. How many friends do you have? What is the age of this/ these friends?

What do you do with your friends out of school?

What can you do on your own? What would you like to do on your own?

What are your future plans? How do you plan to achieve them?

What would help you make your life more enjoyable?

Many young people feel down or sad at times. When did you last feel sad? Who do you go to/talk to when you feel like this? Have you ever felt that life is not worth living? Have you ever thought about harming yourself?

Source: Adapted from Euteach curriculum (www.euteach.com).

questions, which can be used to appropriately elicit important information as a basis for delivering adolescent-centered rheumatology health care.

SKILLS TRAINING FOR YOUNG PEOPLE

Consultations with health professionals can be perceived as opportunities to practice communication, problem-solving, and negotiation skills, all of which are important in the rest of life. The clinic is a safe place to start such skills training, and this can be an effective "sales technique" to encourage parents to allow their son/daughter to be seen alone. "This is a safe place for your son/daughter to practice talking to professionals on their own, which will prepare them for the world of work etc."

To foster such skills, the use of the strategies detailed in Table 6 can be useful.

Table 6   Skills Training in Adolescent Rheumatology

Managing consultations independently
Making own appointments
Self-medication
   Requires education, including rationale, risk-benefit, side effects, monitoring
     requirements, contingency planning for missed medication doses, etc.
Pain self-management techniques
Preparation for spending time away from parental home, e.g., sleepovers, school
   trips, camps, foreign travel
Problem solving (including contingency planning): "What would do if your arthritis
   flared and you were away from home?" "What might you do if your friends are
   drinking alcohol at a party and you are still taking methotrexate ?" "What would
   you do if you didn't get accepted to a university?" "How would you disclose your
   condition to a potential employer?"
Accessing advice from
   Primary care professionals
   The rheumatology team
     Requires knowledge of whom, how, and when to contact
     Requires discernment of elective versus urgent inquiries
Other health resources, such as local sexual health services
Collecting repeat prescriptions
   Requires knowledge of who, how, and when, in addition to any likely change in
     payment criteria, particularly in late adolescence
Goal setting
   Requires negotiation, priority setting.
Working knowledge of rights with respect to health, education, employment,
   disability, etc.
Working knowledge of available resources for young people

Table 7   What Young People Want from Professionals

Treat me like a person
Try to understand
Don't treat me differently
Give me some encouragement
Don't force me
Give me options
Have a sense of humor
Know what you are doing

Source: Adapted from Ref. 57.

SUMMARY

In summary, when you meet young patients in your clinic remember what they want from you as a professional (Table 7). Remember to be empathic, respectful, and non-judgmental. Listen more than you talk. Be patient— teenagers may need further consultations before they trust you enough to open up. Assure confidentiality to the young person, and ensure they understand what it means in practice. Consider seeing or at least preparing to see the young person by themselves as well as with their parents. Be yourself and maintain appropriate boundaries, providing an emotionally and physically safe environment. Consider using interview tools to address the important psychosocial aspects of health, for example, HEADDSS (48,49). If you practice these principles, you are likely to soon experience enhanced job satisfaction and become enthused by adolescent rheumatology health care!

REFERENCES

1. McDonagh JE, Foster H, Hall MA, Chamberlain MA on behalf of the BPRG. Audit of rheumatology services for adolescents and young adults in the UK. Rheumatology 2000; 39:596–602.
2. McDonagh JE, Southwood TR, Shaw KL. Unmet education and training needs of rheumatology health professionals in adolescent health and transitional care. Rheumatology (Oxford) 2004; 43(6):737–43.
3. Shaw KL, Southwood TR, McDonagh JE on behalf of the British Paediatric Rheumatology Group. Transitional Care for Adolescents with Juvenile Idiopathic Arthritis: Results of a Delphi Study. Rheumatology (Oxford) 2004; 43(8):1000–6.
4. Shaw KL, Southwood TR, McDonagh JE. Young people's satisfaction of transitional care in adolescent rheumatology in the UK. Child Care Health Dev 2007; 33(4):368–79.
5. Donovan C, Mellanby AR, Jacobson LD, et al. Teenagers' views on the general practice consultation and provision of contraception. The Adolescent Working Group. Br J Gen Pract 1997; 47(424):715–8.

6. Balding J. Young People in 2003 University of Exeter: Schools Health Education Unit, 2004.

7. Croft CA, Asmussen L. A developmental approach to sexuality education: implications for medical practice. J Adolesc Health 1993; 14(2):109–14.

8. Britto MT, Rosenthal SL, Taylor J, Passo MH. Improving rheumatologists screening for alcohol use and sexual activity. Arch Pediatr Adolesc Med 2000; 154:478–83.

9. Beresford B, Sloper P. Chronically ill adolescents' experiences of communicating with doctors: a qualitative study. J Adolesc Health 2003; 33:172–9.

10. Klostermann BK, Slap G, Nebrig DM, Tivorsak TL, Britto M. Earning trust and losing it: adolescents' views on trusting physicians. J Family Pract 2005; 54 (8):679–87.

11. McPherson A. Primary health care and adolescence. In: MacFarlane A, ed. Adolescent Medicine. London: Royal College of Physicians, 1996:33–41.

12. Cheng TL, Savageau JA, Sattler AL, DeWitt TG. Confidentiality in health care. A survey of knowledge, perceptions and attitudes among high school students. J Am Med Assoc 1993; 269:1404–7.

13. Akinbami LJ, Gandhi H, Cheng TL. Availability of adolescent health services and confidentiality in primary care practices. Pediatrics 2003; 111:394–401.

14. Larcher V. Consent, competence and confidentiality. Br Med J 2005; 330: 353–6.

15. British Medical Association. Consent, Rights and Choices in Health Care for Children and Young People. London: BMJ Books, 2001.

16. Sanci LA, Sawyer SM, Kang MS-L, Haller DM, Patton GC. Confidential health care for adolescents: reconciling clinical evidence with family values. Med J Aust 2005; 183(8):410–4.

17. Shaw KL, Southwood TR, McDonagh JE on behalf of the British Paediatric Rheumatology Group. User perspectives of transitional care for adolescents with juvenile idiopathic arthritis. Rheumatology (Oxford). 2004; 43(6): 770–8.

18. Balding J. Young People into the Nineties. Book 1 Doctor and Dentist. University of Exeter: Schools Health Education Unit, 1991.

19. Robertson LP, Hickling P, Davis PJC, Bailey K, Ryder CAJ, McDonagh JE. A comparison of paediatric vs adult rheumatology clinics. (1) The doctor perspective. Rheumatology 2003; 42:51.

20. Shaw KL, Southwood TR and McDonagh JE on behalf of the British Society of Paediatric and Adolescent Rheumatology. Growing up and moving on in Rheumatology: a multicentre cohort of adolescents with Juvenile Idiopathic Arthritis. Rheumatology 2005; 44: 806–12.

21. Britto MT, Rosenthal SL, Taylor J, Passo MH. Improving rheumatologists screening for alcohol use and sexual activity. Arch Pediatr Adolesc Med 2000; 154:478–83.

22. Zack J, Jacobs CP, Keenan PM, et al. Perspectives of patients with cystic fibrosis on preventive counselling and transition to adult care. Pediatr Pulomonol 2003; 36:376–83.

23. Telfair J, Alexander LR, Loosier PS, et al. Providers' perspectives and beliefs regarding transition to adult care for adolescents with sickle cell disease. J Health Care Poor Underserved 2004; 15:443–61.

24. McDonagh JE, Southwood TR, Shaw KL. The impact of a coordinated transitional care programme on adolescents with juvenile idiopathic arthritis. Rheumatology 2007; 46(1):161–8.

25. Reid GJ, Irvine MJ, McCrindle BW, et al. Prevalence and correlates of successful transfer from pediatric to adult health care among a cohort of young adults with complex congenital heart defects. Pediatrics 2004; 113(3):197–205.

26. Merzel CR, Vandevanter NL, Middlestadt S, Bleakley A, Ledsky R, Messeri PA. Attitudinal and contextual factors associated with discussion of sexual issues during adolescent health visits. J Adolesc Health 2004; 35:108–15.

27. Royal College of Nursing. Chaperoning: the role of the nurse and the rights of patients. Guidance for nursing staff (July 2002). London. Publication code 001 446 (www.rcn.org.uk)

28. American Academy of Pediatrics. The use of chaperones during the physical examination of the pediatric patient. Pediatrics 1996; 98(6):1202.

29. Litt IF. Satisfaction with health care. The adolescent perspective. J Adolesc Health 1998; 23:59–60.

30. Ginsberg KR, Menapace AS, Slap GB. Factors affecting the decision to seek health care: the voice of adolescents. Pediatrics 1997; 100:922–30.

31. Freed LH, Ellen JM, Irwin CE, Millstein SG. Determinants of adolescents' satisfaction with health care providers and intentions to keep follow-up appointments. J Adolesc Health 1998; 22:475–9.

32. Chesney M, Lindeke L, Johnson L, Jukkala A, Lynch S. Comparison of child and parents satisfaction ratings of ambulatory pediatric subspecialty care. J Pediatr Health Care 2005; 19:221–9.

33. Margaret ND, Clark TA, Warden CR, Magnusson AR, Hedges JR. Patient satisfaction in the emergency department — a survey of pediatric patients and their parents. Acad Emerg Med 2002; 9:1379–88.

34. Britto MT, DeVelis RF, Hornung RW, et al. Health care preferences and priorities of adolescents with chronic illnesses. Pediatrics 2004; 114:1272–80.

35. Barlow JH, Shaw KL, Harrison K. Consulting the "experts": children's and parents' perceptions of psycho-educational interventions in the context of juvenile chronic arthritis. Health Educ Res Theory Pract 1999; 14:597–610.

36. Oppong-Odiseng ACK, Heycock EG. Adolescent health services — through their eyes. Arch Dis Child 1997; 77:115–9.

37. Young B, Dixon-Woods M, Windridge KC, Heney D. Managing communication with young people who have a potentially life threatening chronic illness: qualitative study of patients and parents. Br Med J 2003; 325:305–9.

38. Sawyer SM, Tully M-AM, Colin AA. Reproductive and sexual health in males with cystic fibrosis: a case for health professional education and training. J Adoles Health 2001; 28:36–40.

39. Royal College of Paediatrics and Child Health. Bridging the Gap: Health Care for Adolescents. June 2003 (www.rcpch.ac.uk)

40. Kari JA, Donovan C, Li J, Taylor B. Teenagers in hospital: what do they want? Nursing Standard 1999; 13:49–51.

41. Jacobson LD, Wilkinson C, Owen PA. Is the potential of teenage consultations being missed? a study of consultation times in primary care. Family Pract 1994; 11:296–9.

42. Royal College of Paediatrics and Child Health. Coming out of the shadows June 2005 (www.rcpch.ac.uk)

43. Department of Health. *You're welcome quality criteria. Making health services young people friendly.* 2005 (www.dh.gov.uk)

44. Suris JC, Michaud PA, Viner R. The adolescent with a chronic condition. Part 1: developmental issues. Arch Dis Child 2004; 89:938–42.

45. Berry SL, Hayford JR, Ross CK, et al. Conceptions of illness by children with juvenile rheumatoid arthritis: a cognitive developmental approach. J Pediatr Psychol 1993; 18:83–97.

46. Shaw KL, Southwood TR, McDonagh JE What's in a name? Disease knowledge in juvenile idiopathic arthritis (JIA). Arch Dis Child 2004; 89(Suppl. 1):A44.

47. Schubiner H, Eggly S. Strategies for health education for adolescent patients: a preliminary investigation. J Adolesc Health 1995; 17:37–41.

48. Goldenring JM, Cohen E. Getting into adolescent heads. Contemp Pediatr 1988; July: 75–80.

49. McDonagh JE, Kelly DA. Transitioning care of the pediatric recipient to adult caregivers. Pediatr Clin N Am 2003; 50(6):1561–83, xi–xii.

50. Robertson LP, McDonagh JE, Southwood TR, Shaw KL. Growing up and moving on. A multicentre UK audit of the transfer of adolescents with Juvenile Idiopathic Arthritis JIA from paediatric to adult centred care. Ann Rheum Dis 2006; 65:74–80.

51. Yeo MSM, Bond LM, Sawyer SM. Health risk screening in adolescents: room for improvement in a tertiary inpatient setting. Med J Aust 2005; 183(8):427–9.

52. Kowpak M. Adolescent health concerns: a comparison of adolescent and health care provider perceptions. J Am Acad Nurse Pract 1991; 3:122–8.

53. Carroll G, Massarelli E, Opzoomer A, et al. Adolescents with chronic disease: are they receiving comprehensive health care? J Adolesc Health Care 1983; 17: 32–6.

54. McDonagh JE, Southwood TR, Shaw KL. Growing up and moving on in rheumatology: development and preliminary evaluation of a transitional care programme for a multicentre cohort of adolescents with juvenile idiopathic arthritis. J Child Health Care 2006; 10(1):22–42.

55. Palmero TM. Impact of recurrent and chronic pain on child and family daily functioning: a critical review of the literature. J Dev Behav Pediatr 2000; 21: 58–69.

56. Shaw KL, Southwood TR, McDonagh JE. Growing up and moving on in Rheumatology: parents as proxies of adolescents with Juvenile Idiopathic Arthritis. Arthritis Care Res 2006; 55(2):189–98.

57. Woodgate RL. Adolescents' perspectives of chronic illness: "it's hard". J Pediatr Nurs 1998; 13(4):210–23.

5

"When I Remember to ...": Adherence and Chronic Rheumatic Diseases

Fabienne Dobbels

Center for Health Services and Nursing Research, Katholieke Universiteit Leuven, Leuven, Belgium

Karen L. Shaw

School of Health Sciences, University of Birmingham, Birmingham, U.K.

INTRODUCTION

The last few decades have seen impressive advances in treatments for rheumatological conditions. Adolescents with chronic rheumatic diseases can now expect to be prescribed a broad range of pharmacological and nonpharmacological therapies to control pain, improve function, and increase health-related quality-of-life. These can involve significant lifestyle changes, including self-medication (including subcutaneous injection), physical exercise, the wearing and use of orthopedic aids and adaptations, avoidance of risk activities, and regular clinic attendance. In most cases, these changes must be maintained over the long-term and rarely offer immediate benefit. They inevitably impinge upon the adolescent's free-time, limiting leisure and peer activities, and can affect appearance (i.e., through the wearing of splints, use of orthopedic aids or side effects of medication).

It is not surprising therefore, that adherence can be challenging for adolescents who are transitioning towards autonomy and self-identity. Indeed, adolescence is a time of major change, and while striving for independence, adolescents with chronic rheumatic diseases may find that their illness keeps them overly tied to their families, physically, emotionally and financially. Growth and sexual maturation may be delayed, affecting teenager's self-esteem and confidence (1). Disease- and treatment-related changes in physical appearance may cause problems in social functioning in a developmental period in which physical appearance is gaining increased importance (1). This is also at a time where responsibility for managing treatment is expected to shift from the parent to the adolescent.

Review of the literature has shown that adherence is poorest in adolescence and reports overall adherence rates of about 50% among adolescents with long-term conditions (1,2). For the adolescent, poor-adherence may result in increased morbidity, such as exacerbations of symptoms, medical complications, as well as greater mortality (3). An indirect consequence of poor adherence is increased school absenteeism, impacting intellectual and social development, and a decrease in overall health-related quality-of-life (3,4). Pediatricians may also incorrectly attribute poor disease control to inadequacies in treatment rather than to poor adherence, and may decide to prescribe more potent medicines with more serious side effects (3,4). Poor adherence also has implications for providers by inflating health care costs, including the expenses from unused medications, and clinical visits and hospitalizations to treat nonadherence-induced complications (3,5). The cost of poor adherence in the United States has been estimated to reach $100 billion annually (6). It is thought that the reduction of nonadherence will have a far greater effect on health than any further improvements in pharmacological treatment (7).

Thus, the need to improve adherence is crucial, both for the utilization of health resources, and, more importantly, the adolescent's current and future well-being. Indeed, it is likely that the health behaviors established in adolescence will track into their adult life. Health-care providers dealing with adolescents with chronic rheumatic diseases need to fully understand the problems of poor adherence and its associated risk factors in order to be able to develop and implement appropriate interventions to tackle them in daily clinical practice. This chapter reviews and summarizes the state-of-the-art evidence on adherence in adolescents with chronic rheumatic diseases. More specifically, the current knowledge on prevalence, risk factors, and possible interventions to improve adherence is summarized with particular attention for the shortcomings in the present literature.

DEFINITION OF ADHERENCE

According to the World Health Organization (8), adherence can be defined as "the degree to which the person's behavior corresponds with the *agreed* recommendations from a health care provider." The term "compliance" is often used synonymously with "adherence," but often criticized as having coercive and paternalistic connotations (9,10). By contrast, adherence is viewed as an intentional act of commitment to health care that has been agreed by both patient and provider.

Distinct from the concept of adherence is concordance. Whereas adherence focuses upon the adolescent's behavior in accordance with the health professional's recommendations for treatment, concordance is much more concerned with the process of consultation. While most commonly used in relation to prescribing and medicine taking (11), concordance is based upon shared decision-making in which both patient and provider are considered to have different, but equally important expertise. A concordant consultation is therefore one in which the adolescent, their parents, and health professionals all work together to agree when, how, and why the illness should be managed (12,13). Shared decision-making has certainly been identified as an integral part of best practice by adolescents with chronic rheumatic diseases (14) and rheumatology providers (15). However, the concept of concordance is a new one, and while gaining interest in the literature, there is little evaluative research on the impact of this on patient outcome, not least among adolescents with chronic rheumatic diseases. Adherence is therefore the preferred term to be used in this chapter. At this point, it is perhaps important to note that poor adherence can be intentional or involuntary (12). Adolescents face many barriers that may hinder their adherence. However adolescents can also differ from health professionals in their goals for treatment and beliefs about efficacy. Thus, adolescent perceived as non-adherent to a prescribed recommendation may, in fact, be fully adherent to a regimen that they themselves have chosen.

PREVALENCE OF NONADHERENCE

As yet, the bulk of literature in rheumatology has focused on medication adherence with only a limited attention paid to other aspects of the health regimen. Moreover, few articles pertain to adolescents. Pediatric rheumatologists sometimes naïvely think that parental supervision and/or the likelihood of pain will ensure strict adherence (16). As such, magnitude of adherence with pharmacological and nonpharmacological treatment in adolescents with chronic rheumatic disease remains unknown.

The most common methods for assessing adherence include drug assays, electronic monitors, pill counts, physician ratings, and patient or parental reports. A discussion regarding the merits of these is beyond the scope of this review, but can be found in Kroll et al. (17) and Rapoff (4). As yet, there is no single optimal method, and relying on clinical judgment alone is unreliable. Studies have found that the physician's assessment of adherence is no better that that predicted by chance alone (18).

The following paragraphs summarize what is known about adherence in adolescents with chronic rheumatic diseases. The chapter begins with medication adherence, as this includes the most numerous and evaluative studies, and is followed with the non-pharmacological aspects of care, which is largely based upon the findings of more descriptive studies.

Adherence to Pharmacological Therapies

Frequently prescribed medications include non-steroidal anti-inflammatory drugs (NSAIDs), which symptomatically relieve pain and improve joint stiffness, and disease-modifying anti-rheumatic drugs (DMARDs), which can suppress disease activity, improve function and reduce joint damage (19,20). Recently, the introduction of anti–tumor necrosis factor (TNF inhibitors or anti-TNF) has made a profound impact on disease control (20,21).

In general, nonadherence rates of children and adolescents with chronic disease have been reported to vary between 25% and 60% across a range of conditions (22), and appear to peak in adolescence (2), with an average prevalence of 50%. There are limited publications specific to children and adolescents with chronic rheumatic diseases and most pertain to juvenile idiopathic arthritis (JIA). However, review of these all indicate that poor adherence to medication is a significant problem. However, prevalence rates differ according to the method of assessment, the criteria used to interpret adequate adherence, the recommended regimen components, and the setting where adherence is assessed (3). None of the available studies used a clinically validated operational definition that indicates what level of nonadherence is associated with poor outcome. These methodological issues preclude firm conclusions.

Two retrospective studies using serum assays found that 45% of children and adolescents with JRA were non-adherent with medication (23,24). In three case-report studies including 5 patients in total, baseline adherence as assessed by parental observation or pill counts ranged from 38% to 59% (25–27). Parent-reported adherence to medication was 84.9% in a study of Feldman et al. (28). In this study in 118 patients, adherence was evaluated as caregiver's response on a 100-mm visual analogue scale to the question of how often they followed treatment recommendations as prescribed by the health care provider (28). Studies using patient self-report demonstrated that adherence with pharmacological treatment is less than optimal with prevalence ranging from 4% to 89% (1,27,29,30).

The prevalence rates found in adolescents with JIA can be compared with the results of a quantitative review on adherence in acute and chronic patient populations (5). Average nonadherence in 22 studies on arthritis was 18.8%, yet no distinction between pediatric and adult patients was made (5). Average nonadherence rate across different disease populations was 24.8%. Based on the observation that one out of the four patients is nonadherent, it can be estimated that an astonishing number of 112.2 million medical visits will result in poor adherence with prescribed medication (5). In this quantitative review, studies of pediatric patients yield higher nonadherence than studies of adult patients (i.e., 29.4% vs. 25.2%, respectively). Moreover, a trend for higher nonadherence in adolescents compared to younger children was observed.

Adherence to Non-Pharmacological Therapies

Physical therapies commonly used in the treatment of childhood rheumatic diseases include splinting, casting, positioning (e.g., prone lying) and therapeutic exercise of affected limbs (16). They are designed to restore and maintain range of motion, strengthen muscle groups and improve motor skills. Patients with JIA should also regularly attend scheduled clinic appointments and should avoid risk-taking behavior that may hamper their medical condition.

There is a paucity of published literature concerning adherence to non-pharmacological therapies. As such, little is known about the challenges faced by adolescents with JIA or the extent of their nonadherence. It does appear, however, that nonadherence to these non-pharmacological aspects is higher than that to medication (29,31,32) and can cause significant family strain (33).

Physical Therapy

Adherence to exercise is generally suboptimal. Most studies dealing with prescribed exercises rely on interviews that provide quantitative information, such as how many exercises are performed and how often (34). It is questionable whether this is the most valid assessment method. However, the limited studies available have reported overall adherence rates of 53.1% (29) to 67.2% (29,31), and indicated that poor adherence increases with older age (31). Parent-reported prevalence of poor adherence to exercise was 54.1% in the study of Feldman et al. (28). Decreased adherence with physical treatments seems to be associated with school absence (35). The review of Brus et al. (34) reported that exercise adherence ranges between 43% and 65%, but no distinction between adult and pediatric patients was made (34). These numbers appear to be higher compared to the average percentage of adherence for exercise of 72% described in the meta-analysis of DiMatteo (5) on adherence in a variety of chronic diseases, including rheumatoid disorders. Yet, this number should be interpreted with caution, as again no distinction between adolescents and adults has been made.

Occupational Therapy

Adherence in the context of orthopedic aids and adaptations is also under-researched. Studies of adherence with prescriptions for ergonomic measures deal only with the use of wrist splints. Parent-reported nonadherence with splint wearing was 58% in a study of Feldman et al. (28). Similarly, Kyngäs (1) found that less than one-fifth (18%) showed good adherence with wearing splints, and over half (53%) had poor adherence. A study of Rapoff et al. (32) found that 43% of 41 children and adolescents that were prescribed splints had negative reactions to wearing them and cited perceived lack of efficacy and embarrassment among peers as the main reasons. This certainly concords with qualitative data that suggests that children and adolescents with JIA place a premium on peer acceptance and are likely to spurn orthoses and supportive equipment that signal them out as "different," despite understanding the benefits they confer (33). Similar numbers were reported in adult patients with rheumatic disorder (34,36).

Avoidance of Specific Risk Factors

In addition to rehabilitative therapies, adolescents with JIA may also be asked to avoid specific behaviors including socially accepted activities that pose specific risk (e.g., participation in contact sports), and experimental activities that pose both a generic health risk and added threat to those on particular immunosuppressive therapies (e.g., teratogenic effect of methotrexate and increased risk of hepatotoxicity for those who concomitantly use alcohol). Again, there has been little systematic study in this area. This may reflect the fact that general health promotion has not sat within the traditional remit of rheumatology health care (37). However, the seriousness of these issues suggests this is an important part of adherence that should be addressed. Indeed, a study of 9268 adolescents in Switzerland (38) found that those with chronic illness were just as likely to engage in experimental behaviors as their healthy counterparts. Other studies have reposted that while adolescents with chronic illnesses are as sexually active as their healthy peers (39,40), they can have a lower level of knowledge, lower prevalence of contraceptive use, and higher risk of negative outcomes including sexually transmitted infections and sexual abuse (40,41). With respect to JIA, a study in the United Kingdom found that 37.6% of young adults with JIA reported themselves to be sexually active prior to transfer to adult rheumatology care by age 18 years (42). Nash et al. (43) found that 30.7% of adolescents with JIA used alcohol, including 23.5% of those for whom methotrexate was prescribed. The mean age of initiation was 13.6 years. Because of the associated health risk, poor adherence with risk-taking behavior merit further research.

Clinic Attendance

Attention at clinic appointments is essential for reviewing treatment, monitoring adherence, and the early detection of morbidity. Unfortunately, the appointment-keeping behavior of adolescents is less than optimal (44) and may have significant implications for the health and well being of habitual non-attendees. The exact prevalence of poor adherence with appointment-keeping in patients with JIA is unknown, yet it can expected to be high: the meta-analysis of DiMatteo (5) reported an average percentage of nonadherence to appointments of 34.1% for adult and pediatric patients with a variety of chronic diseases. Similarly, there is little research about the contributory factors in non-attendance in rheumatology clinics. Forgetfulness is often cited as the main reason for non-attendance in adolescent patients (44,45).

Telephone reminders have been shown as an effective method to improve their appointment-keeping (45,46). The factors that influence attendance appear wide-ranging and include demographic issues (such as socio-demographic status, geographical distance, access to transport), perceived relevance, the therapeutic relationship, and the clinical environment (44,47,48,49,50).

DETERMINANTS OR RISK-FACTORS FOR NONADHERENCE

Nonadherence is a complex health-related problem that is influenced by multiple factors. The World Health Organization report on nonadherence (8) identified five interrelated, but distinct categories of risk factors for non-adherence with medication taking: socioeconomic factors, patient-related factors, condition-related factors, treatment-related factors, and factors related to the health care system and health care team. These categories can also be used to classify risk factors to adherence with non-pharmacological aspects of treatment. The following paragraphs summarize the evidence on risk factors in patients with JIA, while also providing relevant information found in other populations with chronic illness as well. Table 1 provides an overview of potential risk-factors for poor adherence.

Overall, most evidence is available for risk factors for poor medication adherence. Risk factors for poor adherence to exercise, orthopedic or appointment-keeping are less well documented.

Socioeconomic Factors

Socioeconomic risk factors refer to demographic factors and family-related determinants. A number of demographic factors have been identified that may increase the risk of poor adherence, including ethnicity (i.e., non-white race), onset of disease at a younger age, and the high burden of cost of medication (24). Male adolescents seem to be more prone to poor adherence (5), because they generally exhibit greater risk-taking behavior, putting them at a higher risk for experimentation with their medication, and thus increasing the risk for poor adherence.

Another group of socioeconomic factors are related to social and family functioning. Adolescence implies transition from care provided by the parents to self-care. Active involvement of the parents in the treatment process during this transition process is of particular importance, as adolescents bearing the sole responsibility for medication management, or experiencing little parent supervision are more prone to poor adherence (17,51). Family cohesion, lack of conflict, and good parent-child communication will positively affect adherence (1,51,52). Practical and emotional support from family members can assist patients in adherence and may function as facilitators or cheerleaders (51). In contrast, parents being anxious and concerned about the health and the future of their chronically

Table 1 Potential Risk Factors for Poor Adherence

Socioeconomic factors
    Ethnicity: belonging to minority ethnic group
    Gender: male
    Disease-status: younger age of disease onset
    Economic: greater burden of medication costs
    Family
        Less parental support (practical and emotional)
        Less family cohesion
        Poorer parent-child communication
        Greater conflict
        Greater parental anxiety, parental overprotection
Patient-related factors
    Lower level of cognitive/intellectual functioning
    Lower level of knowledge
    Forgetfulness
    Low self-efficacy
    Negative/incompatible health beliefs
    Low therapeutic motivation
    Emotional disturbance (depression, low self-esteem, body-image disturbance)
Condition-related factors
    Longer disease duration
    Low disease activity
    Less fear of acute problems
Treatment-related factors
    Body-altering/visible treatment effects
    Poly-pharmacy
    Longer duration of treatment regimen
    Greater complexity of regimen
    Unstable efficacy of treatment
Health care system/team
    Less active involvement in decision-making
    Less patient-centered care (i.e., more condition-focused)
    Poor patient-provider communication
    Less follow-up
    Shorter duration of specialist care

ill child may cause parents to become overprotective and controlling, or may render parents unable to give emotional support to the adolescent patient (1,51,52). Moreover, overprotection can compound an adolescent's existing social isolation and peer interaction owing to functional limitations, frequent interruptions of daily activities by treatment requirements, and changed physical appearance (1,51). Friends and peers may help to overcome these feelings of being different by accepting their ill friend with his or her physical limitations (53).

Patient-Related Factors

This category of risk factors has been most extensively studied both in the literature on rheumatic disorders as well as in chronic disease populations in general, clearly indicating a bias as the patient is being seen as the defaulter.

Knowledge about the treatment and the illness is essential for patient's adherence, but information alone is not enough to promote the behavioral changes required as part of the management of the disease (1). Even when patients are given information, they often misunderstand what the doctor says and fail to recall much of the information they are given. Moreover, patients at a lower level of cognitive functioning or with lower intellectual capacities may have difficulties understanding and executing the complex therapeutic regimen. Many patients also stated that forgetfulness was one of the most common reasons for nonadherence (4,24), together with interference of pharmacological and non-pharmacological treatment with the hectic daily life schedules of teenagers.

Adolescents with a chronic disease are often hindered in their striving towards normality and autonomy, which may lead to depression, behavioral disturbances, low self-esteem, or social adjustment difficulties (24,54-56). Patients with recent onset chronic illness must renegotiate their self-identities as formerly well persons. Denial of disease may reflect patients' resistance to accept their illness and medications act as a reminder that they are not "normal," which may consequently result in poor adherence with proposed treatment (54). Myths about arthritis that permeate the public perception may also indirectly contribute to poor adherence. Because arthritis is generally viewed as an inevitable consequence of old age, adolescents can meet disbelief from their environment, which may provoke additional psychological distress.

Another powerful predictor of poor adherence is self-efficacy. Self-efficacy refers to one's confidence in performing a particular behavior (57,58). In a large study by Kyngäs and colleagues, motivation, energy and will power, and feeling arthritis as a threat to their social well being were independent predictors of adherence (53,59).

Patients and their families also have their own ideas about the causes of rheumatic disease, the flare-ups of disease activities, the seriousness of disease, the efficacy of treatment, and the consequences of poor adherence (51,60). Those beliefs are sometimes based on misassumptions or ideas offered by relatives, friends or the lay press, which do not always correspond with the reality (34,51,60-62). It is assumed that health beliefs (i.e., treatment perceptions and illness representations) more strongly influence medication adherence than socio-demographic of clinical factors (63). The self-regulatory theory proposed that patients make the decision to adhere on the basis of a cost-benefit analysis, considering whether their beliefs about the necessity of treatment (e.g., medication taking, exercising) for maintaining health outweigh their concerns about its potential adverse effects (e.g., side effects, muscle pain, having less time for friends) (61,63). Such beliefs are thought to influence families' use of complementary and alternative medicines who may perceive prescribed treatment as "unnatural", fear side effects of conventional medications, or believe them to be inefficacious (64). Feldman et al. (28) suggests that the use of complementary and alternative therapies does not necessarily predict poor adherence with conventional treatments, but may indicate that the adolescent is having problems managing their disease. Questioning the use of complementary and alternative medicines should, therefore, be part of routine clinical assessment. Not only does this enable discussion about health beliefs regarding treatment, but may also open up a discourse regarding the potential side-effects of complementary and alternative medicines and their interactions with medical therapy.

Another study regarding health beliefs on medication adherence in adult patients showed that areas of concern were the potential long-term adverse effect of their medications and the fear of becoming dependent upon medication (65). This study found that concerns of the adherent group were significantly lower than those of the nonadherent group (65). Perception of necessity was not significantly different between both groups. This observation underscores that we should perhaps concentrate more on reassuring patients about the safety of the treatments we prescribe, than on convincing them of the benefits of treatment (65).

Condition-Related Factors

Poor adherence was found to be associated with longer duration of disease (23). Moreover, patients with high disease activity tend to be more adherent with treatment advice than those with low disease activity (66,67). The perception of being in good condition, which is the ultimate goal of rheumatological treatment, may involve a dangerous pitfall, as patients are less likely to take their medications, exercise or wear their splints on a routine basis if they perceive themselves as healthy. Patients' fearful of acute problems were also more likely to be adherent compared to teenagers showing no fear (53).

Treatment-Related Factors

The development of a positive self-concept and body image in adolescents with chronic rheumatic diseases is challenged by the experience of side effects of the medications. NSAIDs and DMARDs are associated with a number of adverse effects, of which gastrointestinal complaints (e.g., nausea, vomiting, diarrhoea, dyspepsia) are most common. Pseudoporphyria or linear facial scarring was estimated to affect 11% of children taking chronic NSAIDs (68). Hepatotoxicity, bone marrow suppression, lung disease, rash, fever may also occur (21). The cosmetic side effects may be particularly troublesome for adolescents and may often lead to poor adherence with medication taking (1).

Polypharmacy may also be a reason for nonadherence. Patients are expected to take not only the agents themselves but also additional therapy such as folic acid and/or calcium supplements to offset medication-related adverse events (16).

Other examples of treatment-related risk factors of poor adherence include longer duration of treatment regimen, complexity of regimen (e.g., taking multiple medications at different times throughout the day, exercising several times a week), and unstable efficacy of treatment (69).

Health Care Setting and Health Care Provider–Related Factors

Health care setting and health care provider–related factors receive too little attention in the literature, yet is recognized by the World Health Organization to be a key determinant in understanding nonadherence (70). This again illustrates the bias in the literature that health care workers prefer to blame the patient for his/her nonadherent behavior, and are reluctant to see themselves as potential contributors of nonadherence.

The amount of direct communication between a doctor and child has been shown to be positively associated with adherence (71). The need for health-related information and effective communication with doctors and other health care providers are major concerns for adolescents (72). Research has shown the relatively passive involvement of young people during consultations, with parent-doctor interactions dominating, and information-giving being directed at the parent as opposed to the young person (73,74). When patients are encouraged to actively participate in decisions concerning their care, they may be more committed to those decisions and ultimately achieve higher levels of adherence (59). In addition, patient-centered care as opposed to condition-focused care will also have a beneficial impact on adherence (61,75). Key features of good doctor-patient interaction are shared goal setting, written management plans and regular follow-up (59,75), i.e. all characteristics that perfectly fit into the concept of "concordance."

Fewer clinic visits and shorter duration of specialist care have also been associated with poor adherence (23). However, support from the health care team may be valuable sources to empower adherence. In a study of Kyngäs et al. (59), the most powerful predictor was support from nurses, with adolescents experiencing support from nurses being 7.28-fold more likely to be adherent compared to teenagers not feeling supported by nurses. Support received from physicians, parents and peers was also extremely important (i.e., odds ratios were 3.42, 2.69, and 2.11 respectively).

The fact that an acute illness model prevails instead of a chronic illness management model could also be seen as a system-related factor contributing to nonadherence. Chronic illness management models that put the patient in the centre of care, provide continuity, address psychosocial, and behavioral issues as much as medical issues, and promote active participation of an informed patient have been shown to enhance the clinical outcomes in a number of chronically ill populations (70,76,77).

ADHERENCE ENHANCING INTERVENTIONS

Traditional outcome research should try to answer the following two questions in future research: (1) does it work under experimental conditions based on randomized clinical trials (efficacy question); and (2) does it work in practice based on quasi-experimental designs (effectiveness question)?

Very few publications on the effectiveness of adherence enhancing interventions in adolescents with chronic rheumatic diseases exist. Few intervention studies to improve adherence in juvenile arthritis have been published (25,26,27,30). All are limited to case reports from the same research group and do not focus exclusively on adolescents. In general, studies have shown evidence for the effectiveness of an intervention that focuses on behavioral strategies, in combination with an educational component (25,26,27,30). A variety of reinforcement-based strategies seem equally effective in enhancing adherence, including a token system and social attention and feedback from family members (25,26,27,30). Randomized controlled trials, however, are scarce. Niedermann et al. (78) performed a literature review to systematically collect randomized controlled trials examining educational and psycho-educational interventions for (adult) patients with rheumatoid arthritis, with focus on their long-term effectiveness. Six educational interventions targeted adherence in various dimensions. There was strong evidence for an increase of long-term adherence in general; yet, the effect for medication taking was moderate (78). Moreover, goals and interventions varied greatly and programmes were organized differently, which made it difficult to determine which were the most successful education interventions (78).

In the absence of good intervention trials, one must rely on meta-analysis and systematic reviews published on other acute and chronic ill patient populations. These reports concluded that educational strategies alone are not effective, and that a high dose combination of educational, behavioral and social support interventions will be most successful (7,79–81).

The limited available evidence in JIA or other adolescent groups with chronic disease on educational, behavioral, psychosocial support, and organizational adherence-enhancing interventions will be discussed in the following section. Table 2 summarizes possible intervention strategies.

Table 2 Interventions to Improve Adherence

Educational interventions
  Provide information on the disease and its treatment
  Use verbal and nonverbal materials
  Use a stepwise approach adapted to the developmental level, when indicated
  Monitor the level of understanding
  Address barriers to adherence and try to find solutions
  Make patient a partner in the educational process
Behavioral interventions
  Use interventions to increase self-efficacy and confidence in self-management
  Reduce the complexity of treatment if possible
  Use tailoring, cueing, reminders, or medication aids
Psychosocial support
  Refer to specialized care in case of psychopathology or dysfunction in the patient
    or the family
  Include peer groups or support groups
  Use modern communication tools (e-mail, internet)
  Encourage the adolescent to actively participate in planning and decision making
Organizational interventions
  Build a trust relationship in which patient is an equal partner in treatment
  Show interest in the person, and not only in the condition
  Offer patient the choice of who is present during the consultation
  Address concerns
  Maintain continuity with follow-up by the same health-care provider

---

Educational Strategies

Knowledge regarding the disease and its treatment is a prerequisite for good medication adherence. Most treatment centers implement some form of patient and family education in their routine clinical practice. The National Arthritis Advisory Board in the United States has developed standards for arthritis patient education (82) and provided the following definition:

> Patient education is planned, organized learning experiences designed to facilitate voluntary adoption of behaviors or beliefs conductive to health. The activities of a patient education program must be designed to attain goals the patient has participated in formulating. The primary focus of these activities includes the acquisition of information, beliefs and attitudes which impact on health status, quality-of-life, and possibly health care utilization.

Careful discussion about the name, purpose, dose, and schedule of prescribed medications is indicated (16). Information regarding possible side effects is necessary (16). The importance of other aspects of treatment should be stressed as well. The health care provider should thereby involve the patient as partner in the educational process, acknowledging patient's previous illness experiences, knowledge and beliefs, rather than providing one-way information (17). Learning formats can be highly variable and can encompass booklets, lectures, role-plays, contracting, goal setting and sharing experiences (83). It is crucial to use a stepwise approach, that is, information must not be overwhelming: pace, amount and presentational style need to be tailored to the child's age, cultural background, and language, as well as their cognitive and intellectual abilities (17). Use short sentences and avoid jargon (4). At the end of the education process, the adolescent can be asked to re-iterate the information, in order to monitor the level of understanding (4). Formal evaluation can be performed by interview, fill-in-the-blank or multiple-choice questionnaires, and situational role-play. Education best can be repeated during clinical follow-up visits, particularly with a disease such as chronic rheumatic diseases in which symptoms wax and wane over time (4). Patients should be encouraged to ask questions (51). Kyngäs et al. (1) thereby suggests that educational programs should be based on an appraisal of each adolescent's needs rather than relying upon the application of a package suitable for all.

Education also provides the opportunity to discuss health beliefs, and to modify wrong beliefs regarding medication effectiveness, and by promoting realistic expectations about risk/benefit ratios (16,84). Barriers to adherence anticipated by the patient and the family and ways to facilitate adherence in the home environment may also be addressed (4,17).

Behavioral Interventions

Knowledge is a prerequisite, but education alone will not guarantee adherence. Behavioral strategies should also be implemented to increase the likelihood of adherence.

The key issue of behavioral interventions is to assist adolescents with rheumatic disease in learning adequate self-management. Self-management can be defined as the individual's ability to manage the symptoms, treatment, physical and psychosocial consequences of lifestyle changes inherent in living with rheumatic disease (83). Efficacious self-management encompasses ability to monitor one's condition and to affect the cognitive, behavioral, and emotional responses necessary to maintain satisfactory quality-of-life. Thus, a dynamic and continuous process of self-regulation is established.

Interventions to increase self-efficacy may help to increase confidence with self-management. Bandura recommended the following four primary strategies for increasing self-efficacy with medication taking (57,85):

1. Try to identify and reinforce the patient's past and present successes or accomplishments.

2. Direct the patient to observe successful behaviors of others.
3. Provide positive feedback for the patient's efforts or encourage people in the patient's social network to do so.
4. Clinicians can try to ensure that their patients do not interpret incorrectly how they are feeling. Assist in emotions hindering adherence with medication taking.

If possible, poly-pharmacy should be avoided by reducing the complexity of treatment (16). Linking medication taking with some other well-established daily activity and tailoring the medication regimen to the lifestyle of the adolescent may assist (16,51). Reminders (e.g., alarm clocks, programming mobile phones, medication calendars, vibrating watches) and self-monitoring strategies (e.g., daily logs) may also helpful. Dispensing incentives for adherence is another behavioral strategy (69).

Interventions to Increase Psychosocial Support

Emotional difficulties or psychopathology displayed by the patients (e.g., depression) or dysfunction in the family (e.g., substance abuse, coercive patterns of interaction) should be identified and specialized care (e.g., psychotherapy or psycho-pharmacological treatment) should be suggested and arranged (69).

Evidence also showed that increased parental supervision is quite effective in the improvement of general adherence (1). Yet, the aim is that adolescents learn to care for themselves (51). Adolescents need frequent support, encouragement, and positive feedback when striving to manage their chronic illness. Health-care providers should involve the family or significant others in care whenever possible and offer them tools to support and reward adherence (1). In addition, adolescents should be encouraged to participate actively in planning and decision-making processes (59). Peer groups may also be valuable sources of emotional support. In addition, support groups for adolescent patients may allow patients to share common problems and to discuss methods of coping and problem solving from peers experiencing the same struggles with medication adherence.

Modern communication tools may help to maintain a level of support between the patient, the parents, and the health care team. Patients can be empowered by e-mail interactions with the health care provider, or phone calls. Clinicians can also provide information about accurate and useful health websites (51).

Organizational Interventions

Organizational strategies emphasize changing clinic and regimen characteristics as a means of promoting adherence such as reducing barriers that limit the interaction between the patient and the health care system (84). The following aspects of an adolescent-doctor consultation may engender effective communication (74): Offer patients the choice of who is present during the consultation and create a sense of equity by using accessible language, with attention being paid to the adolescent as an individual rather than exclusively focusing on the condition. Additional techniques to improve patient-doctor communication are encouraging patients to write down their concerns before each visit, and addressing each concern specifically, yet briefly (86). Continuity of follow-up by organizing contacts with the same health care provider will also increase the likelihood of adherence (69,74).

CONCLUSION

Poor adherence with pharmacological and non-pharmacological treatments is a widespread problem in adolescents with chronic rheumatic diseases, which may result in poor clinical outcome and increased health care costs (Table 3). The detection of poor adherence should be a permanent concern of health care teams dealing with adolescents with JIA. However, research on prevalence, risk factors, and adherence-enhancing interventions in this patient population is scarce. Prospective studies are needed to identify adolescents and families at risk for adherence problems (17). Qualitative research to provide insight in the barriers and facilitators of poor adherence is also needed. Further research is needed to work out the pattern of causal relationships between adherence and clinical outcomes. Finally, the

Table 3   Key Learning Points

Adolescents with chronic rheumatic diseases show poor adherence in pharmacological and non-pharmacological therapies.

Poor adherence is a major cause of suboptimal clinical outcome and may have negative implications for well-being in adulthood.

Poor adherence can be intentional and involuntary.

The determinants of adherence are multifactorial and relate to adolescents' socioeconomic status, psychosocial characteristics, condition, treatment, and the health care system.

Interventions to promote adherence are similarly multifactorial and include education, family support, cognitive-behavioral modifications, and provider characteristics (e.g., adolescent-focused care, improved communication, shared decision-making).

The quality of the therapeutic relationship is an important determinant of adherence, and all health professionals can promote adherence.

There is a dearth of literature concerning the adherence of adolescents with chronic rheumatic diseases, and changing this must be made a priority to improve outcome.

effectiveness of adherence-enhancing interventions should be tested in randomized controlled clinical trials.

REFERENCES

1. Kyngäs HA, Kroll T, Duffy ME. Compliance in adolescents with chronic diseases: a review. J Adolesc Health 2000; 26(6):379–88.
2. Staples B, Bravender T. Drug compliance in adolescents: assessing and managing modifiable risk factors. Paediatr Drugs 2002; 4(8):503–13.
3. Rapoff MA, Lindsey CB, Purviance MR. The validity and reliability of parental ratings of disease activity in juvenile rheumatoid arthritis. Arthritis Care Res 1991; 4(3):136–9.
4. Rapoff MA. Assessing and enhancing adherence to medical regimens for juvenile rheumatoid arthritis. Pediatr Ann 2002; 31(6):373–9.
5. DiMatteo MR. Variations in patients' adherence to medical recommendations: A quantitative review of 50 years of research. Med Care 2004b; 42(3):200–9.
6. Lewis A Noncompliance: a $100 billion problem. Remington Report 1997; 514–5.
7. Haynes RB, Montague P, Oliver T, et al. Interventions for helping patients to follow prescriptions for medications (Cochrane review). The Cochrane Library: Oxford, Update Software, 2000.
8. Sabate E. Adherence to Long-term Therapies: Evidence for Action. Switzerland: World Health Organization, 2003.
9. La Greca AM. Issues in adherence with pediatric regimens. J Pediatr Psychol 1990; 15:423–36.
10. Feinberg J The effect of patient-practitioner interaction on compliance: a review of the literature and application in rheumatoid arthritis. Patient Educ Couns 1988; 11(3):171–87.
11. Stevenson FA, Cox K, Britten N, et al. A systematic review of research on communication between patients and health care professionals about medicines: the consequences for concordance. Health Expect 2004; 7(3):235–45.
12. Marinker M, Shaw J. Not to be taken as directed. Putting concordance for taking medications into practice. Br Med J 2003; 326(7385):348–9.
13. Marinker M, Blenkinsopp A, Bond, C et al., eds. From Compliance to Concordance: Achieving Shared Goals in Medicine Taking. London: Royal Pharmaceutical Society of Great Brittain, 1997.
14. Shaw KL, Southwood TR, McDonagh JE, et al. User perspectives of transitional care for adolescents with juvenile idiopathic arthritis. Rheumatology 2004a; 43 (6):770–8.
15. Shaw KL, Southwood TR, McDonagh JE, et al. Transitional care for adolescents with juvenile idiopathic arthritis: A Delphi study. Rheumatology 2004b; 43(8):1000–6.
16. Akikusa JD, Allen RC. Reducing the impact of rheumatic diseases in childhood. Best Pract Res Clin Rheumatol 2002; 16(3):333–45.
17. Kroll T, Barlow JH, Shaw K. Treatment adherence in juvenile rheumatoid arthritis- a review. Scand J Rheumatol 1999; 28(1):10–8.

18. Goldberg AI, Cohen G, Rubin AH. Physician assessments of patient compliance with medical treatment. Soc Sci Med 1998; 47(11):1873–6.

19. Chikanza IC. Juvenile rheumatoid arthritis: therapeutic perspectives. Pediatr Drugs 2002; 4(5):335–48.

20. Cron RQ. Current treatment for chronic arthritis in childhood. Curr Opin Pediatr 2002; 14(6):684–7.

21. Murray KJ, Lovell DJ. Advanced therapy for juvenile arthritis. Best Pract Res Clin Rheumatol 2002; 16(3):361–78.

22. Costello I, Wong IC, Nunn AJ. A literature review to identify interventions to improve the use of medicines in children. Child Care Health Dev 2004; 30(6): 647–65.

23. Litt IF, Cuskey WR. Compliance with salicylate therapy in adolescents with juvenile rheumatoid arthritis. Am J Dis Child 1981; 135(5):434–6.

24. Litt IF, Cuskey WR, Rosenberg A. Role of self-esteem and autonomy in determining medication compliance among adolescents with juvenile rheumatoid arthritis. Pediatrics 1982; 69(1):15–7.

25. Rapoff MA, Lindsey CB, Christophersen ER. Improving compliance with medical regimens: Case study with juvenile rheumatoid arthritis. Arch Phys Med Rehabil 1984; 65(5):267–9.

26. Rapoff MA, Purviance MR, Lindsey CB. Educational and behavioral strategies for improving medication compliance in juvenile rheumatoid arthritis. Arch Phys Med Rehabil 1988; 69(9):439–41.

27. Rapoff M. Compliance with treatment regimens for pediatric rheumatic diseases. Arthritis Care Res 1989; 2(3):S40–7.

28. Feldman DE, Duffy C, De Civita M, et al. Factors associated with the use of complementary and alternative medicine in juvenile idiopathic arthritis. Arthritis Rheum 2004; 51(4):527–32.

29. Hayford JR, Ross CK. Medical compliance in juvenile rheumatoid arthritis. Arthritis Care Res 1988; 4:190–7.

30. Pieper KB, Rapoff MA, Purviance MR, et al. Improving compliance with prednisone therapy in patients with rheumatic disease. Arthritis Care Res 1989; 2(4):132–5.

31. Duffy CM, De civita M, Gibbon M, et al. Adherence to treatment in juvenile idiopathic arthritis. Pediatr Rheumatol Online J 2003; Abstract 77.

32. Rapoff MA, Lindsley CB, Christophersen ER. Parent perceptions of problems experienced by their children in complying with treatments for juvenile rheumatic arthritis. Arch Phys Med Rehabil 1985; 66(7):427–9.

33. Barlow J, Harrison K, Shaw K. The experience of parenting in the context of juvenile chronic arthritis. Clin Child Psychol Psychiatr 1998; 3(3):445–63.

34. Brus H, van de Laar M, Taal E, et al. Compliance in rheumatoid arthritis and the role of formal patient education. Semin Arthritis Rheum 1997; 26(4): 702–10.

35. Sturge C, Garralda ME, Boissin M, et al. School attendance and juvenile chronic arthritis. Br J Rheumatol 1997; 36(11):1218–23.

36. Spoorenberg A, Boers M, van der Linden S. Wrist splints in rheumatoid arthritis: what do we know about efficacy and compliance? Arthritis Care Res 1994; 7(2):55–7.

37. Britto MT, Rosenthal SL, Taylor J, et al. Improving rheumatologists' screening for alcohol use and sexual activity. Arch Pediatr Adolesc Med 2000; 154 478–83.
38. Miauton L, Narring F, Michaud PA. Chronic illness, life style and emotional health in adolescence: results of a cross-sectional survey on the health of 15–20 year olds in Switzerland. Eur J Pediatr 2003; 162(10):682–9.
39. Suris JC, Parera N. Sex, drugs and chronic illness: health behaviours among chronically ill youth. Eur J Public Health 2005; 15(5):484–8.
40. Suris JC, Resnick MD, Cassuto N, et al. Sexual behavior of adolescents with chronic disease and disability. J Adolesc Health 1996; 19(2):124–31.
41. Valencia LS, Cromer BA. Sexual activity and other high-risk behaviors in adolescents with chronic illness: a review. J Pediatr Adolesc Gynecol 2000; 13 (2):53–64.
42. Packham JC, Hall MA. Long-term follow-up of 246 adults with juvenile idiopathic arthritis: social function, relationships and sexual activity. Rheumatology 2002; 41(12):1440–3.
43. Nash AA, Britto MT, Lovell DJ, et al. Substance abuse among adolescents with juvenile rheumatoid arthritis. Arthritis Care Res 1998; 11(5):391–6.
44. Irwin CE Jr, Millstein SG, Ellen JM. Appointment keeping behaviour in adolescents: factors associated with follow-up appointment-keeping. Pediatrics 1993; 92(1):20–3.
45. Sawyer SM, Zalan A, Bond LM. Telephone reminders and attendance in an adolescent clinic. J Paediatr Child Health 2002; 38(1):79–83.
46. O'Brien G, Lazebnik R. Telephone call reminders and attendance in an adolescent clinic. Pediatrics 1998; 101(6):E6.
47. Nock, MK, Ferriter C. Parent management of attendance and adherence in child and adolescent therapy: a conceptual and empirical review. Clin Child Fam Psychol Rev 2005; 8(2):149–66.
48. Johnson R, Horne B, Feltbower RG, et al. Hospital attendance patterns in long-term survivors of cancer. Arch Dis Child 2004; 89(4):374–7.
49. Freed LH, Ellen JM, Irwin CE Jr, et al. Determinants of adolescents' satisfaction with health care providers and intentions to keep follow-up appointments. J Adolesc Health 1998; 22(6):475–9.
50. Litt IF, Cuskey WR. Satisfaction with health care: A predictor of adolescents' appointment keeping. J Adolesc Health Care 1984; 5(3):196–200.
51. DiMatteo MR. The role of effective communication with children and their families in fostering adherence to pediatric regimens. Patient Educ Couns 2004a; 55(3):339–44.
52. Chaney JM, Peterson L. Family variables and disease management in juvenile rheumatoid arthritis. J Pediatr Psychol 1989; 14(3):389–403.
53. Kyngäs H. Motivation as a crucial predictor of good compliance in adolescents with rheumatoid arthritis. Int J Nurs Pract 2002; 8(6):336–41.
54. Carder PC, Vuckovic N, Green CA. Negotiating medications: patient perceptions of long-term medication use. J Clin Pharm Ther 2003; 28(5):409–17.
55. Barlow JH, Shaw KL, Harrison K. Consulting the 'experts': children's and parents' perceptions of psycho-educational interventions in the context of juvenile chronic arthritis. Health Educ Res 1999; 14(5):597–610.

56. Magen J. Psychiatric aspects of chronic disease in adolescence. J Am Osteopath Assoc 1990; 90(6):521–5.
57. Allegrante JP, Marks R. Self-efficacy in management of osteoarthritis. Rheum Dis Clin N Am 2003; 29(4):747–68.
58. Brus H, van de Laar M, Taal E, et al. Determinants of compliance with medication in patients with rheumatoid arthritis: the importance of self-efficacy expectations. Patient Educ Couns 1999; 36(1):57–64.
59. Kyngäs H, Rissanen M. Support as a crucial predictor of good compliance of adolescents with a chronic disease. J Clin Nurs 2001; 10(6):767–74.
60. Soliday E, Hoeksel R. Health beliefs and pediatric emergency department after-care adherence. Ann Behav Med 2000; 22(4):299–306.
61. Berry D, Bradlow A, Bersellini E. Perceptions of the risks and benefits of medicines in patients with rheumatoid arthritis and other painful musculoskeletal conditions. Rheumatology 2004; 43(7):901–5.
62. Donovan JL, Blake DR, Fleming WG. The patient is not a blank sheet: lay beliefs and their relevance to patient education. Br J Rheumatol 1989; 28(1): 58–61.
63. Horne R, Weinman J. Patients' beliefs about prescribed medicines and their role in adherence to treatment in chronic physical illness. J Psychosom Res 1999; 47(6):555–67.
64. Spigelblatt L, Laine-ammara G, Pless IB, et al. The use of alternative medicine by children. Pediatrics 1994; 94(6 pt 1):811–4.
65. Neame R, Hammond A. Beliefs about medications: a questionnaire survey of people with rheumatoid arthritis. Rheumatology 2005; 44(6):762–7.
66. Brus HL, van de Laar MA, Taal E, et al. Effects of patient education on compliance with basic treatment regimens and health in recent onset active rheumatoid arthritis. Ann Rheum Dis 1998; 57(3):146–51.
67. Owen SG, Friesen WT, Roberts MS, et al. Determinants of compliance in rheumatoid arthritic patients assessed in their home environment. Br J Rheumatol 1985; 24(4):313–20.
68. De Silva B, Banney L, Uttley W, et al. Pseudoporphyria and nonsteroidal antiinflammatory agents in children with juvenile idiopathic arthritis. Pediatr Dermatol 2000; 17(6):480–3.
69. Lemanek KL, Kamps J, Brown Chung N. Empirically supported treatments in pediatric psychology: regimen adherence. J Pediatr Psychol 2001; 26(5):253–75.
70. World Health Organization. Innovative Care for Chronic Conditions: Building Blocks for Action. Switzerland: World Health Organization, 2002.
71. De Winter M, Baerveldt C, Kooistra J. Enabling children: Participation as a new perspective on child-health promotion. Child Care Health Dev 1999; 25(1): 15–25.
72. Jones R, Finlay F, Simpson N, et al. How can adolescents' health needs and concerns best be met? Br J Gen Pract 1997; 47(423):631–4.
73. Tates K, Meeuwesen L. Doctor–parent–child communication. A (re)view of the literature. Soc Sci Med 2001; 52(6):839–51.
74. Beresford BA, Sloper P. Chronically ill adolescents' experiences of communicating with doctors: A qualitative study. J Adolesc Health 2003; 33(3):172–9.

75. Bauman AE, Fardy HJ, Harris PG. Getting it right: why botter with patient-centred care? Med J Aust 2003; 179(5):253–6.
76. Bodenheimer T, Wagner EH, Grumbach K. Improving primary care for patients with chronic illness. J Am Med Assoc 2002; 288(14):1775–9.
77. Bodenheimer T, Wagner EH, Grumbach K. Improving primary care for patients with chronic illness: The chronic care model Part 2. J Am Med Assoc 2002; 288(15):1909–14.
78. Niedermann K, Fransen J, Knols R, et al. Gap between short- and long-term effects of patient education in rheumatoid arthritis patients: A systematic review. Arthritis Rheum 2004; 51(3):388–98.
79. Roter DL, Hall JA, Merisca R, et al. Effectiveness of interventions to improve patient compliance: A meta-analysis. Med Care 1998; 36(8):1138–61.
80. McDonald HP, Garg AX, Haynes RB. Interventions to enhance patient adherence to medication prescriptions. J Am Med Assoc 2002; 288:2868–79.
81. Peterson AM, Takiya L, Finley R. Meta-analysis of trials of interventions to improve medication adherence. Am J Health Syst Pharm 2003; 60(7):657–65.
82. Burckhardt CS, Lorig K, Moncur C, et al. Arthritis and musculoskeletal patient education standards. Arthritis Care Res 1994; 7:1–4.
83. Barlow JH. How to use education as an intervention in osteoarthritis. Best Pract Res Clin Rheumatol 2001; 15(4):545–58.
84. Garcia Popa-Lisseanu MG, Greisinger A, Richardson M, et al. Determinants of treatment adherence in ethnically diverse, economically disadvantaged patients with rheumatoid disease J. Rheumatol 2005; 32(5):913–9
85. Bandura A self-efficacy: the exercise of control New York: WH Freeman and Company, 1997.
86. Daltroy LH. Doctor-patient communication in rheumatological disorders. Baillieres Clin Rheumatol 1993; 7(2):221–39.

6

The Disease Spectrum of Adolescent Rheumatology

Liza J. McCann

Department of Paediatric Rheumatology, Royal Liverpool Children's Hospital, Alder Hey, Liverpool, U.K.

Debajit Sen

University College London Hospital, Middlesex NHS Trust and Great Ormond Street NHS Trust, London, U.K.

INTRODUCTION

The management of rheumatic disease during adolescence involves unique diagnostic and therapeutic challenges to the clinician. Pathogenesis, treatment, and prognosis of many musculoskeletal disorders differ greatly in children compared to adults. Since adolescents can present with manifestations common to either age range, an awareness of differences is essential. The psychological, emotional, and developmental effects of illness in this age group are discussed in Chapter 1. When managing children with chronic rheumatic conditions, knowledge of prognosis, including morbidity, mortality and long-term adverse effects of medications, is paramount, and will be covered in other chapters. This chapter will address the spectrum of disease seen during adolescence, and highlight important differences when compared to pediatric and/or adult populations.

EPIDEMIOLOGY

It is difficult to establish the true epidemiology of musculoskeletal disease in adolescents. There are practical difficulties measuring incidence and prevalence of disease in a patient group that may be under pediatric or adult care and for whom there is no universally accepted age range (Chapter 1).

There is an estimated 2589 incident cases of rheumatic conditions per 100,000 population in the 0–15 age group, and 8935 per 100,000 population in the 16–24 year old age group (1). However, this estimate is not exhaustive, and only covers 10 musculoskeletal conditions selected as the most common or characteristic of their group. Specific adolescent data (10–19 year old age group) are lacking. If this group of 10 conditions is restricted to those requiring continuing secondary health care, (childhood arthritis, SLE, gout, and scleroderma) there is an estimated 129 and 188 prevalent cases per 100,000 population in the 0–15 and 16–24 year old age groups respectively, according to data available (1).

Musculoskeletal symptoms make up the third most common reason for presentation of adolescents in primary care (2). In a nationally representative survey exploring the health status and behaviors of Canadians, adolescent arthritis or rheumatism lasting six months or more, affected seven per 1000 of patients aged 12 to 19 years (3). Chronic back pain, unrelated to arthritis, affected 30 per 1000 adolescents (3).

Epidemiology is complicated by genetic diversity and environment, which play an important part in inflammatory musculoskeletal disease. For example, large regional variations in epidemiology exist among distribution of subsets of juvenile idiopathic arthritis (JIA), probably due to human leucocyte antigen (HLA) alleles and environment (4). Likewise, lupus is three to five times more common in African-American females compared to white females, and twice as common in African-American males (5).

Collection of epidemiological data is difficult in rare diseases, such as juvenile dermatomyositis. For example, the British Paediatric Surveillance Unit found an estimated frequency of new cases in the United Kingdom to be 1.9/million in children less than 16 years (6). This is likely to be an underestimate, since some cases may not have been reported, or may have presented to specialists not included in study (such as adult neurologists). More recent studies in the United States, give estimates up to 4.1/million (7). Reasons for differences are unclear, although, inflammatory myositis has been noted to be more common in Blacks (8) and may be precipitated by high sun intensity (9).

This chapter aims to provide an overview of adolescent rheumatological conditions not represented in other chapters in this book, including vasculitis, juvenile dermatomyositis, scleroderma, musculoskeletal infections, systemic diseases presenting to rheumatology and musculoskeletal malignancies. More unusual presentations, such as periodic fever syndromes and Castleman's disease, are covered briefly.

Caring for adolescents requires an awareness and sensitivity of a patient's developmental and psychological needs. These vary with individuals and differ from those of a child or adult. Some of these needs are addressed and summarized in Table 1. Adolescents appreciate participation in their own care, with their concerns and viewpoints taken seriously (10).

Table 1 Adolescent Issues in Rheumatological Diseases

Specific issues	Possible solutions
Image conscious. Dislike steroids in view of adverse effects, particularly weight gain, striae, and acne. NB: Increased steroid toxicity in peripubertal period	Informed consent prior to use of drugs. Use IV methylprednisolone pulsing to quickly get inflammation under control in order to minimize use of oral steroids. Early use of immunosuppressive medication. Healthy eating advice to limit weight gain. Camouflage nurses may give advice on treatment of stretch marks and makeup use. Early aggressive treatment of JDM may decrease the chance of lipoatrophy and calcinosis, both distressing for adolescents.
Alcohol, drugs, smoking, and risk-taking behavior	Make sure adolescents know about effect of alcohol on methotrexate in the context of health promotion. Assess understanding of information given. Negotiate. Advise taking methotrexate on a day when not binge drinking, and advise an alcohol limit. Ensure awareness of atherosclerosis risk with smoking, particularly in conditions with vasculopathy. Also, implications of decreased ventilatory capacity in JDM and systemic sclerosis. Education is best provided through a multidisciplinary team.
Sexual behavior	Sexual health advice, as given to all young people, to include barrier methods to reduce sexually transmitted infections. Make sure adolescents know about tetarogenic effects of drugs such as methotrexate, and give contraceptive advice. Contraception advice should take into account the presence of anticardiolipin antibodies. Fertility issues with cyclophosphamide should be explained directly to the adolescent in an developmentally and age appropriate manner and sperm/egg storage offered if possible. When adolescent is sexually active, give advice re: regular cervical screening.
Adherence/ concordance	With flare-ups or poor control of disease, always consider nonadherence with treatment. Question in a nonconfrontational way. Decriminalize—"When was the last time you forgot?" Compromise with the adolescent, stressing important treatments and perhaps sacrificing those that are less important (see Chapter 5) Consider once-daily dosing regimens if at all possible.
Disability	Aggressive early treatment (medical and physiotherapy/ occupational therapy) to prevent contractures and deformity. Provide practical help with driving, financial-benefit eligibility, and aids for daily living to promote independence.

(Continued)

Table 1 Adolescent Issues in Rheumatological Diseases (*Continued*)

Specific issues	Possible solutions
Diet and exercise, including bone health	Education regarding healthy eating, taking into account risk of atherosclerosis, osteoporosis, and obesity (particularly if pain and disability is limiting exercise). Discuss weight bearing activities; assess need for calcium and vitamin D supplementation or bishosphonates (see Chapter 12). Educate about the benefits of exercise for building muscle strength and stamina, protecting joints, and preventing mechanical pains secondary to muscle weakness
Schooling, college, university, and work	Good communication with schools and colleges with letters of support as needed. Poor concentration and fatigue is common in inflammatory conditions, making schooling challenging. Career advice may be necessary and practical support for job interviews, including training in disclosure
Holidays without parents and travel abroad	Need knowledge of medications and what to do if become unwell when away. Holiday insurance. Vaccinations. Spare supplies of medication in hand luggage. Informing airline of need to travel with needles. Need awareness that sun exposure may lead to a flare of dermatomyositis or lupus—stress need for sun block, hats and sleeves. Increased risk taking behavior when away with peers
Peer support	Signpost young person to peer support organizations or websites, for example, www.ablelink.org/ www.lehman.cuny.edu/faculty/jfleitas/bandaides/ index.html www.teenagehealthfreak.org www.doctissimo.fr www.ciao.ch www.teenhealthfx.com www.goaskalice.columbia.edu www.childrenfirst.nhs.uk

In order to maximize adherence to medical and physical treatments, a young person needs to be involved in shared decision making within a multi-disciplinary team.

SYSTEMIC VASCULITIS

Although the vasculitides are rare, it is essential that those practicing in the field of rheumatology are familiar with them, as they are potentially fatal and require treatment with potentially toxic therapy. The following section will be limited to the basics essential to the understanding of systemic vasculitis and then focus on the vasculitides most likely to be encountered in adolescents.

Definition

The systemic vasculitides are a group of protean disorders characterized by destructive inflammation of the blood vessel wall. One should note that inflammation around the wall of the blood vessel (perivasculitis) and vasculopathies (referring to disorders of blood vessels in general which may include the vasculitides) should not be confused with the vasculitides.

Classification

Vasculitis may be primary or secondary to a separate pathology, the most common and important of which is infection. The differing terminology used in the classification of the primary systemic vasculitides remains confusing. In 1952, Zeek proposed the classification of the vasculitides according to vessel size (11). Subsequent classification schemes reflected the size of the predominantly affected blood vessels as well as the discovery of the antineutrophil cytoplasmic antibodies. The most recent classification schemes in common use are those developed by the American College of Rheumatology in 1990 (12) and the diagnostic criteria developed at the Chapel Hill Consensus Conference in 1994 (13) as shown in Table 2.

The clinical presentation and histopathology of the vasculitides may overlap. When one considers the potent immunosuppression required to treat the primary systemic vasculitides, it becomes clear that mimics of vasculitis and causes of secondary vasculitis must be excluded (Table 3).

Epidemiology

Estimates of the incidence and prevalence of the vasculitides are fraught with difficulties owing to their rarity, and there is a significant geographical and ethnic variation. There are currently no published data specific to adolescents.

Large Vessel Vasculitis

Takayasu's Arteritis

The ACR classification criteria describe the characteristic features of subclavian or aortic bruit, age <40 years at onset, decreased brachial artery pulse, blood pressure difference of >10 mm Hg between arms, claudication of extremities, and arteriographic evidence of narrowing or occlusion of aorta, its primary branches, or large arteries in the proximal, upper or lower extremities (21). In Japan almost a fifth of cases occur in 10 to 19 year olds

Table 2 Nomenclature of Systemic Vasculitis

		Annual incidence/10^6 population (Ref.)
Large vessel vasculitis		
Giant cell (temporal) arteritis	Granulomatous arteritis of the aorta and its major branches, with a predilection for the extracranial branches of the carotid artery	178 in adults >50 years old (14)
TA	Granulomatous inflammation of the aorta and its major branches	2.6 in adults (15)
Medium vessel vasculitis		
PAN[a]	Necrotising inflammation of medium-sized or small arteries without glomerulonephritis or vasculitis in arterioles, capillaries or venules	9 in adults (16)
KD	Arteritis involving large, medium-sized and small arteries, and associated with mucocutaneous lymph node syndrome	900 in Japanese <5 years old (17) 55 in U.K. children (18)
Small vessel vasculitis		
WG[a]	Granulomatous inflammation involving the respiratory tract, and necrotising vasculitis affecting small to medium-sized vessels (e.g. capillaries, venules, arterioles and arteries)	6 in adults (19)
CSS[a]	Eosinophil-rich and granulomatous inflammation involving the respiratory tract, necrotising vasculitis affecting small to medium sized vessels, and associated with asthma and eosinophilia	
MPA[a]	Necrotising vasculitis, with few or no immune deposits, affecting small vessels (i.e. capillaries, venules or arterioles)	
HSP	Vasculitis, with IgA-dominant immune deposits, affecting small vessels (i.e. capillaries, venules or arterioles)	12 in adults (20) 204 in children (18)

(Continued)

Table 2 Nomenclature of Systemic Vasculitis (*Continued*)

		Annual incidence/10^6 population (Ref.)
Essential cryoglobulinemia vasculitis	Vasculitis, with cryoglobulin immune deposits, affecting small vessels (i.e., capillaries, venules, or arterioles) and associated cryoglobulins in serum	
Cutaneous leukocytoclastic vasculitis	Isolated cutaneous leukocytoclastic angiitis without systemic vasculitis or glomerulonephritis	

Note: Large vessel refers to the aorta and the largest branches directed towards the body; medium vessel refers to the main visceral arteries (e.g., renal, hepatic, coronary, and mesenteric arteries); small vessel refers to venules, capillaries, arterioles, and the intraparenchymal distal arterial radicals that connect with arterioles.
[a] Strongly associated with antineutrophil cytoplasmic antibodies.
Abbreviations: CSS, Churg-Strauss syndrome; HSP, Henoch-Schonlein purpura; KD, Kawasaki disease; MPA, microscopic polyangiitis; PAN, polyarteritis nodosa; TA, Takayasu's arteritis; WG, Wegener's granulomatosis.
Source: Adapted from Ref. 13.

(22) and in the series used to develop the ACR classification criteria, 29% of patients were in this age bracket. In Japanese series a female to male ratio of 9:1 is reported.

The clinical presentation is classically that of an initial non-specific inflammatory disease, before going onto the "pulseless" vascular phase (23). However, the lack of constitutional symptoms and presenting features of hypertension and cardiac failure has been highlighted (24,25). There are no specific laboratory tests. Vascular imaging and histopathological examination may be extremely helpful and indeed essential to diagnosis. It should be noted that a considerable delay in diagnosis has been described in the adolescent population compared to adults (26,27), illustrating the importance of pediatric and adult rheumatologists being alert to this diagnosis. The value of early diagnosis in underscored by the observation that prognosis closely correlates to the initiation of therapy from onset of symptoms (24). Therapy consists of high dose corticosteroids (1 mg/kg/day of prednisolone) (25), tapering once in remission. In the absence of achieving or maintenance of remission, further immunosuppression should be considered, with the best evidence available for the use of methotrexate (28) and cyclophosphamide (29). The use of other immunosuppressive drugs, e.g., azathioprine and the use of immunosuppressive agents in addition to corticosteroids at diagnosis remains controversial. Revascularization of symptomatic occluded vessels

Table 3 Causes of Secondary Vasculitis and Mimics of Vasculitis

Infection	Cause/mimic
Bacterial	Invasive infective arteritis secondary to organisms such as staphylococcus, streptococcus, salmonella, and neiserria
Viral	Hepatitis B–associated PAN
	Hepatitis C–associated cryoglobulinaemia
	CMV, infectious mononucleosis, and rubella may be associated with a small vessel vasculitis
	HIV may be associated with a small to medium-sized vessel vasculitis
Fungal	Aspergillus may be associated with a medium vessel vasculitis and coccidiomycosis with a large vessel vasculitis in immunocompromised patients
Mycobacterial	Tuberculosis may be associated with a vasculitis of any vessel size but typically affects small vessels and venules in particular.
	Leprosy may cause a vasculopathy, perivasculitis, and, only rarely, a vasculitis.
Spirochetal	Syphilis is typically associated with a large to medium vessel arteritis and gonorrhoea with a small vessel vasculitis.
	Lyme disease is rarely associated with a small vessel vasculitis.
Rickettsial	Rocky Mountain spotted fever, epidemic typhus, and scrub typhus may produce a small vessel vasculitis.
Autoimmune rheumatic disease	Inflammatory arthritis (especially rheumatoid factor positive and systemic JIA)
	Dermatomyositis
	Systemic lupus erythematosus
	Sjogren's syndrome
Malignancy	A small-to-medium vessel has been reported in many malignancies.
Drugs	Prescription medications rarely cause a small vessel vasculitis.
	Substance abuse causing predominantly a central nervous system vasculitis has been described with amphetamines, heroin, methylphenidate, etc.
Thromboembolic	Bacterial endocarditis
	Cardiac myxoma
	Antiphospholipid syndrome
Others	Inflammatory bowel disease, serum sickness, transplant- and radiation-associated vasculitis

Abbreviations: JIA, juvenile idiopathic arthritis; PAN, polyarteritis nodosa.

may be undertaken. The reported five-year mortality varies considerably between case series with reports of 94% in North America (25) and 35% in Mexico (24). Considerable morbidity occurs with difficulty in activities of daily living in 74%, and permanent disability in 47% (25). Pregnancy in patients with Takayasu's arteritis is usually successful (25).

Medium Vessel Vasculitis

Kawasaki Disease

The peak age-of-onsetis at one year of age and 80% to 85% of cases occur at less than five years of age. Kawasaki disease (KD) is defined by the presence of fever persisting for at least five days, together with the presence of at least four of the following: changes of extremities (acute: erythema of palms, soles; oedema of hands, feet, and subacute: periungual peeling of fingers, toes in weeks 2 and 3); polymorphous exanthema; bilateral bulbar conjunctival injection without exudates; changes in lip and oral cavity: erythema, lips cracking, strawberry tongue, diffuse injection oral and pharyngeal mucosae; cervical lymphadenopathy (30). Initial treatment is with aspirin and intravenous immunoglobulin and further management is determined by the presence of coronary artery involvement, occurring in 20% to 30% of untreated cases. Although rare in adolescents, it does occur, and may be associated with more cardiovascular morbidity due to late presentation (30).

Polyarteritis Nodosa and Microscopic Polyangiitis

Polyarteritis nodosa (PAN) is observed in children and adolescents, but the peak age-of-onsetis around 50 years. Vasculitis of muscular medium sized vessels is characteristic, with aneurysm formation. Typically patients present with constitutional symptoms, abdominal pain, arthralgia, myalgia, livedo reticularis, peripheral neuropathy, hypertension and renal involvement (31). Angiography may demonstrate characteristic findings (32) but these are not specific to polyarteritis. Treatment is with corticosteroids, which are usually used in high dose to induce remission, and have reduced the five-year mortality from 90% to 50% (33). The addition of further immunosuppresion such as cyclophosphamide improves survival to 20% (34).

Microscopic polyarteritis (MPA) as defined in the CHCC may occur in children and adolescents (35) and may be differentiated from PAN with a clinical presentation of a severe renal-pulmonary syndrome. The characteristic pathologic lesion is necrotizing crescenteric glomerulonephritis without immunoglobulin or complement deposition. There is a strong association with ANCA and treatment is as for adults.

A postinfective vasculitis may present as a cutaneous polyarteritis and should be identified, as it carries a benign prognosis. The typical history is that of an upper respiratory tract infection followed by the appearance of a rash (typically tender nodules over the feet), myalgia, arthralgia/arthritis without internal organ involvement. Treatment is with NSAIDs, steroids and penicillin prophylaxis (34).

Granulomatous Vasculitides

Wegener's Granulomatosis

Wegener's granulomatosis (WG), as defined by the ACR, is a rare disease that is well described in adolescents. As in adults with WG, presentation is with lesions in the respiratory tract, renal involvement, ocular disease, neurological disturbance and cutaneous lesions (Fig. 1). However, the occurrence of subglottic stenosis and saddle-nose deformities is more common in the juvenile population (36). There is a strong association with

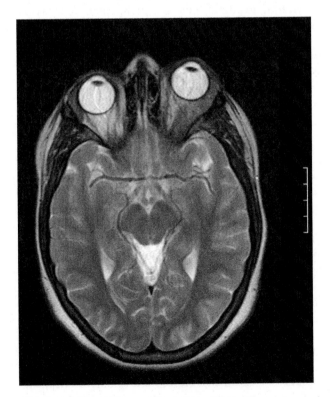

Figure 1 Wegener's granulomatosis. Magnetic resonance image of the brain and orbit of an 18-year-old girl, demonstrating soft-tissue intraorbital infiltration in both orbits, worse on the left, consistent with a granulomatous disorder. Clinical presentation was with left-sided proptosis.

ANCA and treatment is with immunosuppression (steroids, cyclophosphamide and methotrexate). Septrin is commonly used to reduce the remission rate of upper respiratory tract disease (37).

Churg-Strauss Syndrome

Churg-Strauss syndrome (CSS) is extremely rare in the juvenile population and no distinguishing features from adult disease have been identified.

Small Vessel Vasculitis

Henoch-Schonlein purpura (HSP) is the most common juvenile form of small vessel vasculitis. Although HSP is seen in adolescents, the peak age-of-onset is 4–6 years (18). There is an association with preceding infection in up to half of cases (38). HSP presents with the combination of non-thrombocytopenic palpable purpura over the lower extremities, abdominal pain, arthritis, and glomerulonephritis. Pathologically there is IgA deposition in the glomerular mesangium or the dermal vessels (39). HSP is a self-limiting disorder that carries an excellent prognosis. Although 20% to 50% of cases may be associated with renal involvement only 1% progress to chronic renal insufficiency (40). However, it should be noted that this risk is greater in adolescents (41).

Other forms of small vessel vasculitis seen in adolescents include hypersensitivity vasculitis (usually following drugs such as penicillin, antithyroid agents, retinoids) that is treated by removing the offending agent, and cryoglobulinaemic vasculitis that is rarely seen in the context of hepatitis C and intravenous drug abuse.

Miscellaneous

Sarcoid

Sarcoid is a multisystem disorder characterized by non-caseating granuloma. There seems to be two overlapping patterns of clinical presentation in the juvenile population with skin, joint and eye disease in younger children, and lymphadenopathy, weight loss, fever, pulmonary involvement, but no arthritis, in older children and adolescents (42). Sarcoid is more common in the black population and females. Treatment is with steroids and a steroid sparing agent such as methotrexate or azathioprine.

Behçet's Disease

In a study of 1784 Turkish patients with Behçet's disease (BD), 95 were less than 16 years old, most of whom were between 10 and 16 years of age (43). The diagnostic criteria developed by the International Study Group are most widely used to define BD (44). This requires the presence of recurrent oral ulceration and two of: recurrent genital ulceration, eye lesions, skin lesions, and pathery. There are no features of BD that are specific to age-of-onset although the psychological impact of significant genital ulceration during adolescence and the development of a sexual identity should not be underestimated.

SYSTEMIC CONNECTIVE TISSUE DISEASES

Systemic Lupus Erythematosus

For a description of systemic lupus erythematosus refer to Chapter 8.

Juvenile Dermatomyositis and Polymyositis

In children and young people, chronic idiopathic inflammatory myositis is a relatively heterogeneous disorder, where other components of collagen vascular disorders may emerge over time (45). In contrast, adults can be placed in specific subsets of inflammatory myopathy on the basis of clinical, immunological, and epidemiological features. A bimodal distribution for the onset of polymyositis and dermatomyositis has been suggested with a peak in the 5- to 9-year old and 55- to 59-year-old range (46). The disease occurs at least 1.5 times more frequently in females than males in the Western world (7,8,46,47). The ratio is reversed in Japanese and Saudi Arabian studies (48,49), and differs in children and adults (8,48). Inflammatory myositis occurs more frequently in African-American females than in Caucasians, although racial differences are less marked in children (8,46).

Juvenile dermatomyositis (JDM) differs in many aspects from the disease observed in adults, as summarized in Table 4.

Case History

A 14-year-old girl of Caucasian origin was presented to her local hospital with a 2-month history of rash, fatigue and irritability. More recently, she complained of significant weakness and aching with activities. In particular, she had difficulty climbing stairs and brushing her own hair. She had fevers up to 39°C. She became short of breath and had difficulty in swallowing. She had one episode of nasal regurgitation. On examination, she had a typical rash, with heliotrope discoloration over the eyelids, Gottron's patches on her metacarpophalangeal and proximal interphalangeal joints, and some facial swelling with periorbital oedema. The diagnosis of juvenile dermatomyositis was confirmed by a T2-weighted magnetic resonance imaging (MRI) scan of her thigh showing inflammatory changes, and a muscle biopsy consistent with inflammatory myositis. A video fluoroscopy demonstrated swallowing dysfunction and mild aspiration. A CXR, high resolution CT scan, and pulmonary function tests were normal. The girl responded well to methylprednisolone pulses, followed by oral steroid, and

Table 4   Comparison of Childhood and Adult Inflammatory Myopathies

	Juvenile disease (Ref.)	Adult disease (Ref.)
Ratio	DM >> PM; JDM is 20–30× more common in children than polymyositis (6,9,50).	Ratio of DM:PM more even, between 0.3 and 1.5:1 (46,47,51).
Frequency	Dermatomyositis accounts for 85–94% of all inflammatory myositis. Polymyositis accounts for 4–6% of inflammatory myositis (6,9,52). Overlap features with other CTD not unusual. Inclusion body myositis extremely rare (52).	Dermatomyositis accounts for 15–60% of all inflammatory myositis. Polymyositis accounts for 34–50% (46,47,51,52). Disease usually clearly defined. Inclusion body myositis is seen in up to 15% of adult inflammatory myopathies (52).
Presentation	Although presentation can be acute and fulminant, it is more frequently insidious and associated with constitutional symptoms (fatigue, malaise, fever, anorexia, and weight loss) in over 50% children (45,50,53). Irritability is common.	Clinical presentation often acute. Systemic features uncommon (51). Dysphagia and bacterial pneumonia linked to respiratory insufficiency and esophageal impairment is more common in elderly patients (54)
Clinical features	Calcinosis more than 2–3× more frequent in children than adults with DM. Reported in 14–54% of JDM (55–57). Atrophy and contractures more common (45). Raynaud's phenomenon is uncommon (45).	Calcinosis less common, reported in up to 14% (45,57). Interstitial lung disease and cardiac involvement more frequent in adult inflammatory myopathies. Atrophy and contractures less common (45). Raynaud's in 10–20% (45).
Vasculopathy	More vascular inflammation and thrombosis (58). Children more frequently have a multisystem vasculitis that may affect the skin, subcutaneous tissue, gastrointestinal mucosa, viscera, and nerves (59). Vasculopathic ulceration may be fatal if affecting the bowel (59).	Vasculitis and ulceration less commonly seen. In particular, gastrointestinal involvement less frequent (52).

(Continued)

Table 4 Comparison of Childhood and Adult Inflammatory Myopathies (*Continued*)

	Juvenile disease (Ref.)	Adult disease (Ref.)
Malignancy	Very few case reports of malignancy-associated JDM/JPM in children less than 16 years (60–62).	Association with malignancy well recognized, DM > PM, usually within first year of diagnosis, especially in an older age group (54,63,64). Variable risk reported, but probable prevalence of 3–15% for PM and 32–36% for DM (63,64).
Serology	Myositis-specific or myositis-associated autoantibodies present in ~20% children with inflammatory myopathies (52). The possibility of unique myositis-specific antibodies in children is suggested (undefined as yet).	Myositis-specific or myositis-associated antibodies present in ~60% adults. Anti-synthesase antibodies ~2× as common in adults with inflammatory myopathies than children (52).
Muscle biopsy findings	Muscle biopsy shows occlusive thrombosis and muscle infarction with perivascular atrophy (45).	Muscle biopsy has prominent interstitial infiltrate with necrosis of muscle fibres (45).
Prognosis	Once remission is achieved, children achieve good functional outcomes on medium- to long-term follow-up, with the capacity to recover from damage (65).	Adults with myositis report significantly poorer health compared to the general population with less capacity to recover from damage (66).

Abbreviations: DM, dermatomyositis; JDM, juvenile dermatomyositis; JPM, juvenile polymyositis; PM, polymyositis.

methotrexate. However, a few months later, she developed skin ulceration and was given a 6-month course of intravenous cyclophosphamide, 500 mg/m^2 per month.

Key Learning Points

Juvenile dermatomyositis usually presents with a combination of easy fatigue, muscle weakness, and a rash. Presentation may be acute or insidious. Constitutional symptoms with fever, malaise, anorexia, and weight loss are common. Irritability is frequently seen, particularly in the younger age group. Facial swelling and periorbital edema are well recognized early in the disease course. The most typical cutaneous abnormalities of juvenile dermatomyositis are heliotrope discoloration of the eyelids, Gottron's patches and periungual erythema and capillary loop abnormalities (Fig. 2). Gottron's patches are common over proximal interphalangeal, and less commonly, metacarpophalangeal and distal interphalangeal joints. They may also occur over the extensor surface of the knees, elbows and malleoli. Rash can occur the trunk (shawl sign) or extensor surfaces of limbs. Capillary changes are a distinctive, but not pathognomonic, of JDM. Similar changes can occur in scleroderma and other connective tissue diseases.

Muscle weakness is predominantly proximal with weakness in limb-girdle, anterior neck flexors, and abdominal muscles. Moderate muscle pain or stiffness can occur. Joint swelling may be present, although arthralgia is more common than arthritis. Arthritis is usually nonerosive. Restriction in joint range of movement or contractures may occur due to arthritis or, more commonly, secondary to muscle inflammation. Affected muscles may be edematous, indurated, or tender. Muscle weakness may involve pharyngeal, hypopharyngeal, and palatal muscles. Children should always be asked for a history of difficulty swallowing, nasal regurgitation, or change in voice. A speech and language assessment and video fluoroscopy is advisable as aspiration may be present without obvious symptoms.

Diagnostic criteria by Bohan and Peter are the only validated diagnostic criteria to date (59). However, the advancement of noninvasive imaging techniques such as MRI has led to an increasing trend towards using these techniques to aid diagnosis. Increased short tau inversion recovery or fat suppressed, T2-weighted signal intensity MRI images of the

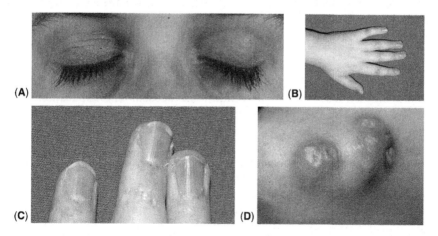

Figure 2 Skin features of juvenile dermatomyositis. (**A**) Eyelid heliotrope discoloration; (**B**) hand demonstrating Gottron's patches over proximal interphalangeal and distal interphalangeal joints; (**C**) nails showing capillary dilatation and drop out; (**D**) elbow showing calcinosis.

thigh can be effectively used to localize muscle inflammation and help in the assessment of disease activity and damage in JDM (67,68). In clinical practice, many centers now use MRI in place of more invasive techniques such as EMG and biopsy (69). MRI may also be used to increase the yield of abnormal results from muscle biopsy or EMG by identifying the affected areas (70).

Despite change in clinical practice, it is important to note that no single test is consistently abnormal in all cases of JDM (6,9,51,50). There is currently interest in revisiting the Bohan and Peter diagnostic criteria for JDM and including investigations such as MRI. At present clinical assessment remains the gold standard for the diagnosis of JDM with most children requiring some combination of investigations to confirm this.

Erythrocyte sedimentation rate, C-reactive protein, and muscle enzymes (CK, LDH, AST, aldolase) correlate poorly with disease activity. Urine spectroscopy for skeletal muscle metabolites (71) and quantitative nail-fold capillaroscopy (72) may be useful tools in a research setting for measuring disease activity. In the absence of these as standard tools, activity is judged on clinical impression (physician's global assessment visual analogue scale) (73) together with manual muscle testing (74) and the Childhood Myositis Assessment Scale (CMAS). The CMAS score is validated up to the age of 18 years as a quantitative assessment of muscle strength, function, and endurance with excellent inter and intra reliability (75,76). Measures of disability and function (CHAQ, HAQ) and quality-of-life questionnaires such as (CHQ and SF36) can be useful in determining degree of disability, psychology, and the presence of chronic pain (77).

Myositis specific antibodies are uncommon in patients with childhood presentation of dermatomyositis (78). When present, they may be more characteristic of an overlap syndrome, such as dermatomyositis and scleroderma overlap.

Treatment of JDM has become more aggressive in order to prevent long-term complications. Despite this, the evidence base remains poor, and head to head trials of different therapies are needed. The implications of therapy during adolescence are detailed in Table 1. Most clinicians would treat a newly diagnosed child or adolescent with JDM with daily oral corticosteroids 1–2 mg/kg/day, combined with intravenous methylprednisolone pulsing. The first line immunosuppressant medication for most rheumatologists is methotrexate, used by SC injection or oral administration. Aggressive early treatment with steroid and methotrexate has been shown to minimize long-term sequalae of JDM, such as calcinosis (79). Ciclosporin A is an alternative treatment, and works quickly (80,81). It may be tolerated with methotrexate (80). However, in the authors' experience, it may not be as good at preventing calcinosis in the long-term, and adverse effects may be unacceptable to many adolescents. There is an international trial in progress comparing methotrexate and ciclosporin in JDM.

Hydroxychloroquine can be used successfully as an adjunctive therapy, particularly in those with prominent cutaneous disease (82). IVIG may be effective in some patients (83). Plasma exchange has been used in severe cases (84,85). with concomitant immunosuppressive therapy. Cyclophosphamide (oral or intravenous) is indicated for vasculitic involvement and skin ulceration, severe lung involvement, gastro-intestinal perforation or CNS disease (86). Our practice is to use intravenous pulses once monthly for six months, with an aim to then change to an alternative disease modifying medication. Infliximab has been used in JDM with success in resistant cases (87). There are early reports of use of B cell depletion with rituximab (88) and we are also participating in an international trial of this. In addition to medication, patients with inflammatory myositis need physiotherapy to prevent joint contractures and rebuild muscle strength (89), as well as occupational therapy and nursing input.

Prognosis of JDM has improved considerably over time. Before the use of corticosteroids, outcome for JDM was poor, with death in one-third of cases and severe permanent physical disability in another third (53). Subsequently, there has been a marked decrease in mortality to less than 10% (90), and an improvement in functional outcomes. The majority of fatalities occur within two years of disease onset, thus early, aggressive therapy may be beneficial in decreasing mortality and improving prognosis (91,92). Decreased bone mineral density may occur in untreated JDM and be augmented by steroid administration (93).

Other causes of myopathy should be considered in adolescents presenting with muscle weakness or pain, including parasitic infections, malignancy-associated myopathy, congenital myopathies or dystrophies, or fibromyalgia.

SYSTEMIC SCLEROSIS AND LOCALIZED SCLERODERMA

The scleroderma spectrum of disorders encompasses a wide variety of disparate conditions whose unifying feature is the clinical presence of hard, tight skin, and pathological deposition of excessive collagen. Children and adolescents with scleroderma make up a very small subgroup of patients seen in a general rheumatology clinic, and the type and pattern of scleroderma is different to that seen in adults. Localized scleroderma is far more common in pediatrics than systemic sclerosis, by a ratio of at least 4:1 (94). There is a significant association with trauma, not seen in adults (94). Childhood-onset scleroderma resembles adult disease in its female predominance, racial predisposition, histological findings, and heterogeneity of clinical expression, but differs in a number of ways. In contrast to the adult disease, childhood onset scleroderma is associated with normal parameters of vascular activation (such as von Willebrand factor, angiotensin-converting enzyme, endothelial-1 and E-selectin), T cell activation (interleukin-2 receptors) and collagen synthesis (carboxy-terminal type I, amino terminal type III). It is also distinguished by a notable lack of anticentromere antibodies, and normal coagulation indices (94). Scleroderma in childhood, particularly the linear form of localized scleroderma, causes growth defects and muscle wasting not seen in adults. In adults, Raynaud's phenomenon occurs in more than 95% of cases, but occurs less commonly in childhood scleroderma, seen in 82% of those with diffuse disease and only 14% of those with localized scleroderma (94).

There have been recent changes in the classification of scleroderma with continued work in this field. Since children with localized scleroderma will have disease into their adolescent or adult years, here follows a description of the juvenile forms.

Localized Scleroderma

Localized scleroderma (*morphea* or *linear scleroderma*) involves the skin and subcutaneous tissue in one area, although there may be involvement of other organ systems. Presentation tends to be indolent, starting with superficial erythema of the skin that gradually spreads. There may be central clearing with a lilac ring appearance. With time, there is hardening of the skin or subdermal structures, leading to an ivory-like appearance of the tissue (95). Loss of hair and anhidrosis is common along with hypopigmentation or hyperpigmentation. Involvement of the deeper structures varies. Classification of localized scleroderma is based on clinical morphological findings and the depth of tissue involved (96,97).

The terms localized scleroderma and morphea have often been used interchangeably, leading to confusion. Morphea is used by most rheumatologists to describe a subgroup of localized scleroderma that presents with oval-shaped patches or plaques characterized by thickening and induration of the skin and subcutaneous tissues without significant internal organ involvement (95,96). Lesions most frequently occur on the trunk, abdomen or proximal extremity (96,98). When active, the edges of the lesions are erythematous and may be warm. Plaques evolve from a sclerotic stage to a non-indurated stage, with skin softening and residual hypopigmentation or hyperpigmentation (95,98). Arthralgias, synovitis, joint contractures, leg-length discrepancy, and carpal tunnel syndrome can occur (96). Widespread dissemination is possible. If there are more than four plaques in two or more sites of the body, the condition tends to be called *generalized morphea* (95).

Linear scleroderma is characterized by one or more linear streaks, most commonly along part or all of a limb, typically affecting a lower extremity (95,96). It can also occur on the trunk or face. When it involves the face or scalp it is called *scleroderma en coup de sabre*. It is usually unilateral and frontoparietal (Fig. 3). Involvement may vary greatly from minor indentation on the forehead to severe hemifacial atrophy. Alopecia

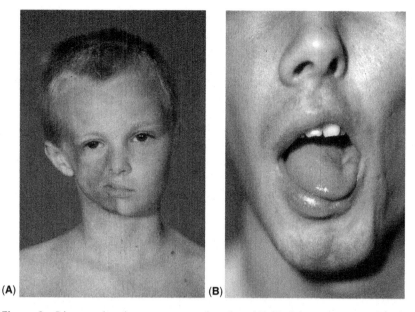

Figure 3 Linear scleroderma en coup de sabre (**A**) Facial appearance with right facial atrophy; (**B**) groove on tongue with and hypoplastic left side.

(with loss of hair from the scalp and eyebrows), ptosis, uveitis, cataract, keratopathy, and seizures may occur (95,96). Atrophy of the tongue and abnormal or stunted growth of the teeth can be seen (95,96). Intracerebral calcification and white-matter changes have been identified on imaging (95,98).

Linear scleroderma is more common in the pediatric/adolescent age group than adults, whereas all other forms are more common in adults (96–98). The appearance of linear scleroderma, especially when involving the face, or associated with localized skeletal growth abnormalities, may be particularly distressing for the adolescent and psychological support may be necessary.

Linear scleroderma usually occurs in children less than 10 years of age with activity lasting a median of 5 years (96). In contrast to morphea, it involves underlying tissues. The sclerodermatous lesions may be warm and erythematous when active, especially at the lesional margins. Lesions may extend at a variable rate, and cause reduced range of movement when crossing joints (95). Contractures of periarticular and ligamentous tissues occur with muscle wasting and significant growth failure of a limb (95). Esophageal involvement has been reported, although rare, and internal organ involvement has been described (67).

Parry-Romberg syndrome is a term used to describe hemifacial atrophy of bone, subcutaneous tissue, and adipose tissue, with relative sparing of the

superficial skin tissues (95,98). It involves dysplasia of the skin and underlying bone of the face and skull unilaterally. Changes are diffuse and uni-
form. Hair is normal. There is greater involvement of the lower face than
there is in en coup de sabre (95). It occurs in the first to second decade of life
and can be associated with neurological deficits, uveitis, and atrophy of the
pinna or tongue on the involved side.

Whether scleroderma en coup de sabre and Parry-Romberg syndrome
are part of the same spectrum or a different entity, remains controversial.
Both can involve neurological, ocular, and vascular abnormalities. CSF
abnormalities can occur with oligoclonal bands, and anti-nuclear antigen
(ANA) can be positive in both (95,98). However there are differences in
histology and distribution. Parry-Romberg can coexist with localized
scleroderma, or can occur as a sequel to various conditions.

Mixed forms of localized scleroderma can occur with the presence of
morphea plaques and linear bands in the same individual.

Investigations

Localized scleroderma is essentially a clinical diagnosis, but investigations
may be supportive. Hypergammaglobulinemia and eosinophilia have
been suggested as indicating active disease. ANA is positive in 28% to
76% of cases of localized scleroderma (94,98). Occasionally, antibodies to
extractable nuclear antigens are seen, such as anti-Ro. Rheumatoid factor
and anti-histone antibodies may also be positive. ESR and CRP are rarely
elevated. Thermography and high frequency ultrasound show promise in
helping clinical decision of ongoing disease activity. MRI can also be useful,
particularly to visualize intraorbital and intracranial lesions (95).

Disease Course and Prognosis

Localized scleroderma tends to be most progressive within the first two
years. It may continue to spread or deepen in involvement for up to 5 to
6 years, but then seems to stop (95,98). Even without treatment, lesions
usually spontaneously enter remission after 3 to 5 years. However, as
children grow, milder lesions may become more evident. Localized
scleroderma very occasionally evolves, or is seen in association with
systemic sclerosis or other connective tissue disorders (98,99).

Management of Localized Scleroderma

One of the major differences in management of young people with scleroderma compared to an adult population is monitoring for associated
growth abnormalities (96,98). Treatments for scleroderma are based on
anecdotal reports, case series and personal experience. Therapies have
included the use of topical corticosteroid creams, topical mycophenolate
mofetil (MMF), intra-lesional steroids and intralesional interferon γ.

Systemic therapies have also been tried including steroids, methotrexate, ciclosporin, MMF, hydroxychloroquine, D-penicillamine, phenytoin, cyclophenyl, vitamin D or vitamin D analogues, vitamin E, vitamin B12 injections, sulphasalazine, bismuth, and etrinate (96,98). The use of ultraviolet light, with or without chemical agents such as psoralen, has been reported as showing some clinical benefit particularly for localized or superficial lesions (95).

It is difficult to know when the disease becomes inactive, but the usual practice in children is to treat with immunosuppressive therapy for a minimum of five years, while weaning prednisolone over six months. Combination therapy may lead to earlier resolution of complicated lesions (98). Physiotherapy and occupational therapy are important when lesions cross joint lines to help prevent or reduce joint contractures, and improve function (95,98). Splints and orthoses may be useful.

Plastic surgery techniques have been used to correct atrophy and scarring (100–103). For best results, surgery should be carried out when lesions are inactive, as otherwise, the imported tissue can become affected in the disease process. If it is imperative to do surgery while the lesion is active, for psychological reasons, surgery should be kept as simple as possible so that reconstructive surgery is possible at a later date. Surgical options include free fat grafting, autologous dermofat grafting, osteotomies, and bony augmentation with soft-tissue expansion and vascularized free-tissue transfer.

Systemic Sclerosis

Pediatric patients make up only 3% of all cases of systemic sclerosis (95). Disease expression is influenced by genetic, ethnic, and environmental factors (97,104). In adults, females out number males, with a ratio of 3–14:1, although sex distribution ratio varies with age (97,104). The disease is more common in African-Americans, with a younger mean age-of-onset and increased risk of diffuse disease (105).

Systemic sclerosis includes diffuse disease (formally known as progressive systemic sclerosis), limited disease (formally known as CREST syndrome) and overlap syndromes with scleroderma (97).

Diffuse disease can evolve rapidly over the first few months and is associated with the presence of anti-Scl 70 antibodies. It tends to involve the proximal extremities and trunk, with rapidly progressive skin involvement and vital organ disease. Risk of malignant phase hypertension, as well as severe cardiac or gastrointestinal involvement, is higher with diffuse disease (97).

Limited systemic sclerosis is associated with the presence of anti-centromere antibody and is confined to the face and extremities, distal to the elbows and knees (97). It tends to progress more slowly and may be stable for several years before the development of pulmonary hypertension. The presence of renal, cardiac or pulmonary disease within the first 5 years is associated with poor outcome.

Investigations

Inflammatory markers such as ESR do not tend to be raised in scleroderma. Anemia may be found due to esophageal blood loss, malabsorption, poor nutrition, and chronic disease. ANA is positive in 80% of adult patients with systemic sclerosis (95). Anti-Scl 70 antibody correlates with diffuse disease and a poor outcome. Anti-centromere antibodies correlate with limited disease and a better outcome (95). Studies in childhood scleroderma report a positive ANA in 22% to 100% of patients, and a positive anti-Scl in 40% of those that are ANA positive. Anti-centromere antibodies are uncommon, reflecting the rarity of limited disease in children (95). The significance of anti-cardiolipin antibodies, found in one-third of patients, is uncertain. Investigations should be done to look for specific organ involvement (Table 5).

Treatment

The management of systemic sclerosis depends on careful monitoring of organ specific manifestations and prompt treatment to avoid irreversible fibrotic tissue damage. In addition to organ-based treatments (Table 5), generalized systemic therapies are directed at the underlying process implicated in the disease. Immune suppression has been tried with various treatments including antithymocyte globulin, mycophenolate mofetil, methotrexate, ciclosporin, and cyclophosphamide (95,106). The association of corticosteroids with hypertensive renal crisis should also be carefully considered. Plasma exchange have also been used (107). The endothelin receptor agonist bosentan, has been tried with some success for digital ulcers and pulmonary hypertension (108,109). Autologous stem cell transplantation has been tried but has an associated mortality (95).

Prognosis

Data for prognosis in children and adolescents with systemic sclerosis are sparse. There is an opinion that the disease progresses towards organ failure and death in the same way as in adults. However, a 95% 5-year survival rate has been reported from a study looking at 135 patients with systemic sclerosis, much better than that reported in adult literature (110). It is not clear whether all patients in this cohort had true systemic sclerosis or scleroderma, and it has been our experience that more aggressive disease may be associated with earlier age of onset.

The fertility rate in patients with scleroderma seems to be similar to that of healthy controls, but there is a higher rate of premature and low birth weight infants. Pregnancy may be dangerous for patients with severe renal, cardiac, or pulmonary disease, and patients may be best advised to avoid pregnancy until the disease stabilizes. Potentially teratogenic medications should be avoided.

Table 5 Clinical Manifestations of Systemic Sclerosis

Organ	Manifestation	Investigations	Treatments
Skin	Peripheral edema, dryness, and pruritis Skin thickening and tightening Eventual softening Pinched nose and loss of facial creases Loss of skin appendages in extremities Hyperpigmentation and hypopigmentation Cutaneous telangiectasis and subcutaneous calcinosis (particularly limited form) Flexor tendon nodules Pitting scars on fingertips and loss of finger pulp Raynaud's phenomenon (90%) Dilatation and dropout of the nailfold capillaries	Serial photographs may be useful. Capillaroscopy, thermography	Lubricants, topical corticosteroids Treatment for Raynaud's: Keep warm; vasodilators or calcium channel blockers Vitamin C and E, fish oils Prostaglandin E1 or prostacylin for peripheral vascular changes Diltiazem for calcinosis Cosmetic issues
Joints	Joint stiffness, loss of range-of-movement, and contractures secondary to skin tightening and fibrosis of the joint capsule Synovial inflammation less common Erosions rare Osteoporosis	USS or MRI to detect subclinical synovitis DEXA scan	NSAID; physio- and occupational therapy Podiatry Intraarticular steroid injections for synovitis Advice re: physical exercise
Gut	Xerostomia (salivary gland fibrosis or overlap with Sjogren's) Dental loosening and tongue atrophy	Dental reviews pH studies	Artificial tears and oral sprays Prokinetic agents Proton pump inhibitors

(Continued)

Table 5 Clinical Manifestations of Systemic Sclerosis (*Continued*)

Organ	Manifestation	Investigations	Treatments
	Restricted mouth opening from progressive skin tightening	Plain abdominal X-ray, USS, barium follow-through or video capsule studies	Intermittent antibiotics
	Abnormalities of the lower esophageal sphincter and fibrosis of the lower two-thirds of the esophagus, resulting in poor propulsion and "lower dysphagia"		Stool softeners and enemas
			Total parenteral nutrition
		Loss of colonic haustra and pseudo-diverticular can be seen radiologically	Surgery or laser therapy for vascular bleeds
	Stricture formation; Barrett's esophagus		
	Esophageal carcinoma	Fecal fats	
	Severe gastroesophageal reflux	Endoscopy may be indicated	
	Delayed gastric emptying +/- severe atony		
	Pseudo-obstruction from reduced motility of small intestine with bloating and cramping		
	Diarrhea and malabsorption from bacterial overgrowth		
	Constipation from large bowel involvement		
Pulmonary disease	Present in the vast majority of patients	Pulmonary function tests with TLCO	Corticosteroids, cyclophosphamide, azathioprine, calcium channel blockers, vasodilators, D-penicillamine
	Pulmonary hypertension and interstitial fibrosis	High-resolution CT scan and high-resolution X-rays	
	Onset usually insidious, with shortness of breath, dry cough, fatigue, and reduced energy		Ambulatory prostacyclin or bosentan
	Clubbing is rare	BAL or DTPA scanning	Warfarin
	Asymptomatic pleural effusions common		Advice re: smoking
	Aspiration from severe gastroesophageal reflux		

Organ	Clinical features	Investigations	Management
Heart	Progressive fibrosis with small vessel obliterative disease, ischemia and re-perfusion, restrictive cardiomyopathy and congestive cardiac failure Pulmonary hypertension and cor pulmonale secondary to lung disease Myocarditis (rare) associated with polymyositis	ECG and ECHO Thallium scanning Right heart catheterization for pulmonary hypertension	Calcium channel blockers, anti-arrhythmic agents, corticosteroids Transplantation Advice re: smoking
Kidneys	Mild proteinuria, progresses with a decrease in creatinine clearance Can be associated with hypertension Malignant hypertension, often accompanied by microangiopathic hemolytic anemia, occurs in up to 20%	Urine dipstick and urine albumin creatinine ratio GFR	Maintain good perfusion ACE inhibitors Anti-hypertensives Avoid steroids Dialysis where needed
CNS	Central nervous system involvement rare, but neuropathies can occur	Imaging Nerve conduction studies Biopsy	Corticosteroids Physiotherapy and occupational therapy
Endocrine	Glandular fibrosis can occur resulting in hypothyroidism	Thyroid function tests	Thyroxine as needed

Abbreviations: ACE, angiotensin converting enzyme; BAL, bronchoalevolar; DEXA, dual-energy X-ray absorptiometry; ECG, electrocardiogram; ECHO, echocardiogram; GFR, glomerular filtration rate; NSAID, nonsteroidal anti-inflammatory drug; USS, ultrasound scan.

Overlap Syndromes

Children and adolescents can present with signs and symptoms that are characteristic of more than one connective tissue or inflammatory disorder. This occurrence is more common in children and adolescents compared to adults. In our experience, children's signs and symptoms may evolve over time from those of one connective tissue disease to another. For example, combinations of features of JIA, systemic lupus erythematosus, juvenile dermatomyositis, scleroderma, and vasculitis are seen. These children are best described as having "overlap syndromes" or "undifferentiated connective tissue disease." Treatment should be tailored to organ involvement and underlying pathophysiology rather than be disease specific.

MUSCULOSKELETAL DISORDERS RELATED TO INFECTION OR INFLAMMATORY TRIGGERS

Infections Presenting as Musculoskeletal Disorders

Musculoskeletal infections in adolescents, although uncommon, represent a unique therapeutic challenge (Table 6). The pathogenesis and prognosis of musculoskeletal infections differs in children and adults due to behavioral differences, bone growth and changing vascularity. For example, in children less than 8 months of age, the metaphysis is traversed by capillaries, allowing spread of infection. In contrast, the growth plate in older children and adolescents is avascular and, together with the thicker bony cortex and more adherent fibrous periosteum, it acts as a barrier to spread of infection (111). Hence, osteomyelitis in adolescents is more likely to spread via purulent debris into the cortical lamellae, and less often into the joint, than in younger children. Once the growth plate closes late in adolescence, hematological osteomyelitis often begins in the diaphysis and can spread to involve the whole intramedullary canal. Adolescents will generally have minimal restriction of movement in the affected extremity, in contrast to the pseudo-paralysis seen in young children with osteomyelitis. Contiguous osteomyelitis, describing bone infections caused by extension of infection from adjacent soft tissues, is most common in adults, but rare in children and adolescents.

Adolescents can exhibit manifestations of infection common to children and adults. The main difference from childhood is the increased frequency of arthritis secondary to sexually transmitted disease. Other entities seen in childhood, but less commonly in adulthood, such as rheumatic fever, remain prevalent in adolescence.

Chronic Recurrent Multifocal Osteomyelitis and Synovitis, Acne, Pustulosis, Hyperostosis, and Osteitis Syndromes

Chronic recurrent multifocal osteomyelitis (CRMO) is a sterile inflammatory disorder that usually occurs at multiple sites, e.g., long bones, spine,

Table 6 Musculoskeletal Infections in Adolescents

Musculoskeletal complaint (cause)	Pattern of arthritis	Clinical characteristics
Gonococcal arthritis (*Neisseria gonorrhoea*)	40% mono-arthritis 30% oligo-arthritis 30% polyarticular Asymptomatic tenosynovitis in 2/3, especially dorsum of hands and wrists	Frequent cause of acute septic arthritis in adolescence. Arthritis occurs as part of the disseminated phase of the disease in 1–3% of patients with symptomatic infection and in up to 0.3% of asymptomatic carriers. Initial presentation is with systemic features, dermatitis, tenosynovitis, and migratory polyarthralgia or polyarthritis (bacteraemic phase). This is followed by a progressive localization of joint symptoms and effusions in one or more joints (septic joint phase).
Bacterial arthritis and osteomyelitis (*Staphylococcus, Streptococcus, Pseudomonas aeroginosa*, gram-negative infections)	Mono-arthritis, usually lower limb	Septic arthritis usually occurs in a single joint, most commonly the hip, knee, or ankle. Osteomyelitis should be suspected in the presence of fever and severe bone pain extending beyond joint margins, with or without local swelling or pseudoparalysis, particularly in immunocompromised patients.
Reactive arthritis (*Salmonella, Shigella, Yersinia*)	Asymmetrical lower limb oligo-arthritis most common	Reactive arthritis secondary to enteric organisms is relatively common. The arthritis can be very painful, but is usually short-lived. The presence of HLA B27 increases the risk of the arthritis being more prolonged and is positive in nearly 2/3 of adults and adolescents with reactive arthritis. Less commonly, non-gonococcal urethritis can cause a reactive arthritis. In adolescents, there is a greater involvement in the upper limb (mainly wrist) compared to adults

(Continued)

Table 6 Musculoskeletal Infections in Adolescents (*Continued*)

Musculoskeletal complaint (cause)	Pattern of arthritis	Clinical characteristics
Lyme disease (*Borrelia burgdorferi*)	Arthritis is mono-articular in 70% of patients and oligo-articular in 25%	Endemic in parts of the United States, Europe, and Asia. Higher prevalence in children and adolescents (22–60%). Intermittent arthritis may appear weeks to months after infection, and may be the only clinical manifestation. Large effusions tend to occur with warmth of the joint, but little pain
Viral arthritis (rubella, mumps, parvovirus B19, HIV, hepatitis B and less commonly EBV, CMV, coxsackie B, adenovirus 7, herpes simplex, varicella zoster, and echoviruses) Small- and large-joint arthritis	Symmetrical polyarthritis, oligo arthritis or arthralgia	Reactive arthritis can occur after viral infections or after vaccinations. Joint symptoms occur more frequently in adolescence compared to childhood following rubella and mumps infections. Small- and large-joint involvement occurs. A variety of musculoskeletal presentations are recognized in up to 75% of patients with HIV, including a mild polyarticular arthralgia, incomplete Reiter's syndrome, mono-articular or oligo-articular arthritis. Following hepatitis B infection, a disease resembling serum sickness can be seen in up to 20% adults with a polyarthritis and rash. Another 40% can get arthralgia.
Rheumatic fever group A streptococcal infection. Migratory arthritis, often short-lived.	Migratory polyarthritis of large joints	Remains endemic in the developing world, with increasing incidence in the developed world. A non-erosive arthritis occurs in 47–100% of patients and is the presenting feature in 14–42%.

Brucella (small, gram-negative coccibacilli transmitted to humans via contact with infected animals or their secretions)	Mono-articular arthritis in 70%. Oligo-articular in 30%	Rarely seen in developed countries, but remains an important cause of septic arthritis in the third world and Middle East in all age groups. Most common method of infection is through the consumption of unpasteurized goat's milk. The disease is characterized by multi-system involvement. Arthritis is the second most common manifestation after fever and is seen in 33–40% of patients. In adolescents, oligo-articular disease is seen more frequently, and the spine and small joints are usually spared.
Postinfectious myositis (influenza A and B, coxsackie B virus or others)	Myositis	A transient viral myositis can follow viral infections, particularly influenza or coxsackie. Other infections that can cause a myositis include toxoplasmosis, trichinosis, schistosomiasis, and trypanosomiasis
Pyomyositis (*Staphylococcus aureus*, *Staph. epidermidi*, group A *Streptococcus*)	Myositis	More common in the developing world. Presents initially with an insidious onset of dull, cramping pain, with or without low-grade fever. This is followed by an increased magnitude of symptoms accompanied by systemic signs (supportive phase)

Abbreviations: CMV, cytomegalovirus; EBV, Epstein-Barr virus.
Source: Adapted from Refs. 111–113.

and pelvic bones. It occurs mainly in children and adolescents. It is characterized by prolonged, fluctuating and recurrent episodes of pain over several years. Although histopathological and laboratory findings are non-specific they are essential to exclude an infective or malignant process. Plain radiographs usually reveal changes consistent with a chronic osteomyelitis. Metabolically active lesions may be detected on a radioisotope bone scan and MRI may be extremely helpful (114). NSAIDs form the base of the treatment pyramid with glucocorticoids reserved for non-responders. Nonresponders to steroid therapy or those on unacceptably high doses may be treated with second line agents e.g., sulphasalazine, methotrexate or pamidronate. Pustulosis is more common in multifocal cases (115), reinforcing the concept that synovitis, acne, pustulosis, hyperostosis and osteitis (SAPHO) syndrome may be part of the same disease spectrum as CRMO. Treatment is with a similar hierarchy of drugs (116).

OTHER CAUSES OF MUSCULOSKELETAL SYMPTOMS

Inflammatory Bowel Disease

Approximately 2% of all patients with inflammatory bowel disease (IBD) present before the age of 10 years, but 30% present between the age of 10 and 19 years (117). Diagnosis is easy when patients present with the classical triad of bloody diarrhea, abdominal pain, and weight loss, but not infrequently, young people will present with extraintestinal manifestations such as arthritis, cutaneous disease, uveitis, depression, and growth or pubertal delay. These extraintestinal expressions are more common in Crohn's disease, but are also well recognized in ulcerative colitis. Rarely, these manifestations, particularly arthritis, can be the only initial symptom for months to years in children with IBD (117). Usually, arthritis develops after diagnosis of bowel disease and is seen in 7% to 21% of children with IBD (118,119). The most typical pattern of disease is peripheral polyarticular presentation particularly affecting lower limbs (118,119). This form of arthritis tends to improve with treatment of bowel disease. Treatments may include enteral diet (for Crohn's disease), aminosalicylates, methotrexate (for articular manifestations) and infliximab (for the more severe end of the spectrum; being particularly effective for those with axial involvement). More unusually, a HLA-B27 positive sacroiliitis with enthesitis and lower limb oligo-arthritis occurs, that bears no relationship to bowel symptoms, and tends to persist (118,119). Vasculitis has been reported in patients with IBD and arthritis (119).

Systemic Disease Causing Musculoskeletal Symptoms

Musculoskeletal symptoms may be due to an underlying systemic disease such as nutritional abnormalities (such as rickets, scurvy, hypervitaminosis), haemoglobinopathies, metabolic abnormalities, cystic fibrosis, endocrine disorders, hyperostosis, and sphingolipidosis (120). A description of musculoskeletal presentations of these disorders is beyond the scope of this book.

Tumors of the Musculoskeletal System

Malignancies may present with musculoskeletal symptoms in the context of primary tumors of bone, fibrous or soft tissue, metastases to bone or leukemia. In the younger child leukemia must always be considered and excluded, however, this is generally not pertinent to the adolescent group. Fortunately metastatic bone disease is very rare. It occurs most commonly in younger children with neuroblastoma (121).

"Red flags" that should alert the clinician to consider this group of disorders include pain quality (e.g., night pain), swelling and tenderness in the absence of trauma, and the presence of systemic features. A brief synopsis of this group of disorders follows. If the reader is considering any of these diagnoses the support of colleagues in radiology and orthopedics with an expertise in this field should be sought.

Benign Tumors

Benign musculoskeletal tumors may occur in the juvenile population. Osteoid osteoma is a tumor of bone that is most common in the second decade of life. It is more common in boys and typically occurs in the neck and intertrochanteric area of the femur. Diagnosis is achieved radiographically and treatment is tailored to achieve pain relief. Osteochondroma is the most common tumor of cartilaginous origin. It has an equal sex distribution and occurs more frequently in adolescents (122). It presents as a painless exostotic mass with symptoms from secondary pressure effects. Common sites include the knee and elbow. Other benign musculoskeletal tumors include chondroma, chondroblastoma and chondromyxoid fibroma, juvenile fibromatosis, ossifying fibroma, fibrous dysplasia, and nonossifying fibroma. The latter is relatively common in adolescence and may be confused with malignant pathology.

Benign soft tissue tumors that may present in adolescents include pigmented villonodular synovitis, synovial hemangioma, and synovial chondromatosis. Clinical suspicion of the former is raised by obtaining a bloody knee aspirate.

Malignant Tumors

Malignant musculoskeletal tumors occur relatively commonly in the second decade of life. Osteosarcoma accounts for 60% of all bone tumors in the juvenile population with 75% of cases occurring between 8 and 25 years of age (122). Tumors arise in the metaphyses (60% around the knee) and metastasize early. Even in expert hands the prognosis may be poor with five-year disease free survival of 65% (123). Rhabdomyosarcoma is the most common soft tissue sarcoma in children and is relatively uncommon in adolescents. Tumors arise in striated muscle most commonly in the head and neck area. They may arise in the extremities in about 20% and this tends to be more prevalent in adolescents (122). Ewing's sarcoma is the most malignant of bone tumors. It occurs most frequently in white males in their second decade. Tumors arise in the diaphysis of long bones with a characteristic radiographic appearance. The 5-year survival varies from 50% to 80% depending on the site of the primary tumor and the presence of metastases.

UNCOMMON CHRONIC SYSTEMIC INFLAMMATORY DISORDERS

Periodic Fever Syndromes

Hereditary periodic fever syndromes are a group of rare inherited disorders defined by recurrent attacks of self limited inflammation for which no infections or autoimmune cause can be identified. The membranous synovial and serosal linings are particular targets resulting in articular and abdominal pain. A family history is useful but often lacking. A useful indication of hereditary periodic fever syndrome as opposed to persistent inflammation is the presence of normal inflammatory markers between episodes with normal growth and development. There are clinical similarities between diseases in this category, but also clear distinctions between mode of inheritance and characteristic features. Life threatening amyloidosis can occur in a percentage of cases of periodic fever syndromes, and despite improved diagnostic methods and therapeutic interventions, it remains the most frequent cause of death (124,125). Familial Mediterranean fever (FMF) is the most prevalent periodic fever syndrome worldwide. It frequently presents in adolescence, and will hence be covered. Syndromes that tend to present earlier in childhood will not be covered, e.g., muckle-wells syndrome; familial cold autoinflammatory syndrome (FCAS); chronic neurologic and cutaneous articular syndrome (CINCA); tumor necrosis factor receptor associated periodic syndrome (TRAPS); and hyperimmunoglobulinemia D periodic fever syndrome.

Familial Mediterranean Fever

Familial Mediterranean fever is defined by recurrent febrile episodes accompanied by abdominal pain (95%), serositis (25–80%), synovitis (75%), and an erysipelas-like rash (7–40%) and splenomegaly (126). Each attack lasts for 12 to 72 hours at intervals of days to months. Between attacks, children or adolescents are asymptomatic and their inflammatory markers are normal. Onset of symptoms occurs within the first decade of life in 50% of individuals (126). It is common in countries surrounding the eastern Mediterranean sea (particularly in Sephardic and Iraqi Jews, Armenians, and Levantine Arabs) and rare in North America and Northern Europeans. A more severe form is seen in North African Jews correlated with homozygosity for M694V (126). FMF has a favorable response to treatment with colchicine, with reduction in the frequency of attacks or preventing them completely. Treatment should be continued for life, but without treatment or with inadequate treatment, amyloidosis is frequent. Early diagnosis using genetic analysis, followed by early treatment with colchicines, will reduce the risk of renal failure secondary to amyloidosis. TNF receptor inhibitors such as etanercept also provide a rational approach to treatment.

Castleman's Disease (Angiofollicular Lymph Node Hyperplasia)

Castleman's disease is a rare atypical lymphoproliferative disorder characterized by enlarged lymph nodes with striking vascular proliferations. It is separated into localized disease, usually observed in young patients, and multicentric disease, more common in older patients. Localized disease has a good prognosis with surgery. Multicentric disease can be associated with other systemic disorders such as HIV, AIDS, malignant lymphoma, and rheumatoid arthritis. Diagnosis depends on biopsy. Treatment options include surgery, chemotherapy, anti-herpetic treatments, antiretroviral therapy and monoclonal antibodies against IL-6 and CD20 (127). Prognosis depends on the underlying disorder.

CONCLUSION

This chapter covers a spectrum of disease seen in adolescent rheumatology. Other presentations are covered in detail elsewhere in this book. It is no means exhaustive, but gives an idea of the challenges that face those caring for adolescents within the field of rheumatology and related areas. Along with clinical acumen, an appreciation of the special needs of adolescents is required, particularly when dealing with schooling issues, career choices, and evolving sexual and risk-taking behavior. For good holistic care, multidisciplinary input is essential.

REFERENCES

1. Symmons D, Asten P, McNally R, Webb R. Healthcare needs assessment for musculoskeletal diseases. Arthritis Research Campaign Epidemiology Unit, University of Manchester 2002. Available from: URL: www.arc.org.uk
2. Churchill R, Allen J, Denman S, Williams D, Fielding K, von FM. Do the attitudes and beliefs of young teenagers towards general practice influence actual consultation behaviour? Br J Gen Pract 2000; 50(461):953–7.

3. Adam V, St-Pierre Y, Fautrel B, Clarke AE, Duffy CM, Penrod JR. What is the impact of adolescent arthritis and rheumatism? Evidence from a national sample of Canadians. J Rheumatol 2005; 32(2):354–61.

4. Thomson W, Barrett JH, Donn R, et al. Juvenile idiopathic arthritis classified by the ILAR criteria: HLA associations in UK patients. Rheumatology (Oxford) 2002; 41(10):1183–9.

5. McCarty DJ, Manzi S, Medsger TA Jr, Ramsey-Goldman R, LaPorte RE, Kwoh CK. Incidence of systemic lupus erythematosus. Race and gender differences. Arthritis Rheum 1995; 38(9):1260–70.

6. Symmons DP, Sills JA, Davis SM. The incidence of juvenile dermatomyositis: results from a nation-wide study. Br J Rheumatol 1995; 34(8):732–6.

7. Mendez EP, Lipton R, Ramsey-Goldman R, et al. US incidence of juvenile dermatomyositis, 1995–1998: results from the National Institute of Arthritis and Musculoskeletal and Skin Diseases Registry. Arthritis Rheum 2003; 49(3): 300–5.

8. Medsger TA Jr, Dawson WN Jr, Masi AT. The epidemiology of polymyositis. Am J Med 1970; 48(6):715–23.

9. Ramanan AV, Feldman BM. Clinical features and outcomes of juvenile dermatomyositis and other childhood onset myositis syndromes. Rheum Dis Clin N Am 2002; 28(4):833–57.

10. Britto MT, DeVellis RF, Hornung RW, DeFriese GH, Atherton HD, Slap GB. Health care preferences and priorities of adolescents with chronic illnesses. Pediatrics 2004; 114(5):1272–80.

11. Zeek PM. Periarteritis nodosa; a critical review. Am J Clin Pathol 1952; 22(8): 777–90.

12. Hunder GG, Arend WP, Bloch DA, et al. The American College of Rheumatology 1990 criteria for the classification of vasculitis. Introduction. Arthritis Rheum 1990; 33(8):1065–7.

13. Jennette JC, Falk RJ, Andrassy K, et al. Nomenclature of systemic vasculitides. Proposal of an international consensus conference. Arthritis Rheum 1994; 37(2):187–92.

14. Salvarani C, Gabriel SE, O'Fallon WM, Hunder GG. The incidence of giant cell arteritis in Olmsted County, Minnesota: apparent fluctuations in a cyclic pattern. Ann Intern Med 1995; 123(3):192–4.

15. Weyand CM, Goronzy JJ. Molecular approaches toward pathologic mechanisms in giant cell arteritis and Takayasu's arteritis. Curr Opin Rheumatol 1995; 7(1):30–6.

16. Michet CJ. Epidemiology of vasculitis. Rheum Dis Clin N Am 1990; 16(2): 261–8.

17. Yanagawa H, Yashiro M, Nakamura Y, Kawasaki T, Kato H. Epidemiologic pictures of Kawasaki disease in Japan: from the nationwide incidence survey in 1991 and 1992. Pediatrics 1995; 95(4):475–9.

18. Gardner-Medwin JM, Dolezalova P, Cummins C, Southwood TR. Incidence of Henoch-Schonlein purpura, Kawasaki disease, and rare vasculitides in children of different ethnic origins. Lancet 2002; 360(9341):1197–202.

19. Cotch MF, Hoffman GS, Yerg DE, Kaufman GI, Targonski P, Kaslow RA. The epidemiology of Wegener's granulomatosis. Estimates of the five-year

period prevalence, annual mortality, and geographic disease distribution from population-based data sources. Arthritis Rheum 1996; 39(1):87–92.

20. Watts RA, Carruthers DM, Scott DG. Epidemiology of systemic vasculitis: changing incidence or definition? Semin Arthritis Rheum 1995; 25(1): 28–34.
21. Arend WP, Michel BA, Bloch DA, et al. The American College of Rheumatology 1990 criteria for the classification of Takayasu arteritis. Arthritis Rheum 1990; 33(8):1129–34.
22. Lindsley CB. Takayasu's arteritis. In: Cassidy J, Petty R, eds. Textbook of Pediatric Rheumatology. 4th ed. philadelphia: WB Saunders, 2001:614–5.
23. Hall S, Barr W, Lie JT, Stanson AW, Kazmier FJ, Hunder GG. Takayasu arteritis. A study of 32 North American patients. Medicine (Baltimore) 1985; 64(2):89–99.
24. Morales E, Pineda C, Martinez-Lavin M. Takayasu's arteritis in children. J Rheumatol 1991; 18(7):1081–4.
25. Kerr GS, Hallahan CW, Giordano J, et al. Takayasu arteritis. Ann Intern Med 1994; 120(11):919–29.
26. Hoffman GS. Takayasu arteritis: lessons from the American National Institutes of Health experience. Int J Cardiol 1996; 54(Suppl.):S99–102.
27. Vanoli M, Daina E, Salvarani C, et al. Takayasu's arteritis: A study of 104 Italian patients. Arthritis Rheum 2005; 53(1):100–7.
28. Hoffman GS, Leavitt RY, Kerr GS, Rottem M, Sneller MC, Fauci AS. Treatment of glucocorticoid-resistant or relapsing Takayasu arteritis with methotrexate. Arthritis Rheum 1994; 37(4):578–82.
29. Shelhamer JH, Volkman DJ, Parrillo JE, Lawley TJ, Johnston MR, Fauci AS. Takayasu's arteritis and its therapy. Ann Intern Med 1985; 103(1):121–6.
30. Newburger JW, Takahashi M, Gerber MA, et al. Diagnosis, treatment, and long-term management of Kawasaki disease: a statement for health professionals from the Committee on Rheumatic Fever, Endocarditis, and Kawasaki Disease, Council on Cardiovascular Disease in the Young, American Heart Association. Pediatrics 2004; 114(6):1708–33.
31. Lightfoot RW, Jr, Michel BA, Bloch DA, et al. The American College of Rheumatology 1990 criteria for the classification of polyarteritis nodosa. Arthritis Rheum 1990; 33(8):1088–93.
32. Ewald EA, Griffin D, McCune WJ. Correlation of angiographic abnormalities with disease manifestations and disease severity in polyarteritis nodosa. J Rheumatol 1987; 14(5):952–6.
33. Frohnert PP, Sheps SG. Long-term follow-up study of periarteritis nodosa. Am J Med 1967; 43(1):8–14.
34. Dillon MJ, Ansell BM. Vasculitis in children and adolescents. Rheum Dis Clin N Am 1995; 21(4):1115–36.
35. Lhote F, Guillevin L. Polyarteritis nodosa, microscopic polyangiitis, and Churg–Strauss syndrome. Clinical aspects and treatment. Rheum Dis Clin N Am 1995; 21(4):911–47.
36. Rottem M, Fauci AS, Hallahan CW, et al. Wegener granulomatosis in children and adolescents: clinical presentation and outcome. J Pediatr 1993; 122(1):26–31.

37. Stegeman CA, Tervaert JW, de Jong PE, Kallenberg CG. Trimethoprim-sulfamethoxazole (co-trimoxazole) for the prevention of relapses of Wegener's granulomatosis. Dutch Co-Trimoxazole Wegener Study Group. N Engl J Med 1996; 335(1):16–20.

38. Masuda M, Nakanishi K, Yoshizawa N, Iijima K, Yoshikawa N. Group A streptococcal antigen in the glomeruli of children with Henoch-Schonlein nephritis. Am J Kidney Dis 2003; 41(2):366–70.

39. Giangiacomo J, Tsai CC. Dermal and glomerular deposition of IgA in anaphylactoid purpura. Am J Dis Child 1977; 131(9):981–3.

40. Stewart M, Savage JM, Bell B, McCord B. Long term renal prognosis of Henoch-Schonlein purpura in an unselected childhood population. Eur J Pediatr 1988; 147(2):113–5.

41. Goldstein AR, White RH, Akuse R, Chantler C. Long-term follow-up of childhood Henoch-Schonlein nephritis. Lancet 1992; 339(8788):280–2.

42. Pattishall EN, Strope GL, Spinola SM, Denny FW. Childhood sarcoidosis. J Pediatr 1986; 108(2):169–77.

43. Sarica R, Azizlerli G, Kose A, Disci R, Ovul C, Kural Z. Juvenile Behcet's disease among 1784 Turkish Behcet's patients. Int J Dermatol 1996; 35(2): 109–11.

44. Criteria for diagnosis of Behcet's disease. International Study Group for Behcet's Disease. Lancet 1990; 335(8697):1078–80.

45. Pachman LM, Cooke N. Juvenile dermatomyositis: a clinical and immuno-logic study. J Pediatr 1980; 96(2):226–34.

46. Oddis CV, Conte CG, Steen VD, Medsger TA Jr. Incidence of polymyositis-dermatomyositis: a 20-year study of hospital diagnosed cases in Allegheny County, PA 1963–1982. J Rheumatol 1990; 17(10):1329–34.

47. Hanissian AS, Masi AT, Pitner SE, Cape CC, Medsger TA Jr. Polymyositis and dermatomyositis in children: an epidemiologic and clinical comparative analysis. J Rheumatol 1982; 9(3):390–4.

48. Hiketa T, Ohashi M. Juvenile dermatomyositis – statistical observation of 105 patients with dermatomyositis. Nippon Hifuka Gakkai Zasshi 1991; 101(8): 825–30.

49. Shehata R, al-Mayouf S, al-Dalaan A, al-Mazaid A, al-Balaa S, Bahabri S. Juvenile dermatomyositis: clinical profile and disease course in 25 patients. Clin Exp Rheumatol 1999; 17(1):115–8.

50. Pachman LM, Hayford JR, Chung A, et al. Juvenile dermatomyositis at diagnosis: clinical characteristics of 79 children. J Rheumatol 1998; 25(6): 1198–204.

51. Bohan A, Peter JB, Bowman RL, Pearson CM. Computer-assisted analysis of 153 patients with polymyositis and dermatomyositis. Medicine (Baltimore) 1977; 56(4):255–86.

52. Rider LG, Miller FW. Idiopathic inflammatory muscle disease: clinical aspects. Baillieres Best Pract Res Clin Rheumatol 2000; 14(1):37–54.

53. Bitnum S, Daeschner CW Jr, Travis LB, Dodge WF, Hopps HC. Deramtomyositis. J Pediatr 1964; 64:101–31.

54. Marie I, Hatron PY, Levesque H, et al. Influence of age on characteristics of polymyositis and dermatomyositis in adults. Medicine (Baltimore) 1999; 78(3): 139–47.
55. Sallum AM, Kiss MH, Sachetti S, et al. Juvenile dermatomyositis: clinical, laboratorial, histological, therapeutical and evolutive parameters of 35 patients. Arq Neuropsiquiatr 2002; 60(4):889–99.
56. Spencer CH, Hanson V, Singsen BH, Bernstein BH, Kornreich HK, King KK. Course of treated juvenile dermatomyositis. J Pediatr 1984; 105(3):399–408.
57. Muller SA, Winkelmann RK, Brunsting LA. Calcinosis in dermatomyositis; observations on course of disease in children and adults. AMA Arch Derm 1959; 79(6):669–73.
58. Banker BQ, Victor M. Dermatomyositis (systemic angiopathy) of childhood. Medicine (Baltimore) 1966; 45(4):261–89.
59. Bohan A, Peter JB. Polymyositis and dermatomyositis (first of two parts). N Engl J Med 1975; 292(7):344–7.
60. Martini G, Calabrese F, Biscaro F, Zulian F. A child with dermatomyositis and a suspicious lymphadenopathy. J Rheumatol 2005; 32(4):744–6.
61. Sherry DD, Haas JE, Milstein JM. Childhood polymyositis as a paraneoplastic phenomenon. Pediatr Neurol 1993; 9(2):155–6.
62. Falcini F, Taccetti G, Trapani S, Lippi A, Bartolozzi G. Acute lymphocytic leukemia with dermatomyositis-like onset in childhood. J Rheumatol 1993; 20(7):1260–2.
63. Wakata N, Kurihara T, Saito E, Kinoshita M. Polymyositis and dermatomyositis associated with malignancy: a 30-year retrospective study. Int J Dermatol 2002; 41(11):729–34.
64. Hill CL, Zhang Y, Sigurgeirsson B, et al. Frequency of specific cancer types in dermatomyositis and polymyositis: a population-based study. Lancet 2001; 357(9250):96–100.
65. Huber AM, Lang B, LeBlanc CM, et al. Medium- and long-term functional outcomes in a multicenter cohort of children with juvenile dermatomyositis. Arthritis Rheum 2000; 43(3):541–9.
66. Sultan SM, Ioannou Y, Moss K, Isenberg DA. Outcome in patients with idiopathic inflammatory myositis: morbidity and mortality. Rheumatology (Oxford) 2002; 41(1):22–6.
67. Maillard SM, Jones R, Owens C, et al. Quantitative assessment of MRI T2 relaxation time of thigh muscles in juvenile dermatomyositis. Rheumatology (Oxford) 2004; 43(5):603–8.
68. Hernandez RJ, Sullivan DB, Chenevert TL, Keim DR. MR imaging in children with dermatomyositis: musculoskeletal findings and correlation with clinical and laboratory findings. AJR Am J Roentgenol 1993; 161(2):359–66.
69. Brown V, Halkon E, Pilkington C, et al. Revision of diagnostic criteria for juvenile dermatomyositis [abstract]. Clin Exp Rheumatol 2004; 22:528.
70. Pitt AM, Fleckenstein JL, Greenlee RG Jr, Burns DK, Bryan WW, Haller R. MRI-guided biopsy in inflammatory myopathy: initial results. Magn Reson Imaging 1993; 11(8):1093–9.

71. Chung YL, Wassif WS, Bell JD, Hurley M, Scott DL. Urinary levels of creatine and other metabolites in the assessment of polymyositis and dermatomyositis. Rheumatology (Oxford) 2003; 42(2):298–303.

72. Smith RL, Sundberg J, Shamiyah E, Dyer A, Pachman LM. Skin involvement in juvenile dermatomyositis is associated with loss of end row nailfold capillary loops. J Rheumatol 2004; 31(8):1644–9.

73. Rider LG, Feldman BM, Perez MD, et al. Development of validated disease activity and damage indices for the juvenile idiopathic inflammatory myopathies: I. Physician, parent, and patient global assessments. Juvenile Dermatomyositis Disease Activity Collaborative Study Group. Arthritis Rheum 1997; 40(11):1976–83.

74. Miller LC, Michael AF, Baxter TL, Kim Y. Quantitative muscle testing in childhood dermatomyositis. Arch Phys Med Rehabil 1988; 69(8):610–3.

75. Lovell DJ, Lindsley CB, Rennebohm RM, et al. Development of validated disease activity and damage indices for the juvenile idiopathic inflammatory myopathies. II. The Childhood Myositis Assessment Scale (CMAS): a quantitative tool for the evaluation of muscle function. The Juvenile Dermatomyositis Disease Activity Collaborative Study Group. Arthritis Rheum 1999; 42(10):2213–9.

76. Huber AM, Feldman BM, Rennebohm RM, et al. Validation and clinical significance of the Childhood Myositis Assessment Scale for assessment of muscle function in the juvenile idiopathic inflammatory myopathies. Arthritis Rheum 2004; 50(5):1595–603.

77. Takken T, Elst E, Spermon N, Helders PJ, Prakken AB, van der NJ. The physiological and physical determinants of functional ability measures in children with juvenile dermatomyositis. Rheumatology (Oxford) 2003; 42(4): 591–5.

78. Feldman BM, Reichlin M, Laxer RM, Targoff IN, Stein LD, Silverman ED. Clinical significance of specific autoantibodies in juvenile dermatomyositis. J Rheumatol 1996; 23(10):1794–7.

79. Fisler RE, Liang MG, Fuhlbrigge RC, Yalcindag A, Sundel RP. Aggressive management of juvenile dermatomyositis results in improved outcome and decreased incidence of calcinosis. J Am Acad Dermatol 2002; 47(4):505–11.

80. Reiff A, Rawlings DJ, Shaham B, et al. Preliminary evidence for cyclosporin A as an alternative in the treatment of recalcitrant juvenile rheumatoid arthritis and juvenile dermatomyositis. J Rheumatol 1997; 24(12):2436–43.

81. Heckmatt J, Hasson N, Saunders C, et al. Cyclosporin in juvenile dermatomyositis. Lancet 1989; 1(8646):1063–6.

82. Olson NY, Lindsley CB. Adjunctive use of hydroxychloroquine in childhood dermatomyositis. J Rheumatol 1989; 16(12):1545–7.

83. Al-Mayouf SM, Laxer RM, Schneider R, Silverman ED, Feldman BM. Intravenous immunoglobulin therapy for juvenile dermatomyositis: efficacy and safety. J Rheumatol 2000; 27(10):2498–503.

84. Dau PC. Plasmapheresis in idiopathic inflammatory myopathy. Experience with 35 patients. Arch Neurol 1981; 38(9):544–52.

85. Anderson L, Ziter FA. Plasmapheresis via central catheter in dermatomyositis: a new method for selected pediatric patients. J Pediatr 1981; 98(2):240–1.

86. Riley P, Maillard SM, Wedderburn LR, Woo P, Murray KJ, Pilkington CA. Intravenous cyclophosphamide pulse therapy in juvenile dermatomyositis. A review of efficacy and safety. Rheumatology (Oxford) 2004; 43(4):491–6.
87. Maillard S, Wilkinson N, Beresford MW, Davidson JE, Murray KJ. The treatment of persistent severe idiopathic inflammatory myositis with anti-TNF therapy. [abstract]. Arthritis Rheum 2002; 44:S307.
88. Levine TD. A pilot study of rituximab therapy for refractory dermatomyositis. [abstract]. Arthritis Rheum 2002; 46:S488.
89. Maillard SM, Jones R, Owens CM, et al. Quantitative assessments of the effects of a single exercise session on muscles in juvenile dermatomyositis. Arthritis Rheum 2005; 53(4):558–64.
90. Sullivan DB, Cassidy JT, Petty RE. Dermatomyositis in the pediatric patient. Arthritis Rheum 1977; 20(Suppl. 2):327–31.
91. Miller LC, Michael AF, Kim Y. Childhood dermatomyositis. Clinical course and long-term follow-up. Clin Pediatr (Phila) 1987; 26(11):561–6.
92. Bowyer SL, Blane CE, Sullivan DB, Cassidy JT. Childhood dermatomyositis: factors predicting functional outcome and development of dystrophic calcification. J Pediatr 1983; 103(6):882–8.
93. Alsufyani KA, Ortiz-Alvarez O, Cabral DA, et al. Bone mineral density in children and adolescents with systemic lupus erythematosus, juvenile dermatomyositis, and systemic vasculitis: relationship to disease duration, cumulative corticosteroid dose, calcium intake, and exercise. J Rheumatol 2005; 32(4):729–33.
94. Vancheeswaran R, Black CM, David J, et al. Childhood-onset scleroderma: is it different from adult-onset disease. Arthritis Rheum 1996; 39(6):1041–9.
95. Murray KJ, Laxer RM. Scleroderma in children and adolescents. Rheum Dis Clin N Am 2002; 28(3):603–24.
96. Peterson LS, Nelson AM, Su WP, Mason T, O'Fallon WM, Gabriel SE. The epidemiology of morphea (localized scleroderma) in Olmsted County 1960–1993. J Rheumatol 1997; 24(1):73–80.
97. Mayes MD. Classification and epidemiology of scleroderma. Semin Cutan Med Surg 1998; 17(1):22–6.
98. Uziel Y, Krafchik BR, Silverman ED, Thorner PS, Laxer RM. Localized scleroderma in childhood: a report of 30 cases. Semin Arthritis Rheum 1994; 23(5):328–40.
99. Soma Y, Tamaki T, Kikuchi K, Abe M, Igarashi A, Takehara K, et al. Coexistence of morphea and systemic sclerosis. Dermatology 1993; 186(2): 103–5.
100. Lapiere JC, Aasi S, Cook B, Montalvo A. Successful correction of depressed scars of the forehead secondary to trauma and morphea en coup de sabre by en bloc autologous dermal fat graft. Dermatol Surg 2000; 26(8):793–7.
101. Eguchi T, Harii K, Sugawara Y. Repair of a large "coup de sabre" with soft-tissue expansion and artificial bone graft. Ann Plast Surg 1999; 42(2):207–10.
102. Sengezer M, Deveci M, Selmanpakoglu N. Repair of "coup de sabre," a linear form of scleroderma. Ann Plast Surg 1996; 37(4):428–32.
103. Katarincic JA, Bishop AT, Wood MB. Free tissue transfer in the treatment of linear scleroderma. J Pediatr Orthop 2000; 20(2):255–8.

104. Steen VD, Oddis CV, Conte CG, Janoski J, Casterline GZ, Medsger TA Jr. Incidence of systemic sclerosis in Allegheny County, Pennsylvania. A twenty-year study of hospital-diagnosed cases, 1963–1982. Arthritis Rheum 1997; 40 (3):441–5.

105. Mayes MD, Lacey JV, Jr, Beebe-Dimmer J, et al. Prevalence, incidence, survival, and disease characteristics of systemic sclerosis in a large US population. Arthritis Rheum 2003; 48(8):2246–55.

106. Stratton RJ, Wilson H, Black CM. Pilot study of anti-thymocyte globulin plus mycophenolate mofetil in recent-onset diffuse scleroderma. Rheumatology (Oxford) 2001; 40(1):84–8.

107. Cozzi F, Marson P, Rosada M, et al. Long-term therapy with plasma exchange in systemic sclerosis: effects on laboratory markers reflecting disease activity. Transfus Apher Sci 2001; 25(1):25–31.

108. Korn JH, Mayes M, Matucci CM, et al. Digital ulcers in systemic sclerosis: prevention by treatment with bosentan, an oral endothelin receptor antagonist. Arthritis Rheum 2004; 50(12):3985–93.

109. Giannelli G, Iannone F, Marinosci F, Lapadula G, Antonaci S. The effect of bosentan on matrix metalloproteinase-9 levels in patients with systemic sclerosis-induced pulmonary hypertension. Curr Med Res Opin 2005; 21(3): 327–32.

110. Foeldvari I, Zhavania M, Birdi N, et al. Favourable outcome in 135 children with juvenile systemic sclerosis: results of a multi-national survey. Rheumatology (Oxford) 2000; 39(5):556–9.

111. Waagner DC. Musculoskeletal infections in adolescents. Adolesc Med 2000; 11(2):375–400.

112. Hashkes PJ, Biro F, Glass D. Infection, arthritis and adolescence. In: Isenberg DA, Miller J, eds. Adolescent Rheumatology. 1st ed. London: Martin Dunitz; 2005:45–70.

113. Cassidy JT, Petty RE. Arthritis Related to Infection. Textbook of Pediatric Rheumatology. 4th ed. Philadelphia: Saunders; 2001:640–711.

114. Jurik AG. Chronic recurrent multifocal osteomyelitis. Semin Musculoskelet Radiol 2004; 8(3):243–53.

115. Girschick HJ, Raab P, Surbaum S, et al. Chronic non-bacterial osteomyelitis in children. Ann Rheum Dis 2005; 64(2):279–85.

116. Kerrison C, Davidson JE, Cleary AG, Beresford MW. Pamidronate in the treatment of childhood SAPHO syndrome. Rheumatology (Oxford) 2004; 43(10):1246–51.

117. Buller HA. Problems in diagnosis of IBD in children. Neth J Med 1997; 50(2): S8–11.

118. McDonagh J. Juvenile spondyloarthropathies and other causes of back pain. In: Isenberg DA, Miller J, eds. Adolescent Rheumatology. 1st ed. London: Martin Dunitz, 1999:99.

119. Petty RE, Cassidy JT. Arthropathies of inflammatory bowel disease. In: Cassidy JT, Petty RE, eds. Textbook of Pediatric Rheumatology. 4th ed. Philadelphia: WB Saunders, 2001:357–61.

120. Cassidy J, Petty R. Primary and Acquired Disorders of Bone and Connective Tissue. Textbook of Pediatric Rheumatology. 4th ed. Philadelphia: WB Saunders, 2001:726–54.

121. Leeson MC, Makley JT, Carter JR. Metastatic skeletal disease in the pediatric population. J Pediatr Orthop 1985; 5(3):261–7.

122. Cassidy JT, Petty RE. Skeletal malignancies and related disorders. In: Cassidy JT, Petty RE, eds. Textbook of Pediatric Rheumatology. 4th ed. Philadelphia: WB Saunders, 2001:763–78.

123. Bacci G, Longhi A, Bertoni F, et al. Primary high-grade osteosarcoma: comparison between preadolescent and older patients. J Pediatr Hematol Oncol 2005; 27(3):129–34.

124. McDermott MF, Frenkel J. Hereditary periodic fever syndromes. Neth J Med 2001; 59(3):118–25.

125. Hull KM, Drewe E, Aksentijevich I, et al. The TNF receptor-associated periodic syndrome (TRAPS): emerging concepts of an autoinflammatory disorder. Medicine (Baltimore) 2002; 81(5):349–68.

126. Ben-Chetrit E, Levy M. Familial Mediterranean fever. Lancet 1998; 351 (9103):659–64.

127. Waterston A, Bower M. Fifty years of multicentric Castleman's disease. Acta Oncol 2004; 43(8):698–704.

7

The Young Adult with Juvenile Idiopathic Arthritis

Jon C. Packham

Staffordshire Rheumatology Centre, Haywood Hospital, Stoke on Trent,
and Primary Care Musculoskeletal Research Centre, Keele University,
Staffordshire, U.K.

INTRODUCTION

Juvenile idiopathic arthritis (JIA) is a heterogeneous group of diseases with a variable clinical course and outcome. It affects approximately 1 in 1000 children in the United Kingdom, with 58 prevalent cases of JIA per 100,000 15- to 24-year-olds (1). These children have a significant risk of long-term morbidity, with at least one-third of children continuing to have active inflammatory disease into adulthood (2–4). Up to 60% of all patients continue to have some limitation of their activities of daily living (3–6).

JIA AND THE RELATIONSHIP TO ADULT ARTHRITIDES

A WHO/International League Against Rheumatism (ILAR) report in 1995 (7,8) proposed the now widely accepted classification based on clinical patterns, including seven different subtypes of JIA. These subtypes include: systemic onset arthritis, oligo-arthritis and extended oligo-arthritis, rheumatoid factor positive polyarthritis, rheumatoid factor negative polyarthritis, enthesitis-related arthritis and psoriatic arthritis (Table 1). An eighth category "other" is also included in the classification. The criteria that exclude an individual from one of the subtypes above and place them in the "other" category have been the cause of some debate. Exclusion criteria include specific disease states causing joint inflammation, such as systemic lupus erythematosus, rheumatic fever, septic arthritis and neoplasia.

Table 1   The Frequencies of JIA Subsets Observed in the United Kingdom

JIA subset	Frequency %
Persistent oligo-arthritis JIA	50
Extended oligo-arthritis JIA	
Polyarthritis (RhF –ve) JIA	17
Systemic onset JIA	11
Enthesitis-related JIA	10
Psoriatic JIA	7
Polyarthritis (RhF +ve) JIA	3

Source: Adapted from Ref. 1.

Oligo-Arthritis and Extended Oligo-Arthritis JIA

Oligoarticular JIA is the most common subtype of JIA, representing 50% of all JIA (1). Oligo-arthritis affects young girls at least six times more frequently than boys, with a peak incidence below 3 years of age. The prevalence is between 20 and 30 per 100,000, and most ethnic groups are affected (9). Children with this form of JIA have four or fewer joints affected within the first six months of disease, although as many as one-third may subsequently progress to polyarticular involvement (10). Those that subsequently have a cumulative involvement of five or more joints are reclassified into the extended oligo-arthritis subtype. Specific exclusions include a positive family history of psoriasis or spondyloarthropathy and a positive rheumatoid factor. Children who remain oligoarticular for five years are unlikely to progress to extended oligo-arthritis.

This group of patients are classically associated with antinuclear antibody (ANA; 40–75%), usually in low titre (less than 1 in 640) with a homogeneous or sometimes speckled pattern. A positive ANA is important in identifying those children at highest risk of developing chronic anterior uveitis, which is the most serious potential consequence of oligo-arthritis JIA (11).

Onset of oligo-arthritis JIA becomes less and less common through adolescence and by adulthood there is no convincing evidence of an adult counterpart of this disease. Although oligo-arthritis does occur in adulthood, this is usually HLA-B27 related; it falls under the spondyloarthropathy category and has no ANA or occult uveitis associations.

Rheumatoid Factor Negative Polyarthritis JIA

This subtype is classified as a polyarthritis affecting five or more joints during the first six months of disease in the absence of a consistently raised rheumatoid factor. Onset is most frequently in girls below the age of seven. There is a much lower risk and severity of erosive changes on X ray and extra-articular manifestations than in rheumatoid factor positive JIA and prognosis is less severe. There is an association to chronic asymptomatic anterior uveitis, but with a lower incidence than in the oligo-arthritis JIA subset, but there is a similar association with ANA positivity.

In adults with rheumatoid arthritis, there is a subgroup of 25% of patients who are rheumatoid factor negative. In this adult seronegative subgroup, erosive joint damage and extra-articular manifestations are less common than in rheumatoid factor positive disease. The occult anterior uveitis and ANA positivity associations seen in juveniles are not, however, seen in adult disease.

Systemic Onset Juvenile Idiopathic Arthritis

Previously known as Still's disease this form of childhood arthropathy carries the most adverse prognosis, with a significant mortality (up to 10% in studies prior to aggressive immunomodulatory therapies) (12). The adult version of this disease still carries the label of "adult Still's disease," despite the changes in terminology in the pediatric form. It is unusual for patients to present over the age of 35 years. The latter is similar in presentation, drug responsiveness, and increased amyloidosis risk, but much rarer than the juvenile form affecting 0.16 per 100,000 (13).

Adult and pediatric disease are characterized by a daily spiking fever and an evanescent, non-fixed, macular erythematous rash that is most pronounced at the height of fever and arthritis. If arthritis is not present (as may be the case in early disease), the diagnosis may still be made in the presence of organ involvement, such as serositis (pericarditis or pleurisy), generalized lymphadenopathy, splenomegaly, or hepatomegaly. These features, coupled with a neutrophilia (greater than $13 \times 10^9/L$ in 75% or more of patients) and elevated acute-phase reactants, may suggest infection, particularly if the arthropathy is not evident at disease onset with systemic features. Specific diseases in addition also require consideration and exclusion (Table 2).

The mean duration of active disease is five years, although a minority of juvenile patients have persistent disease into adult life. This is in contrast

Table 2 Differential Diagnoses Requiring Exclusion in Systemic Onset JIA

Infection
Malignancy (particularly neuroblastoma and leukemia)
Neonatal onset multisystem inflammatory diseases
FAPA syndrome (fever, aphthous ulceration, pharyngitis, and adenopathy)
Hyper IgD syndrome
Periodic syndromes (familial Mediterranean fever, TRAPS, etc.)
Kawasaki disease
Drug hypersensitivity

to adult-onset Still's disease where only 25% to 5% of patients achieve remission in their disease course (14,15). In some patients the systemic features, including the fever and malaise, respond well to nonsteroidal anti-inflammatory drugs. In most patients, particularly those with persistent polyarticular arthritis and severe systemic features (such as serositis), corticosteroids and disease modifying drugs may be necessary. The established practice has become the early use of low-dose methotrexate (0.3–0.5 mg/kg/ week, orally or ideally, subcutaneously) administered weekly, since most other disease modifying antirheumatic drugs (gold, sulphasalazine, etc.) have not been shown to be of proven benefit. In the past, AA amyloidosis was relatively common (7–11%) (16) in this subtype but is decreasing in frequency probably due to improved therapies, especially when commenced early. The use of chlorambucil has dramatically improved the outcome of amyloidosis, but in view of its potential toxicity, particularly neoplasia in the longer term, anti-TNF therapy is becoming the preferred therapeutic option (17,18). The systemic onset subset of JIA appears to be the least responsive subset to treatment with etanercept; systemic features, rather than joint inflammation appear to be particularly unresponsive. In systemic JIA there also appears to be a progressive loss of efficacy of etanercept with long term use (17).

Enthesitis-Related Arthritis

This subset was previously referred to as either juvenile ankylosing spondylitis or type II pauciarticular arthritis. It is a spondyloarthropathy usually manifesting as a predominantly lower limb arthritis and enthesitis (inflammation of the insertions of tendon, ligament, or joint capsule into bone). It is the only form of JIA to show a male preponderance (19), usually occurring in the early teens.

There is a reduced incidence of sacroiliitis, with 23.4% of enthesis-related JIA showing radiological changes at diagnosis, compared to 100% of patients with adult ankylosing spondylitis as demanded by New York classification criteria. However, there is also likely to be significant overlap of enthesitis-related JIA with adult undifferentiated spondyloarthropathy where radiological sacroiliitis is not a cardinal diagnostic feature.

If enthesitis is absent, then the diagnosis can still be made if arthritis and two other spondyloarthropathy-related features are present as described by the ILAR criteria for enthesitis-related arthritis (Table 3) (8).

As seen in adults with spondyloarthropathies, acute painful anterior uveitis is a prominent extra-articular feature, usually occurring as an acute unilateral anterior uveitis with a high frequency of recurrence, sometimes in the contralateral eye. Anterior uveitis in these cases is likely to be extremely painful and therefore not liable to go undetected, in contrast to the uveitis associated with oligo-arthritis JIA.

Table 3 ILAR (International League Against Rheumatism) Criteria for Enthesitis-Related JIA

Arthritis *and* enthesitis *or*
Arthritis *and* at least one of the following:
Sacroiliac joint tenderness
Inflammatory spinal pain
HLA-B27
Positive family history of at least one of the following:
Anterior uveitis
Spondyloarthropathy confirmed by a rheumatologist
Inflammatory bowel diseases

In juvenile enthesitis-related arthritis there is a higher rate of peripheral arthritis and enthesitis at presentation when compared to adult onset ankylosing spondylitis (19), and more enthesitis when compared to other subtypes of JIA (Table 4) (21). The rate of patients being HLA-B27 positive are similar in enthesis-related JIA and ankylosing spondylitis.

Psoriatic JIA

Psoriatic arthritis is classified as arthritis associated with psoriasis or arthritis and at least two of the following: dactylitis [i.e., when the whole digit (toe or finger) is swollen as a result of inflammation in the digital joints and associated tendon sheaths], nail pitting or onycholysis, and/or psoriasis in a first-degree relative. Arthritis may predate the onset of psoriasis by many years in the juvenile form. Even if psoriasis is present, it may be limited in its extent (e.g., natal cleft or scalp).

There are differences between juvenile- and adult-onset psoriatic arthritis in terms of association with chronic anterior uveitis in the juvenile

Table 4 Comparison of Enthesitis-Related Arthritis and Related Adult Disorders

	Disorder			
Characteristics	Enthesitis-related JIA	Ankylosing spondylitis	Psoriatic arthritis	Colitis-related arthritis
HLA-B27 positive	85%	90%	~50%	~50%
Sacroiliitis	<50%	100%	20%	<20%
Peripheral joint involvement	90%	25%	95%	20%

Source: Adapted from Ref. 20.

form and HLA associations (22,23). It is more likely that psoriasis is present either before or at the onset of joint symptoms (90%) in the adult form than in the juvenile form.

Rheumatoid Factor Positive Polyarthritis JIA

This is classified as an arthritis involving five or more joints during the first six months of disease associated with a rheumatoid factor positive test on at least two occasions at least three months apart. This subtype is generally considered to be the juvenile form of erosive adult rheumatoid arthritis (RA) although erosions are often late due to the greater amount of cartilage the younger the patient. The peak age of onset is in mid to late adolescence although it can develop in much younger children. As in adult RA, there is a female predominance. Rheumatoid nodules and classical vasculitis are seen only in this group, in which all extra-articular manifestations found in adult RA may occur, including ocular, cardiac and pulmonary involvement. There are no major differences known between juvenile- and adult-onset arthritis pathological processes. There are however differences in outcome related to effects of joint inflammation occurring in a growing skeleton and the psychosocial impact of having arthritis in childhood.

The genetic associations of both juvenile and adult rheumatoid factor positive arthritis are strongly linked to the "shared epitope" HLA-DRB1 *01401/*01404 (24). Interestingly in adult RA, this association is stronger with a younger onset of adult onset disease (25).

OUTCOMES

Disease Activity

The proportion of patients with active disease in long-standing JIA ranges between 31% and 55% (2,3,6,26–32), depending upon the selection and severity of the population studied.

There does not appear to be a reduction in disease activity as disease duration increases. Continuing high levels of inflammation (CRP/ESR) are related to poor physical function (HAQ) (Table 5) (3).

Systemic onset JIA is associated with the highest levels of inflammation in the pediatric population and the worst long-term functional outcome. However, in adulthood the levels of clinical inflammation are significantly lower than any other subset (2,3). This suggests that the concept of arthritis "burning out" may hold true in this specific subtype.

Osteoporosis

Osteoporosis occurs more commonly in JIA and is associated with an increased risk of bony fracture. It is covered more thoroughly in Chapter 12.

Table 5 Hospital-Based Studies of Long-Term Disease Activity in JIA

Author (year) (Ref.)	Length of follow-up (years)	Active disease %
Laaksonen (1966) (27)	>15	41
Ansell (1976) (26)	>15	31
Hanson (1977) (28)	>10	55
Calabro (1989) (29)	>25	35
Wallace and Levinson (1991) (30)	>15	45
David (1994) (2)	>10	48
Zak (2000) (6)	>20	37
Packham (2002) (3)	>25	54 (CRP)
		43 (clinical)
Minden (2002) (31)	>15	53
Foster (2003) (32)	>20	39

Surgery

The inflammation related to juvenile arthritis is sufficient that in poorly controlled disease, it can cause such severe joint damage that patients require prosthetic joint replacement, often at a young age. In one long-term study group (3), prosthetic joint replacement was common, with 49% of the patient group having at least one major prosthetic joint replacement. The frequencies of joint replacement with JIA subset are shown in Table 6. The subgroups of systemic JIA, rheumatoid factor positive and negative polyarticular disease had highest risk of requiring orthopedic interventions. Other joint replacements were comparatively infrequent (shoulder 4.9%, elbow 3.3%, wrist 1.6%, and ankle 1.6%).

Predisposing factors were disease duration, poor function, presence of growth defects, height retardation, and continuing active inflammation. The need for prosthetic joint replacement increases with severity and time. However, the correlation of the need for prosthetic joint surgery with growth defects and height retardation, highlights the influence of severe disease in childhood and the importance of disease control from an early age. With the recent introduction of more effective immunosuppressive agents and earlier aggressive intervention, the proportion of these patients who go on to require surgery is likely to significantly reduce in the future.

Uveitis and Visual Impairment

Ocular involvement in JIA is a particular problem and can take many forms. An acutely painful red eye may be seen in the anterior uveitis associated with enthesis-related JIA. Sicca syndrome is known to be associated with

Table 6   Percentage of Patients in Each Subset with Prosthetic Joints

| | Total % patients with | | |
JIA subset	Any large joint prosthesis	Hip prosthesis	Knee prosthesis
Systemic	75.0	59.6	30.8
Oligo-arthritis	13.3	13.3	6.6
Extended oligo-arthritis	38.1	32.7	23.6
RhF –ve polyarthritis	56.1	51.2	34.1
RhF +ve polyarthritis	64.9	61.3	40.5
Enthesis-related	34.4	28.1	9.4
Psoriatic	15.4	15.4	7.7
All JIA	49.4	43.1	25.6

Source: Adapted from Ref. 3.

rheumatoid factor positive polyarthritis JIA, as it is in adult rheumatoid arthritis. The most common problem in the oligo-arthritis JIA subset is occult anterior uveitis, which affects around 20% of individuals. Because it is asymptomatic, it can easily be missed without appropriate screening with slit lamp examination. Untreated, it can cause blindness in up to 10% of affected patients. Topical corticosteroids and mydriatics are effective in the majority of patients, but intra-ocular injections or systemic corticosteroids are often required to prevent the formation of posterior synechiae between the lens and the iris. In severe refractory cases, immunosuppressive drugs such as methotrexate may be necessary to control the uveitis.

About 80% to 90% of patients with uveitis are positive for ANA. ANA-positive girls presenting with oligo-articular disease below the age of two years have up to a 95% likelihood of developing chronic anterior uveitis. Uveitis can cause other forms of eye pathology such as glaucoma and cataracts. Iatrogenic cataract formation from long-term steroid use may also be troublesome in patients requiring oral corticosteroids for disease control.

Physical Ability

Long-term outcome studies of JIA show huge variation, with between 2% and 48% of JIA patients developing severe functional limitation (Steinbrocker classes III and IV or HAQ score > 1.5) (33). The length of follow-up strongly influences long-term outcome. In adult RA, Scott (34) prospectively followed up aggressively DMARD treated patients at 5, 10, and 20 years. Although function initially improved, it deteriorated considerably between 10 and 20 years. These findings are mirrored in JIA; in 1966

Laaksonen (27) demonstrated that the natural history of JIA is for poor physical function to increase from 12% at 3 to 7 years after onset, to 48% after 16 or more years.

However, over the past 40 years the impact of JIA upon long-term physical function appears to have reduced, probably related to improving treatments. Figure 1 shows the improvement in function seen when publications on long-term outcome in JIA (35) are grouped together into each decade in which disease onset occurred.

Disease subtype has a strong impact upon long-term functional outcome. Systemic onset JIA and rheumatoid factor negative polyarthritis JIA are related to poor functional outcome and persistent oligoarticular and enthesis-related JIA are associated with relatively few functional problems (Table 7) (3).

Social Functioning

Adolescence is also a time of social change when a young person has to establish self-identity and relationships outside the family (see Chapters 2 and 5) . Body image is important to all adolescents (36,37) and may be detrimentally affected in JIA. Generalized growth failure and pubertal retardation (38) are seen in severe JIA. Some local growth anomalies (e.g., a short digit) are often mild but may cause concern to the patient, while other anomalies, such as micrognathia, can profoundly change facial appearance. Drug therapy in JIA may also have detrimental effects. Oral corticosteroids alter the distribution of fat stores and can change skin appearance with acne, striae and hirsuitism. Chlorambucil and cyclophosphamide may cause

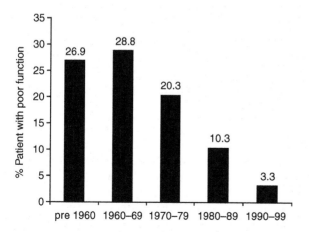

Figure 1 Percentage of patients with poor functional outcome (Steinbrocker III or IV or HAQ score >1.5) related to decade of disease onset.

Table 7   Long-Term Disability Related to JIA Subset

JIA subset	% Patients with poor long-term (28-year) functional outcome (HAQ > 1.5)
Systemic onset JIA	62.5
Oligo-arthritis JIA	0
Extended oligo-arthritis	42
Polyarthritis (RhF −ve)	50
Polyarthritis (RhF +ve)	52.8
Enthesis-related	16.1
Psoriatic JIA	25
All subsets	42.9

Source: Adapted from Ref. 3.

gonadal failure, which can have a profound effect on an individuals' perception of their sexuality.

Difficulties with relationships may persist into adulthood because of delayed social maturation. If the individual is physically dependant, there will be more reliance on friends and sexual partners to act as carers. Relationships with sexual partners may take longer to establish (39), possibly because the relationship is not just partner-to-partner but also potentially carer-to-dependant. However, a number of adults with JIA have long-term relationships with other disabled people.

Limited mobility can affect an individual's ability to participate in socializing activities and gain independence (40,41), (i.e., having to rely on parents for transport when friends are able to use a bus or train independently). The attitudes of society to physical deformity may also affect social interaction. Social life may be affected because of the restrictions on alcohol intake related to methotrexate prescription. Despite this, most children and adolescents with JIA perceive themselves as socially competent (42) and are remarkably similar to case controls on measures of social functioning and behavior (43). In adulthood, social activity reduces in the majority of patients. This becomes more marked those patients with significant physical disability (44).

Psychological Morbidity

There are features of JIA that suggest that young people may be at high risk of psychological complications, these include: pain, disability and physical deformity. A number of studies have shown that psychological problems, particularly depression, are higher in adults with inflammatory arthritis compared to the general population (45,46). The major psychological difference between adult-onset inflammatory arthritis and JIA is that coping strategies are not fully developed in childhood and that adolescence has to be negotiated with a chronic disease. This may affect the long-term psychological health of the individual and the ability to cope with disability in adulthood (see Chapter 2).

David et al. (2) reported clinical depression in 21% of 43 adults with polyarticular JIA, the rate increasing with the degree of disability. Anxious and helpless responses were seen more commonly in patients whose arthritis started in adolescence, possibly because adolescents have less time to adapt and develop alternative coping strategies compared to those with arthritis from early childhood. Aasland et al. (47) found that 17% of 52 adult JIA patients had a psychiatric diagnosis, often anxiety, but none had a depressive disorder. Peterson et al. (5) studying a cohort with predominantly oligoarticular JIA, suggested they ".... were not emotionally impaired and were able to perform social activities similar to controls."

Packham et al. (48) reported a 32% anxiety and 5% depression incidence in 246 adult JIA patients. Patients with systemic onset JIA had significantly higher levels of anxiety 41.7% and depression 10.7%, and those with oligoarticular JIA had lower levels of anxiety 7.7% compared to patients in the other JIA subsets. Depression was most commonly seen when the age at onset of JIA was between 6 and 12 years (11.1%) compared to early (2.7%) or late (0%) onset JIA. Those patients in the late onset group over 12 years of age had the highest risk of developing anxiety-related problems (41.5%, $p < 0.05$), compared to the mid (29.6%) and early (28.7%) groups. The age at onset of disease may have a later effect on the effectiveness of learned coping strategies to avoid anxiety or depression. The apparent benefit to psychological health in the early onset group may be related to a lack of sufficient cognitive development (49) to comprehend the potential effects of arthritis. In the mid and late onset groups there may be a more pronounced effect on the development of self-identity and self-confidence.

Previous depression is common (21%) (48), often occurring first in the late teens or early twenties. At this age individuals tend to leave home and seek independence, consequently this is the time when coping techniques are being finalized and also put under the most strain. Depressive episodes become less common in later life, suggesting that experience enables patients to learn to cope with their disease more effectively. This supports the hypothesis suggested by Timko et al. (50) that psychosocial adjustments continue with time as an individual adapts to the disease. There is an important role for transitional care from pediatric to adult care at this time to ensure that at a time of change in care and an increase in patients' responsibility for their own care, they have acquired sufficient personal tools and strategies to cope with the demands of their situation. Transition is discussed further in Chapter 16.

There is little influence from physical disease–related factors on mood. Two important causes of anxiety and depression are a lack of satisfaction with social support and poor body image. In both anxiety and depression, the most important predictive factor is self-efficacy, patients' belief that they can achieve a specific behavior or control a specific symptom. This measure may indicate either less predictability of symptoms in those patients or difficulty coping with similar levels of symptoms experienced by other patients. Self-management courses, with specific techniques being learned and practiced, not only improve self-efficacy but also benefit adult patients' health outcomes (51). Similar studies have yet to be conducted in adolescent populations.

Sexual and Reproductive Health

Establishing a sexual identity is a key task of adolescent development, and addressing sexual and reproductive health issues during adolescence and adulthood are important aspects of management.

Women with JIA have similar levels of sexual activity and relationships when compared to healthy controls. However, this group has a higher rate of gynecological problems than controls; these include increased incidence of menorrhagia, pelvic inflammatory disease, difficulty in conceiving, and a higher-than-normal rate of miscarriage. These may all reflect hormonal imbalances including luteinizing hormone hypersecretion (52).

There is an increased risk (at least 3.4%) of premature ovarian failure in women with JIA compared to the general population (53). There are significant implications for women with JIA in terms of when they should consider starting a family, as delay may put them at risk of infertility. Early loss of ovarian function has both significant physical sequelae (amenorrhoea, breast atrophy, mucosal dryness, fatigue, and loss of libido) and psychosocial sequelae (exclusion from "motherhood," loss of self-esteem, and poor body image). It also has major health implications, with a nearly two-fold, age-specific increase in mortality rate (54).

Sexuality includes the adoption of certain gender roles (55). Society's definition of masculinity traditionally identifies the male as strong, practical, and the main "bread winner" in a family. The corresponding role for a woman traditionally identifies her as a wife, homemaker, attentive mother, and, more recently, an income provider. Arthritis may interfere with an individual's capacity to meet these expectations. Men with JIA are less sexually active and have greater difficulty establishing a permanent partnership than both healthy males and women with JIA (52). Poor body image, low self-esteem, social isolation, and fears of being unable to support a family or to fill the social role expected from a male in a relationship may all have contributed to this finding.

Despite high levels of disability, most patients are sexually active. A significant minority (37%) of adolescents become sexually active while still under the care of a pediatric rheumatologist (44). As potentially teratogenic drugs are increasingly used in the pediatric population, the need to address sex education and contraception in adolescent clinics becomes essential. Delay in the onset of sexual activity tends to be related to poor body image and decreased mobility that limits social activities (56–59).

Sexual activity can be adversely affected by arthritis, with pain, the fear of pain, fatigue, depression, and anxiety all potentially reducing libido (60,61). Many patients who are sexually active experience difficulties related to their disease. Although the majority of adverse effects are related to the physical effects of arthritis (pain and physical restriction), a significant minority of patients experience body image or self-confidence problems (44).

Family

JIA often has significant implications for family structure and dynamics (see Chapter 14). The effect on the family can be at many levels, such as financial, emotional, and with intra-family relationships. There may also be a negative effect on the siblings of a child with JIA.

Financially, the family may incur additional expenses in travel and health care costs. A parent or partner may be restricted in the ability to work, because of their role as carer. Adults with JIA are more likely to be unemployed or paid lower salaries than their able-bodied peers. If a patient has poor mobility, this may necessitate mobility aid provision or home remodeling. It may also influence choice of accommodation. This is particularly the case with access to the upper storey of a house: in adult patients with JIA (62), 58% of patients have difficulty climbing stairs, 33% choose to live in ground-floor accommodations, and 22% of those with stairs required assistance in the form of stair rails or a stair lift.

Families (and sometimes professionals) can become overprotective to an individual with JIA. This often leads to a family having lower expectations and setting less demanding goals for an individual. This may have a detrimental effect on transition, with lack of career maturity and work experience linked to a parent's view that work experience should occur at an average of 16 years (much later than their nondisabled peers) (63). The same research also indicates that parents often have lower expectations of their child's educational potential, despite young people with JIA either matching or outperforming their able-bodied peers' educational achievements (5,62,64).

Young people with poor self-confidence and JIA are much more likely to spend time with their family rather than with their friends/peers. This can lead to social impoverishment, loneliness, and social isolation for the individual. It can also impact on the socialization of the family, which may become more insular and inward looking as a result of the social dependence of the disabled individual within it.

Families need to develop resilient traits such as balancing illness and family needs effectively, maintaining flexibility in the family unit, remaining socially integrated, maintaining clear family boundaries, and developing collaborative rather than dependant relationships with health professionals (65). These traits are equally valuable in families where the patient is a child living with parents or an adult living with another adult. They are needed to prevent opportunities being lost for healthy family members and to avoid the dissolution of the family unit. Up to a three-fold increase of divorce in families of children with JIA has been reported (66).

Employment

Unemployment impacts the financial security and independence of the individual. There is also a cost implication for society, with patients who become more dependent upon the state, requiring more financial support. The majority of state support is related to the increased disability in the unemployed group, which necessitates a higher level of care and mobility support. However, a proportion of these costs would fall if patients were able to return to employment.

Ansell and Wood (26) found that 83% of 243 patients were in education, employment or married and running a home at 15 years follow-up. Miller (64) followed up 44 patients for an average of 16.1 years and showed that patients received a similar level of education to their siblings and the local population. Poor physical function was more common in those adults staying in education or becoming "homemakers," compared to those entering the workplace.

The employment rate tends to fall, with longer follow-up periods. Foster (67) found that 21% of 180 patients at 18.7-years follow-up were unemployed, despite good academic attainment. David et al. (2) studied 43 patients with a mean disease duration of 19.7 years. Sixty-six percent of patients were employed, but 30% were not working as a direct result of their disease. Peterson et al. (5) reported in a cohort study performed on 44 patients with an average follow up of 24.7 years, that they had similar educational achievement to controls, but a significantly lower level of employment (70.5% vs. 87.3%). In their cohort, Oen et al. (67) showed that the overall unemployment rate in JIA was similar to the general population, but the rate in the 20 to 24 age group was significantly increased. This might suggest that young adults with JIA find it harder to initially enter the workplace at a key time in career development.

Packham and Hall (62) described a 28% unemployment rate in 246 patients with an average disease duration of 28 years. Despite being a well-educated patient group, unemployment was much higher than in the general population. The majority of patients without work attribute their unemployment to the disabling effects of their disease. Physical disability is not as severe in employed patients compared to those without work. The unemployed patients who had never entered the workplace tended to be less disabled than those who could no longer work, suggesting the factors that govern successful transition from education to employment are not solely related to physical ability. Poor educational achievements and limited physical function predict unemployment as one would expect, but the presence of poor coping strategies also correlates strongly with unemployment. This suggests that an individual's ability to successfully cope with their arthritis has a large impact on their success in entering competitive employment.

Appropriate vocational planning and support can facilitate the transition from school to work in adolescence. White and Shear (69) reviewed a group of 242 patients (72% with JIA) who had been given specific prevocational assistance. They reported an employment rate of 72% with a further 15% of patients still attending university. The unemployment rate was just 6%, while 6% were full time housewives and mothers. Twenty-seven percent completed university compared to just 7% of the control population.

Many individuals feel that they are discriminated against at work (62). Discrimination is by nature subjective, enmeshed irrevocably with the perceptions patients have of the environment they live in. If an individual feels he has been discriminated against, it does not necessarily follow that the events leading to that perception were discriminatory. Conversely, the unthinking actions of others may amount to discrimination by omission. Most workplace discrimination occurs around job interviews, with problems split between a failure to be interviewed initially and a perception of unreasonably high levels of failure once interviewed. Once in a job, discrimination tends to be more covert, with access problems and delays in promotion predominating. Only a small proportion of people experience overt negative or discriminatory attitudes towards them. If discrimination does occur, it often originates from direct superiors, rather than being institutional in nature.

SUMMARY

As young people JIA patients progress into adulthood, their disease can have a widespread impact upon many of the facets of normal life. The challenges young people with JIA face do not stop when they stop being adolescent. Adulthood often brings additional stressors and strains that add to the burden of illness they experienced as a child. Pediatric rheumatology care providers must be aware of the impact of JIA in adulthood and ensure that their patients have an appropriate transition to adult care.

It is equally important for adult rheumatology care providers to recognize the differences in childhood onset inflammatory arthritis as compared to disease starting in adulthood. The simple fact that they have had to pass through adolescence with a chronic disease sets adult patients with JIA apart from patients of a similar age with adult-onset inflammatory arthritis.

REFERENCES

1. Symmons D, Jones M, Osbourne J, et al. National Diagnostic Index: Paediatric Rheumatology in the United Kingdom. Data from the British Paediatric Rheumatology Group National Diagnostic Register. J Rheumatol 1996; 23: 1975–80.
2. David J, Cooper C, Hickey L, et al. The functional and psychological outcomes of juvenile chronic arthritis in young adulthood. Br J Rheumatol 1994; 33: 876–81.
3. Packham JC, Hall MA. Long term follow up of 246 adults with juvenile idiopathic arthritis: functional outcome. Rheumatology 2002; 41:1428–35.
4. Gare BA, Fasth A. The natural history of juvenile chronic arthritis: a population based cohort study. II. Outcome. J Rheumatol 1995; 22:308–19.
5. Peterson LS, Mason T, Nelson AM, O'Fallon WM, Gabriel SE. Psychosocial outcomes and health status of adults who have had juvenile rheumatoid arthritis. Arthritis Rheum 1997; 49(12):2235–40.
6. Zak M, Pedersen FK. Juvenile chronic arthritis into adulthood: a long-term follow-up study. Rheumatology 2000; 39:198–204.
7. Fink CW. A proposal for the development of classification criteria for the idiopathic arthritides of childhood. J Rheumatol 1995; 22:1566–9.
8. Petty RE, Southwood TR, Manners P, et al. International League of Associations for Rheumatology Classification of Juvenile Idiopathic Arthritis: Second Revision, Edmonton 2001. J Rheumatol 2004; 31:390–2.
9. Andersson Gare B, Fasth A, Andersson J, et al. Incidence and prevalence of juvenile chronic arthritis: a population survey. Ann Rheum Dis 1987; 46(4): 277–81.
10. Sherry DD, Mellins ED, Wedgewood RJ. Decreasing severity of chronic uveitis in children with pauciarticular arthritis. Am J Dis Child 1991; 145(9):1026–8.
11. Leak AM and Ansell BM. The relationship between ocular and articular disease activity in juvenile rheumatoid arthritis complicated by chronic anterior uveitis. Arthritis Rheum 1987; 30(10):1196–7.
12. Svantesson H, Akesson A, Eberhardt K, Elborgh R. Prognosis in juvenile rheumatoid arthritis with systemic onset. A follow-up study. Scand J Rheum 1983; 12:139–44.
13. Magadur-Joly G, Billaud E, Barrier JH, et al. Epidemiology of adult Still's disease: estimate of the incidence by a retrospective study in West France. Ann Rheum Dis 1995; 54:587–90.
14. Ohta A, Yamaguchi M, Kaneoka H, Nagayoshi T, Hiida M. Adult Still's disease: review of 228 cases from the literature. J Rheumatol. 1987; 14:1139–46.
15. Pouchet J, Sampalis JS, Beaudet F, et al. Adult Still's disease: manifestations, disease course and outcome in 62 patients. Medicine (Baltimore) 1991; 70: 118–36.
16. David J, Vouyiouka O, Ansell BM, Hall A, Woo P. Amyloidosis in juvenile chronic arthritis: a morbidity and mortality study. Clin Exp Rheumatol 1993; 11:85–90.
17. Russo RAG, Katsicas MM, Zelazko M. Etanercept in systemic juvenile idiopathic arthritis. Clin Exp Rheumatol 2002; 20(5):723–6.

18. Quartier P, Taupin P, Bourdeaut F, et al. Efficacy of etanercept for the treatment of juvenile idiopathic arthritis according to onset type. Arthritis Rheum 2003; 48(4):1093–101.
19. Burgos-Vargas R, Pacheco-Tena C, Vazquez-Mellado J. Juvenile onset spondyloarthropathies. Rhem Dis Clin N Am 1997; 23:569–98.
20. Arnett FC, Khan MA, Wilkens RF. A new look at ankylosing spondylitis. Patient Care 1989; 23(Nov):82–101.
21. Burgos-Vargas R, Vazquez-Mellado J. The early clinical recognition of juvenile-onset ankylosing spondylitis and its differentiation from juvenile rheumatoid arthritis. Arthritis Rheumatism 1995; 38(6):835–44.
22. Paiva ES, Macaluso DC, Edwards A, Rosenbaum JT. Characterisation of uveitis in patients with psoriatic arthritis. Ann Rheum Dis 2000; 59(1):67–70.
23. Hamilton ML, Gladman DD, Shore A, Laxer RM, Silverman ED. Juvenile psoriatic arthritis and HLA antigens. Ann Rheum Dis 1990; 49:694–7.
24. Murray KJ, Moroldo MB, Donnelly P, et al. Age specific effects of juvenile rheumatoloid arthritis-associated HLA alleles. Arthritis Rheum 1999; 42(9): 1843–53.
25. Macgregor A, Ollier W, et al. HLA-DRB1 *01401/*01404 genotype and rheumatoid arthritis: increased association in men, young age at onset and disease severity. J Rheumatol 1995; 22:1032–36.
26. Ansell BM, Wood PHN. Prognosis in juvenile chronic polyarthritis. Clin Rheum Dis 1976; 2:397–412.
27. Laaksonen A. A prognostic study of juvenile rheumatoid arthritis: analysis of 544 cases. Acta Paediatr Scand 1966; 166(Suppl. 1):23–30.
28. Hanson V, Kornreich H, Bernstein B. Prognosis of juvenile rheumatoid arthritis. Arthritis Rheum 1977; 20:279–84.
29. Calabro JJ, Marchesano JM, Parrino GR. Juvenile rheumatoid arthritis:long-term management and prognosis. J Musculoskeletal Med 1989; 6:17–32.
30. Wallace CA, Levninson JE. Juvenile rheumatoid arthritis: outcome and treatment for the 1990s. Rheum Dis Clin N Am 1991; 17:891–905.
31. Minden K, Niewerth M, Listing J, et al. Longterm outcome in patients with juvenile idiopathic arthritis. Arthritis Rheum 2002; 46:2392–401.
32. Foster HE, Marshall N, Myers A, Dunkley P, Griffiths ID. Outcome in adults with juvenile idiopathic arthritis. Arthritis Rheum 2003; 48:767–75.
33. Steinbrocker O, Traeger CH and Battman RG. Therapeutic criteria in rheumatoid arthritis. J Am Med Assoc 1949; 140:659–62.
34. Scott DL, Coulton BL and Symmons DPM. Long term outcome of treating rheumatoid arthritis: results after 20 years. Lancet 1987; 1:1108–11.
35. Packham JC. Health status of adults with chronic arthritis since childhood: a clinical, functional and psychological assessment. 2004. MD thesis, University of Southampton).
36. Strax TE. Psychosocial issues faced by adolescents and young adults with disabilities. Pediatr Ann 1991; 20:501–6.
37. Selekman J, McIlvain-Simpson G. Sex and sexuality for the adolescent with a chronic condition. Pediatr Nursing 1991; 17:535–8.
38. Fraser PHS, Erlandson D, et al. The timing of menarche in juvenile rheumatoid arthritis. J Adolescent Health Care 1988; 9:483–7.

39. Hamilton A. Sexual problems in arthritis and allied conditions. Int Rehab Med 1980; 3:38–42.

40. Rapoff MA. Psychosocial aspects of pediatric rheumatic diseases. Curr Opin Rheumatol 2001; 13(5):405–9.

41. Wilkinson VA. Juvenile chronic arthritis in adolescence: facing the reality. Int Rehab Med 1981; 3(1):11–7.

42. Huygen ACJ, Kuis W, Sinnema G. Psychological, behavioural and social adjustment in children and adolescents with juvenile chronic arthritis. Ann Rheum Dis 2000; 59:276–82.

43. Noll RB, Kozlowski K, Gerhardt C, Vannatta K, Taylor J, Passo M. Social, emotional and behavioural functioning of children with juvenile rheumatoid arthritis. Arthritis Rheumatism 2000; 43(6):1387–96.

44. Packham JC, Hall MA. Long term follow up of 246 adults with juvenile Idiopathic arthritis: social function, relationships and sexual activity. Rheumatology 2002; 41:1440–3.

45. Creed F. Psychological disorders in rheumatoid arthritis: a growing consensus? Ann Rheum Dis 1990; 49:808–12.

46. Baum J. A review of the psychological aspects of rheumatic diseases. Semin Arthritis Rheum 1982; 11:352–61.

47. Aasland A, Flato B, Vondivik LH. Psychosocial outcome in juvenile chronic arthritis: a nine year follow-up. Clin Exp Rheumatol 1997; 15:561–8.

48. Packham JC, Hall MA, Pimm TC. Long term follow-up of 246 adults with juvenile idiopathic arthritis: predictive factors for mood and pain. Rheumatology 2002; 41:1444–9.

49. Brainerd CJ. Piaget's Theory of Intelligence. New Jersey: Prentice Hall, Inc. 1978.

50. Timko C, Stovel KW, Moos Rh, Miller JJ. Adaptation to juvenile rheumatic disease: A controlled evaluation of functional disability with a one-year follow-up. Health Psychol 1992; 11:91–100.

51. Lorig K, Chastain R, Ung E, et al. Development and evaluation of a scale to measure perceived self-efficacy in people with arthritis. Arthritis Rheum 1989; 32:37–44.

52. Ostensen M, Almberg K, Koksvik HS. Sex, reporduction and gynaecological disease in young adults wiht a history of juvenile chronic arthritis. Rheumatol. 2000: 27:1783–7.

53. Packham JC, Hall MA. Premature ovarian failure in adults with JIA Clin Exp Rheum 2003; 21(3):347–50.

54. Snowdon DA, Kane RL, Beeson WL, et al. Is early natural menopause a biologic marker of health and aging? Am J Public Health 1989; 79:709–14.

55. Majerovitz SD, Revenson TA. Sexuality and rheumatoid disease: the significance of gender. Arthrit Care Res 1994; 7:29–34.

56. Ungerer JA, Horgan B, Chaitow J, et al. Psychosocial functioning in children and young adults with juvenile arthritis. Pediatrics 1988; 81:195–202.

57. Herstein A, Hill RH, Walters K. Adult sexuality and juvenile rheumatoid arthritis. J Rheumatol 1977; 4:35–9.

58. Hill RH, Herstein A, Walters K. Juvenile rheumatoid arthritis: follow-up into adulthood—medical, sexual and social status. Can Med Assoc J 1976; 76:790–5.

59. Yoshimo S, Uchida S. Sexual problems of women with rheumatoid arthritis. Arch Phys Med Rehabil 1981; 62:122–3.
60. Blake DJ, Maisiak R, Alarcon GS, Holley HL, Brown S. Sexual quality-of-life of patients with arthritis compared to arthritis-free controls. J Rheumatol 1987; 14:570–6.
61. Panush RS, Mihailescu GD, Gornisiewicz MT, Sutaria SH. Sex and Arthritis. Bull Rheum Dis 2000; 49(7):1–4.
62. Packham JC, Hall MA. Long-term follow-up of 246 adults with juvenile idiopathic arthritis: education and employment. Rheumatology 2002; 41: 1436–9.
63. White PH, Gussek DG, Fisher B, et al. Career maturity in adolescents with chronic illness. J Adolesc Health Care 1990; 11:372.
64. Miller JJ. Psychosocial factors related to rheumatic diseases in childhood. J Rheumatol 1993; 20(Suppl. 38):1–11.
65. Patterson JM. Family resilience to the challenge of child's disability. Pediatr Ann 1991; 20:501–6.
66. Henoch MJ, Batson JW, Baum J. Psychosocial factors in juvenile rheumatoid arthritis. Arthritis Rheum 1978; 21:229–33.
67. Foster HE, Martin K, Marshall N. Juvenile idiopathic arthritis: Functional development, educational achievement and employment. Ann Rheum Dis 1999; 33 [XIV EULAR Congress (6–11 June)] Abstract 1427.
68. Oen K, Malleson PN, Cabral DA, Rosenberg AM, Petty RE, Cheang M. Disease course and outcome of juvenile rheumatoid arthritis in a multicentre cohort. J Rheumatol 2002; 29:1989–99.
69. White PH, Shear ES. Transition/job readiness for adolescents with juvenile arthritis and other chronic illness. J Rheumatol 1992; 19(Suppl. 33):23–27.

8

The Young Person with Systemic Lupus Erythematosus

Lori B. Tucker

Division of Rheumatology, Centre for Community Child Health Research, BC Children's Hospital, Vancouver, British Columbia, Canada

INTRODUCTION

Systemic lupus erythematosus (SLE) is a severe, chronic, autoimmune disease, in which widespread inflammation can result in damage to a broad range of organ systems. The prognosis for patients with SLE has dramatically improved over the past 30 years so that the majority of patients will survive 10 to 20 years or longer with their disease; however, morbidity is high due to intermittent disease flares and treatment-related toxicity. Although the onset of SLE is most common in the age range of 20 to 40 years, a significant number of patients have onset of SLE in childhood and adolescence.

EPIDEMIOLOGY

Among the conditions seen in the pediatric rheumatology clinic population, SLE is relatively rare, and accurate data of incidence and prevalence are minimal. However, at least 15% of patients with SLE have the onset of their disease in childhood or adolescence. Several studies, from Canada, Finland, and Japan have estimated the annual incidence rate for juvenile onset SLE as between 0.36 and 0.9 per 100,000 children (1–3). There is a peak of incidence in the pubertal and immediate postpubertal period. SLE is a disease seen predominantly in women in the adult onset cases, with a female to male ratio of 9:1 in nearly all case series (6). The female to male ratio is generally lower in the pediatric onset cases, with an overall female to male ratio of 4–5:1 reported from most case series (4,5). The average age at diagnosis of juvenile SLE ranges from 11 to 14 years (6) and therefore this disease is primarily seen in adolescents.

It is well-known that SLE is more common among Hispanic and non-Caucasian ethnic groups, and this is true in juvenile onset SLE as well (7). Children and adolescents who are Afro-Caribbean, African American, Asian, or Native American are overrepresented in juvenile SLE (8,9).

MANAGEMENT OF JUVENILE SLE—GENERAL CONCEPTS

Juvenile SLE is a chronic disease characterized by flares and remissions, often with long periods of active disease requiring intensive treatment. At times, the disease or its complications can result in severe problems needing urgent and aggressive care. Juvenile SLE can certainly be life threatening, particularly if there is inadequate treatment or poor compliance with treatments.

The treatment of juvenile SLE should incorporate medical management with pharmacologic agents, and attention to general health issues such as diet, sun exposure, exercise, and participation in school, and peer activities. Education for the adolescent and family is a very important consideration. Optimal care for the adolescent with SLE should include the family and patient as an active member of the health care team, with a pediatric rheumatologist, clinical nurse specialist, psychologist, nutritionist, physiotherapist, and occupational therapist as part of the team. The health care providers involved with the adolescent should not only have expertise in the area of lupus treatment but should also have expertise and interest in the care of adolescents with chronic health conditions.

Compliance with a long-term and complicated medical program is a frequent difficulty in adolescents with SLE. Some adolescents with renal disease may not feel particularly ill. They may therefore have difficulty understanding the reason for taking medications or following an intensive treatment program. The medications that are the mainstay of treatment for SLE have side effects that adolescents find objectionable. For example, high-dose prednisone will result in weight gain, skin striae, and acne. Many adolescents will either refuse to take the medication once they have experienced these side effects, or not take the medication as prescribed to try to avoid the side effects. Finally, adolescents who have had SLE for many years may develop "treatment fatigue." They become tired of being ill, attending doctor appointments, and taking medications and simply decide to stop. Their adolescent developmental stage leads them to believe that nothing bad will happen to them. It is critical for health care providers for adolescents with SLE be aware of these potential issues, and to keep alert for signs of noncompliance with treatment, as this may have disastrous results for the patient. (For further discussion of adherence, see Chapter 5.)

General Health Issues or "But I Want to Hang Out in the Sun, in a Tiny Bikini, Smoking Cigarettes and Drinking with My Friends"!

Exposure to sunlight (UVB radiation) should be avoided by adolescents with SLE. Some patients with SLE will develop scarring photosensitive rashes on UV exposure, and this exposure may also lead to an increase in SLE symptoms. Adolescents should be advised to use a sunscreen with SPF over 30 every day. Although particular care should be taken on sunny days, even a walk to school on an overcast day can be a problem. Use of a hat for facial protection is also advised. Certainly, suntanning is not recommended, and attending a tanning salon is definitely not advised.

Diet is often a concern among adolescents with SLE. This is a particular problem with respect to excessive weight gain frequently seen with high-dose steroid treatment, and poor calcium intake for adolescents on steroids. The use of high-dose corticosteroids is nearly universal when SLE is active, with an increase in appetite and weight gain extremely common. Nutritional counseling, done when the steroids are begun, has been shown to limit the total weight gain for children and adolescents on high-dose steroids (10). This counseling can include recommendations of increasing calcium intake as well. However, physicians and nurses caring for adolescents with SLE should be aware that the weight gain associated with steroids is generally the issue of highest concern to these patients, and desire to avoid weight gain is a frequent contributor to poor compliance with medical recommendations.

Many adolescents may already be tobacco smokers or are exposed to tobacco smoking through friends and family. Smoking can be detrimental to adolescents with SLE for several reasons: it may exacerbate Raynaud's phenomenon; it is not recommended for anyone with pulmonary disease; it provides additional risk for cardiovascular disease; and there is evidence that it may be associated with decreased efficacy of medications such as hydroxychloroquine (11). In one study, patients with SLE who were cigarette smokers had significantly higher disease activity scores, suggesting that exposure to cigarettes should be avoided for all SLE patients (12). Health-care providers should ask adolescents about possible cigarette use in a confidential setting, and provide options for tobacco cessation if the adolescent is a smoker.

The use of alcohol, marijuana, and other illegal drugs is common amongst adolescents and experimentation is common even amongst those who are not regular users. It is important to establish a nonjudgmental confidential environment in which the health care provider can ask about use of these substances, and provide clear guidance about health implications to the adolescent. For many adolescents, providing factual information about the risks of drug use in the context of their illness is adequate in helping them to make good health choices. (For further discussion of communication strategies with adolescents, see Chapter 4.)

Medications

The medical treatment of juvenile SLE is complex, and should be highly individualized to each particular patient's needs. It is rare that a patient with juvenile SLE will not require medications at some point in the disease course, and most adolescents will require treatment with multiple immunosuppressant medications over long periods of time. Children and adolescents have more severe and active SLE than adult patients, and therefore studies have shown that they are treated with higher doses of corticosteroids and more likely to have had other immunosuppressants such as cyclophosphamide (13,14). Table 1 lists the common medications used in the treatment of adolescents with SLE.

The mainstay of treatment for active juvenile SLE is corticosteroids, given orally or intravenously when disease is quite active. High-dose (≥ 1 mg/kg/day) prednisone is generally effective in getting rapid disease control; a gradual tapering of the dose is required to prevent flaring. Nearly all adolescents who take corticosteroids will experience some side effects and toxicity, and these side effects are frequently very disturbing to the patients. The corticosteroid side effects which are most concerning to adolescents include increased acne, facial hair growth, and striae. Attention should be

Table 1   Medications Used in the Management of SLE in Adolescents

Nonsteroidal anti-inflammatory drugs
   Control of musculoskeletal symptoms, i.e., arthritis
Corticosteroids
   Control of active disease
     May require intravenous dosing to achieve rapid disease control,
       followed by oral dosing
     Split high-dose oral prednisone 1–2 mg/kg/day recommended for rapid
       control of active disease, followed by a slow weaning. Schedule based on
       clinical and laboratory response
Hydroxychloroquine
   Adjunctive treatment with corticosteroids and immunosuppressives
   Control of mucocutaneous disease
Immunosuppressives
   Control of active disease and maintenance of quiescent disease
     Azathioprine
     Mycophenolate mofetil
     Cyclophosphamide
     Rituximab
Anticoagulation
   Prevention of recurrent thromboses in patients with high titer
     antiphospholipid antibodies who have had previous thrombosis
   Use of long-term low-dose aspirin to prevent thrombosis controversial

directed to providing adequate treatment for the acne, with the involvement of a dermatologist if necessary. Facial hair growth should resolve as doses of steroid are tapered. Some patients develop severe widespread striae; this is not preventable, and there is no effective treatment for them once present. Infectious complications relating to steroids in combination with other immunosuppressants are frequent and require careful attention. Adolescents with SLE on steroids may be at increased risk for developing avascular necrosis. In some cases, there may be avascular necrosis in multiple sites. Careful evaluation should be done when an adolescent with SLE has persistent complaints of hip, knee, or other musculoskeletal pain that are not explained.

The immunosuppressant treatment for SLE will vary depending on the patient's clinical characteristics. Medications commonly used include azathioprine, mycophenolate mofetil, and intravenous cyclophosphamide (15). Many pediatric rheumatology centers will use intravenous cyclophosphamide for treating active lupus nephritis and other serious organ involvement of SLE (16). IV cyclophosphamide is generally given as a once monthly treatment for 6 to 7 months, with further treatments dependant on response. Among the many possible side effects of cyclophosphamide is thinning hair or significant hair loss; this is often very distressing to the patients.

The other important possible side effect of cyclophosphamide is impaired future fertility. Premature ovarian failure is a well-known possible complication of chemotherapy. In patients with SLE, the risk of developing premature ovarian failure after chemotherapy treatment seems to be lowest for children and adolescents. It is reported that 100% of those over age 30 years who receive cyclophosphamide will develop it, compared with about 50% of patients between ages 20 and 30 years and only 13% of patients younger than 20 years (17). However, this still is a significant concern for many patients. More recently, some centers have explored the possibility of using gonadotropin-releasing hormone analogs during the cyclophosphamide course to protect against premature ovarian failure. Somers et al. (18) showed a significant reduction in ovarian failure using this approach in a group of young adult women treated with monthly leuprolide acetate, a synthetic gonadotropin-releasing hormone analog.

It is very important, however, to stress with adolescents that they can still become pregnant while taking cyclophosphamide or afterwards—being on cyclophosphamide is not an effective form of contraception! In our clinic, we counsel adolescents about the need for regular and effective contraception while taking cyclophosphamide due to the possible negative effects on a developing fetus if there is an unplanned pregnancy. Recent evidence has shown that low-dose oral contraceptive pills are safe for women with lupus and are not associated with increased flares (19). Use of depo-provera injections for contraception, although highly effective, has been shown to have a negative impact on bone density if used over a long time (20). In adolescents with SLE, whose bone density is already impacted by chronic use of steroids, this side effect must be balanced with the need for contraceptive efficacy. The decision of which contraceptive is best should be an individual decision by the adolescent, rheumatologist, family doctor, and possibly a gynecologist.

Staying Active in a Normal Teen Lifestyle: School, Friends, Sexual Health, and Family

School

As much as possible, it is important for adolescents with SLE to be encouraged to remain a part of their usual school, family, and social setting. Completing education is important for these patients, whose disease will continue into adulthood. Involvement of appropriate vocational counseling during the high school years may be helpful in providing advice and directing towards available resources for post-secondary education or job training. The pediatric rheumatology team may need to become directly involved with the patient's school if the patient is ill enough to require time off school to attend appointments, requires hospital admissions, or modification of their school program. Young adults may need to take a reduced course load at college or university in order to to succeed.

Friends

To adolescents, the most important group of individuals is their friends (see Chapter 5). For adolescents with SLE, many issues relating to friends and peer experiences come up; for example, "Should I tell my friends I have SLE?" Adolescents may become depressed, either due to their disease or effects of treatment such as weight gain, etc. and this may lead to withdrawal from friends and further depression. Careful attention should be paid to these issues by the pediatric rheumatology team. Involving a social worker, psychologist, or nurse who can get to know the patient may be an important way to allow the young person to express their concerns in a private, nonjudgmental setting and to get good advice.

Sexual Health

One of the important developmental tasks of adolescence is the development of sexual identity. In addition to the physical changes that occur during this time, the adolescent will often seek out information and may engage in experimenting and/or early sexual behaviors. For adolescents with SLE, their disease provides additional challenges to this developmental trajectory.

Adolescents with SLE may have delay in pubertal development (21); this may be the effect of active disease and/or medications. Slowed growth is also a significant side effect of corticosteroids, and this may be an added concern in adolescents, who are normally preoccupied with their body image. Slow pubertal development and growth may isolate an adolescent from peers and can be a significant area of distress.

Other concerns which should be considered in the care of adolescents with SLE include: irregular or absent menses resulting from active disease, the need for modification of contraceptive choices due to disease, risks of impaired fertility due to cyclophosphamide treatment, risks of unplanned pregnancy or pregnancy occurring during active disease to the mother and baby. The pediatric rheumatology team should begin to address these issues proactively.

Family

Family-centered, comprehensive care should be the goal for adolescents with SLE, as with all pediatric rheumatology patients. Parents of an adolescent with a chronic illness such as SLE have enormous challenges in surmounting the usual tasks of parenting an adolescent as well as helping their teen learn independent health behaviors. The pediatric rheumatology team should work to support parents through this process as well as adolescents (see Chapter 14).

MORBIDITY IN ADOLESCENTS WITH SLE

As mortality from SLE has decreased over the past decades (9,22), it has been noted that morbidity from the disease and treatments has become a significant problem for patients. (23). Infections related to immunosuppression are quite common among patients with SLE, and care must be taken to treat these quickly to avoid serious or life-threatening situations. Several important or emerging problems for adolescents with SLE entering adulthood are discussed in the following sections.

Bone Health in SLE

The use of long-term corticosteroids to control SLE activity has detrimental effects on bone health, leading to decreased bone mass (24). This is of particular concern in the adolescent, as adolescence and young adulthood are an important time to develop optimal peak bone mass (25). In adults, a low bone mineral density (BMD) is associated with an increase in risk for osteoporotic fractures. Although the magnitude of the fracture risk for adolescents with low BMD due to SLE and steroid treatment is not known, it is a concern for long-term morbidity. Current strategies employed are to measure BMD with dual energy X-ray absorptiometry and to encourage supplemental calcium and vitamin D. The use of bisphosphonates in adolescents is controversial at the present time (see Chapter 12).

Cardiovascular Health

Premature atherosclerosis and coronary heart disease (CHD) are long-term adverse events that occur at much greater frequency among patients with SLE than would be expected. Patients with SLE have a five- to six-fold increased risk of CHD, and in young women between 20 and 40 years, this risk is reported to be as high as 50-fold greater than peers (26). Although the actual risk of a cardiac event related to atherosclerosis is relatively low in adolescence, clearly the process of accelerated atherosclerosis may begin during this time. The etiology of early CHD in patients with SLE involves both classic risk factors as well as factors relating to disease such as chronic inflammation, autoantibodies such as antiphospholipid antibodies, and vascular perturbation by vasculitis (27). Table 2 lists risk factors for early atherosclerosis in patients with SLE. Certain classic cardiovascular disease risk factors are more common among patients with SLE, such as diabetes, hypertension, and hypercholesterolemia. This concern provides more evidence for the importance of controlling hypertension, and monitoring for elevated lipids and diabetes among adolescents with SLE.

One method of measuring the earliest development of accelerated atherosclerosis is by examining the carotid intimal-media wall thickness using sophisticated ultrasonagraphy. In one study of pediatric patients with SLE, patients were shown to have a significantly higher carotid intimal-wall thickness (IMT) compared with healthy controls (28). Children with nephrotic range proteinuria were found to have the highest IMT measurements. These data suggests that aggressive attempts should be undertaken to treat children and adolescents with nephrotic lupus nephritis, in order to help prevent later CHD.

Mental Health and Psycheducational Functioning

Central nervous system (CNS) involvement with SLE is a common event for children and adolescents, reported to occur in 20% to 95% of patients (29).

Table 2 Risk Factors for Accelerated Atherosclerosis in SLE

Traditional risk factors
   Hypertension
   Hypercholesterolemia
   Diabetes
   Smoking
   Obesity
   Family history of CHD
Potential disease-related risk factors
   Proteinuria related to nephrotic syndrome
   Chronic inflammation
   Long-term corticosteroid treatment

Although some CNS events, such as seizure or neuropathies, may be relatively isolated with few long-term sequelae, many CNS events, such as stroke, transverse myelitis, psychosis, or depression, may result in a long-term impact on functional ability. In addition, there is data to suggest that many patients with SLE have subtle cognitive disturbances, which can impact memory (30). These disturbances may result in significant difficulties for adolescents with SLE in school and work, even if they have not had evidence of a major CNS insult.

In one study of a cohort of pediatric SLE patients, 48% were found to have neuropsychiatric SLE, which included depression, concentration or memory problems and psychosis (31). Some patients had more than one CNS manifestation. Although a good outcome was reported in these patients, with 90% reported to have recovery, this was analyzed over a short time period. The gradual and subtle long-term impact on neuropsychological functioning of these insults has never been adequately studied.

LONG-TERM OUTCOMES OF JUVENILE ONSET SLE

Juvenile onset SLE can be life threatening during childhood and adolescence, can cause significant organ damage with subsequent long-term implications, and will continue to require monitoring and treatment into adult life. Therefore, this disease almost certainly has a significant long-term impact on affected children and adolescents. However, outcomes can be optimized with careful attention to factors relating to lupus disease activity, medication side effects, and healthy lifestyle choices (Table 3).

Mortality of juvenile onset SLE, as measured in the "short term" (5- and 10-year survival), has most certainly improved greatly over the last decades. Survival for children and adolescents with SLE is excellent in most pediatric rheumatology centers, with recent data showing 5-year survival of 100%, and 10-year survival of 85% in a cohort of patients followed in the British Columbia Children's Hospital Pediatric Rheumatology Program. (9). In a cohort of pediatric SLE patients with nephritis followed in Toronto

Table 3 Modifiers for Improved Outcomes in SLE

Weight reduction
Increased physical activity
No smoking
Monitoring lipid levels and consideration of medical treatment
Vigilant treatment of hypertension
Screening for bone density and treatment of patients with low density
Aggressive treatment of lupus disease activity

Canada, survival was 94% at an average of 11 years follow-up (32). A report of a similar cohort of pediatric SLE patients with nephritis from Italy showed 75% patient survival at 10 years (37). These data compare with survival rates in the 1970's of less than 40% at 10 years for pediatric patients with SLE and renal disease, and 75% at 10 years for pediatric patients treated with immunosuppressive medications (33).

One method of measuring impact of SLE over time is to use a standardized tool which measures organ damage due to SLE and its treatments. The Systemic Lupus International Collaborative Clinics/American College of Rheumatology Damage Index (SDI) has been developed to measure irreversible damage in a variety of organ systems due to SLE or its treatments(34,35). This tool has been used in a number of outcome studies of children and adolescents with SLE, uniformly showing gradual increase in disease damage scores over time. Of interest, most studies show that children and adolescents appear to accumulate damage more quickly than adults with SLE (14,22,36,37), with higher scores after a similar period of disease. These data suggest that the long-term impact of SLE for adolescents will be significant over their lives, as the accumulated damage to kidneys, central nervous system, musculoskeletal system and other organs will certainly cause functional problems for these patients.

CONCLUSION

Systemic lupus erythematosus is a relatively rare autoimmune disease, which may present during adolescence. This disease can be severe, involving multiple organ systems, and the treatments required for disease control have potential side effects and long-term toxicity as well. The development of a disease such as SLE during adolescence is a challenge to the healthy social development of the adolescent, and the involvement of a supportive multidisciplinary pediatric rheumatology team is important in assisting the adolescent and his/her family.

REFERENCES

1. Malleson PN, Fung MY, Rosenberg AM. The incidence of pediatric rheumatic diseases: results from the Canadian Pediatric Rheumatology Association Disease Registry. J Rheumatol 1996; 23(11):1981–7.
2. Fujikawa S, Okuni M. A nationwide surveillance study of rheumatic diseases among Japanese children. Japonica 1997; 39(242):244.
3. Kaipiainen-Sappanen O, Savolainen A. Incidence of chronic juvenile rheumatic diseases in Finland during 1980–1990. Clin Exp Rheumatol 1996; 14:441–4.
4. Cassidy JT, Sullivan DB, Petty RE, Ragsdale C. Lupus nephritis and encephalopathy Prognosis in 58 children. Arthritis Rheum 1977; 20(Suppl. 2): 315–22.

5. King KK, Kornreich HK, Bernstein BH, Singsen BH, Hanson V. The clinical spectrum of systemic lupus erythematosus in childhood. Arthritis Rheum 1977; 20(Suppl. 2):287–94.

6. Petty RE, Laxer RM. Systemic lupus erythematosus. In: Cassidy JT, Petty RE, Laxer RM, Lindsley CB, eds. Textbook of Pediatric Rheumatology. Philadelphia: Elsiever Saunders, 2005: 342–91.

7. Sutcliffe N, Clarke AE, Gordon C, Farewell V, Isenberg DA. The association of socio-economic status, race, psychological factors and outcome in patients with systemic lupus erythematosus. Rheumatology (Oxford) 1999; 38(11):1130–7.

8. Meislin AG, Rothfield NF. Systemic lupus erythematosus in childhood: analysis of 42 cases with comparative data in 200 adult cases followed concurrently. Pediatrics 1968; 42:37–49.

9. Miettunen PM, Ortiz-Alvarez O, Petty RE, et al. Gender and ethnic origin have no effect on longterm outcome of childhood onset systemic lupus erythematosus. J Rheumatol 2004; 31(8):1650–4.

10. Tekano J, Tucker LB, Khattra P. Limiting obesity in children with rheumatic diseases requiring corticosteroid. Arthritis Rheum 2006; 54(Suppl. 9): Abstract.

11. Jewell ML, McCauliffe DP. Patients with cutaneous lupus erythematosus who smoke are less responsive to antimalarial treatment. J Am Acad Dermatol 2000; 42(6):983–7.

12. Ghaussy NO, Sibbitt W Jr, Bankhurst AD, Qualis CR. Cigarette smoking and disease activity in systemic lupus erythematosus. J Rheumatol 2003; 30(6): 1215–21.

13. Tucker LB, Menon S, Schaller JG, Isenberg DA. Adult- and childhood-onset systemic lupus erythematosus: a comparison of onset, clinical features, serology, and outcome. Br J Rheumatol 1995; 34(9):866–72.

14. Tucker LB, Uribe AG, Fernandez M, et al. Clinical differences between juvenile and adult onset patients with systemic lupus erythematosus (SLE): Results from a multiethnic longitudinal cohort. Arthritis Rheum 2006; 54(6):S162.

15. Carreno L, Lopez-Longo FJ, Gonzalez CM, Monteagudo I. Treatment options for juvenile-onset systemic lupus erythematosus. Pediatr Drugs 2002; 4(4): 241–56.

16. Lehman TJ. Modern treatment of childhood SLE. Clin Exp Rheumatol 2001; 19(5):487–9.

17. Blumenfeld Z, Shapiro D, Shteinberg M, Avivi I, Nahir M. Preservation of fertility and ovarian function and minimizing gonadotoxicity in young women with systemic lupus erythematosus treated by chemotherapy. Lupus 2000; 9: 401–5.

18. Somers EC, Marder W, Christman GM, Ognenovski V, McCune WJ. Use of a gonadotropin-releasing hormone analog for protection against premature ovarian failure during cyclophosphamide therapy in women with severe lupus. Arthritis Rheum 2005; 52(9):2761–7.

19. Petri M, Kim MY, Kalunian K, et al. Combined oral contraceptives in women with systemic lupus erythematosus. New Engl J Med 2005; 353(24):2550–8.

20. Cromer BA, Scholes D, Berenson A, et al. Depot medroxyprogresterone acetate and bone mineral density in adolescents — the Black Box warning: a

Position Paper of the Society for Adolescent Medicine. J Adolesc Health 2006; 39(2):296–301.

21. Silva CA, Leal MM, Leone C, et al. Gonadal function in adolescent and young women with juvenile systemic lupus erythematosus. Lupus 2002; 11: 419–25.

22. Brunner HI, Silverman ED, To T, Bombardier C, Feldman BM. Risk factors for damage in childhood-onset systemic lupus erythematosus: cumulative disease activity and medication use predict disease damage. Arthritis Rheum 2002; 46(2):436–44.

23. Lacks S, White P. Morbidity associated with childhood systemic lupus erythematosus. J Rheumatol 1990; 17(7):941–5.

24. Trapani S, Civinini R, Ermini M, Paci E, Falcini F. Osteoporosis in juvenile systemic lupus erythematosus: a longitudinal study on the effect of steroids on bone mineral density. Rheumatol Int 1998; 18(2):45–9.

25. Rouster-Stevens KA, Klein-Gitelman M. Bone health in pediatric rheumatic disease. Curr Opin Pediatr 2005; 17(6):703–8.

26. Bruce IN. 'Not only..but also': factors that contribute to accelerated atherosclerosis and premature coronary heart disease in systemic lupus erythematosus. Rheumatology (Oxford) 2005; 44(12):1492–502.

27. de Leeuw K, Freire B, Smit AJ, Bootsma H, Kallenberg CG, Bijl M. Traditional and non-traditional risk factors contribute to the development of accelerated atherosclerosis in patients with systemic lupus erythematosus. Lupus 2006; 15(10):675–82.

28. Falaschi F, Ravelli A, Martignoni A, et al. Nephrotic-range proteinuria, the major risk factor for early atherosclerosis in juvenile-onset systemic lupus erythematosus. Arthritis Rheum 2000; 43(6):1405–9.

29. Sibbitt W Jr, Brandt JR, Johnson CR, et al. The incidence and prevalence of neuropsychiatric syndromes in pediatric onset systemic lupus erythematosus. J Rheumatol 2002; 29:1536–42.

30. Wyckoff PM, Miller LC, Tucker LB, Schaller JG. Neuropsychological assessment of children and adolescents with systemic lupus erythematosus. Lupus 1995; 4:217–20.

31. Steinlin MI, Blaser SI, Gilday DL, et al. Neurologic manifestations of pediatric systemic lupus erythematosus. Pediatr Neurol 1995; 13(3):191–7.

32. Hagelberg S, Lee Y, Bargman J, et al. Longterm followup of childhood lupus nephritis. J Rheumatol 2002; 29(12):2635–42.

33. Walravens PA, Chase P. The prognosis of childhood systemic lupus erythematosus. Am J Dis Child 1976; 130:929–33.

34. Gladman DD, Urowitz MB, Goldsmith CH, et al. The reliability of the Systemic Lupus International Collaborating Clinics/American College of Rheumatology Damage Index in patients with systemic lupus erythematosus. Arthritis Rheum 1997; 40(5):809–13.

35. Gladman DD, Ginzler E, Goldsmith CH, et al. The development and initial validation of the Systemic Lupus International Collaborating Clinics/American College of Rheumatology damage index for systemic lupus erythematosus. Arthritis Rheum 1996; 39:363–9.

36. Bandeira M, Buratti S, Bartoli M, et al. Relationship between damage accrual, disease flares and cumulative drug therapies in juvenile-onset systemic lupus erythematosus. Lupus 2006; 15:515–20.
37. Ravelli A, Duarte–Salazar C, Buratti S, et al. Assessment of damage in juvenile-onset systemic lupus erythematosus: a multicenter cohort study. Arthritis Rheum 2003; 49(4):501–7.

9

Adolescent Chronic Pain

Jacqui G. Clinch

*Adolescent Pain Management Service, Royal National Hospital
for Rheumatic Diseases, Bath, U.K.*

INTRODUCTION

Pediatricians, particularly pediatric rheumatologists, review a large number of adolescents who have a wide variety of pains (1,2). Many of these pains do not have an inflammatory or other obvious disease process driving them but have a significant impact on the physical and emotional well-being of the young person and their family (2).

Unfortunately in pediatrics these patients tend to be passed from one specialist to another in order to find a cause and a cure; there can be "over-medicalization" and further increase in the pain associated disability. It is important for physicians and allied health professionals to recognize chronic pain conditions and move forward, starting appropriate treatment plans addressing physical and emotional health and also including the family.

EPIDEMIOLOGY

Epidemiological studies provide data crucial to the understanding of the etiology, natural history, impact, aggregation, and transmission of a disease or condition.

Pain is a health care problem that carries severe personal and economic consequences. The Nuprin Pain Report (3), conducted in the United States, estimated that half a billion dollars were lost directly because of pain among those employed full time. Pain in adolescents does not create the same economic hardship as adult pain, thus, to date, motivation to gain a more comprehensive understanding of pain in the adolescent population is lacking. It is, however, widely appreciated that significant numbers of adolescents who report pain go on to suffer pain and pain-associated disability in adulthood. Studies have concluded that since pain reports in childhood and early adolescence seem to be associated with the report of pain in early adulthood, more attention should be given to the way ill health is managed in the vulnerable adolescent group. (4).

It has been estimated that 15% to 25% of all children and adolescents suffer from recurrent or chronic pain conditions (5,6). A study in Germany showed that of 749 school age children, 83% had experienced pain during the preceding three months. A total of 30.8% of the children and adolescents stated that the pains had been present for over six months. Musculoskeletal pains accounted for 64% of all pain reported (7). It is widely recognized to be more common in girls (8–11) but recent studies have shown that the incidence in boys may actually be increasing (7). In a large Scandinavian study the prevalence of childhood pain was slightly higher in low-educated or low-income families compared to those of high status. Children living in low educated, low-income, worker families had approximately a 1.4-fold increased chance of having pain (9). It is generally believed that chronic pain is much more prevalent in developed countries, although there is little current research that shows this. There is, however, recognition that cultural background should certainly be taken into account when planning rehabilitation (12).

There have been some recent epidemiological studies looking at complex regional pain syndrome (CRPS). Prior to the 1970s, CRPS was seldom reported in adolescents. More recently, however, hundreds of pediatric patients have been reported (13–15). CRPS is seen most commonly around puberty although there are a few cases reported below the age of 10. CRPS type 1 is more commonly seen in girls with a ratio of 4:1 (female to male) (15). Unlike adults, the lower extremities are more commonly affected. Like the other pain conditions, CRPS 1 is seen predominantly in Caucasian populations.

ETIOLOGY AND PATHOGENESIS OF CHRONIC PAIN IN ADOLESCENTS

Idiopathic pain syndromes, in adolescents, seem to be related (either singularly or in combination) to illness, injury, psychological distress, and environmental factors (2). There is a lot of interest in the physiology of chronic pain conditions, particularly looking at the autonomic system.

Illness

In many of the diffuse pain conditions, there is a history of a preceding illness including glandular fever, tonsillitis, and influenza. Diffuse and localized chronic pains can also complicate almost any other chronic childhood illness (16) including juvenile arthritis, inflammatory bowel disease (17), cerebral palsy, cancer (18), sickle cell disease (19), muscular dystrophies (20) and cystic fibrosis (21).

It is difficult to know whether the direct infectious or inflammatory condition has effect on the evolution of chronic pain or whether the pain is a consequence of the immobility, medical therapies, environmental changes, etc. There is a strong association between joint hypermobility and diffuse pain (22).

Injury

It is not unusual for an adolescent with a localized chronic pain to recall a sporting injury, operation or other trauma around the time that the chronic pain commenced (23,24). Hypermobility has also been associated with falls and subsequent pain problems. There may often be a period of enforced immobilization; this may be an additional factor in the development of a chronic pain syndrome.

Psychosocial Factors

Although it is often tempting to cite psychosocial distress as a trigger to chronic pain in adolescents, the data are lacking (25). Undoubtedly, the pain- associated disability and the impact on lifestyle that follows has an enormous effect on psychosocial well-being (26–29).

Genetics

There is some evidence that CRPS may have a genetic predisposition (30) in Caucasian women, but the underlying genomics are far from clear. There have also been reports chronic idiopathic musculoskeletal pains in siblings (31–33) and parent-child pairs (34).

Environmental

There is often a family member who has suffered pain or disability. The social history may show a recent life event (moving house/school, illness, or death) (29,35,36). It has been reported that girls have lower pain thresholds, poor sleep patterns, and a tendency to hypermobility when compared with boys (37–39). This may, in part, explain the female preponderance in diffuse idiopathic pain (DIP).

Pathophysiological

Once more there are few data on the pathophysiology of childhood chronic pain. It has been widely postulated that, in childhood CRPS, there is either overactivity of the sympathetic nervous system or under-responsiveness of the alpha adrenergic pathways. Despite a lot of studies in adults with fibromyalgia there has been no convincing evidence to suggest a definitive pathophysiological pathway.

There is some interest in related proteomes found in adult fibro-myalgia, but this is very early pilot data (40).

Pain sensitivity varies substantially among humans. A significant part of the human population develops chronic pain conditions that are characterized by heightened pain sensitivity. A group in North Carolina recently showed that catecholamine-O-methyltransferase (COMT) activity substantially influences pain sensitivity, and the three major haplotypes determine COMT activity in humans that inversely correlates with pain sensitivity and the risk of developing a chronic pain condition. This again is early work, but it underlines the need to continue research in this area (41). There has also been interest in the preliminary findings that pain sensitivity may be higher in adolescents who were born prematurely (42).

CLINICAL PRESENTATION OF CHRONIC PAIN IN ADOLESCENTS

Pain conditions may present insidiously or acutely. Often in adolescents they follow a mild injury, operative procedure, or illness. Pains that would be expected to subside become more intrusive and disabling. In some cases these lead to severe pain associated disability and significant reduction of quality of life.

It is important to identify young people who are developing signs and symptoms attributable to a chronic pain syndrome as early as possible. This allows appropriate multidisciplinary intervention and rehabilitation.

GENERAL FEATURES OF CHRONIC PAIN

It is not unusual for the pains to start in a localized area of the body (e.g., lateral aspect of the ankle following sporting injury) (43). The pains quickly intensify and there is reluctance to mobilize. Often the painful area expands, radiating in time to involve larger areas of the body. In describing the pain, words such as "stabbing, throbbing, burning, or aching" are used. The discomfort increases and becomes constant. As the pains continue the young person shies away from using the area of body affected, this leads to muscular spasms, odd positioning or gait, and greatly reduced fitness. This in turn further amplifies the pain.

Unfortunately pain has a direct affect on other systems, leading to symptoms that can be as disabling as the pain itself. These include the following:

1. *Hypersensitivity and allodynia*: Allodynia describes a hypersensitivity that is significantly more than the initial insult would indicate. Young people describe unbearable pain with minimal skin contact. Often they

do not allow any touch and, when severe, do not wear clothing over the affected area. Some young people cannot even bear a draught.

2. *Perceived thermodysregulation*: Young people complain of feeling cold, even in warm climates. Limbs are particularly cool and mottled. Occasionally there will be areas that are very red and hot to touch on a background of the mottled skin. This mild thermodysregulation is in no way life threatening but can cause misery and be compounded by reduced movement and poor sleep. There may also be an abnormal perception of temperature (44) with an increase in thermal pain sensitivity (45).

3. *Autonomic dysfunction*: Pain is a powerful stressor. Continuous pain signals, immobility, and fatigue act directly on the autonomic system (46). In an environment of physical and emotional anxiety the sympathetic system is more active. This leads to tachycardia, hyperventilation (compounded with panic attacks), cold sweats, blurred vision, abdominal pain, and extreme pallor. Nausea, dizziness and occasional blackouts are other generalized symptoms that are not uncommon.

4. *Musculoskeletal disequilibrium*: Pain is a powerful sensation that stops us from moving or touching an affected area. When a painful limb is not moved, the brain has an altered image of that area. Proprioceptive signals from the joints are reduced and the limb is held in a rigid, fixed position. It is not unusual for legs to "give way," knees and hips to be held flexed, feet to be inverted and hands clenched with flexed wrists. These positions are often described as the most comfortable. Unfortunately muscles and tendons quickly tighten, and this complicates the pain and disability. One must also remember that these young people are still growing, often in their peripubertal growth spurt, and this can have dire effects on the final positioning.

Back pain, particularly lower lumber and cervical pain, commonly complicates chronic pain conditions where the pains start are elsewhere. The adaptive positioning of a young person with leg or abdominal pains particularly affect the gait and resting positions and thus alter the loads on the spine and pelvis.

During pain flares young people may describe blurred vision, nausea, dizziness, blackouts, hyperacusis, and extreme cold. Conversion symptoms such as paralysis, blindness, loss of speech (or hoarse voice), or bizarre gaits are also not uncommon in this population.

Classification of Chronic Pain Syndromes

While chronic pain and pain-associated disability can complicate any chronic illness, there are certain pain syndromes that are recognized in children. These have been mentioned previously.

Diffuse Idiopathic Pain Syndromes (Juvenile Fibromyalgia)

The onset of pain in diffuse idiopathic pain (DIP) syndromes (47) is often gradual. There may have been an initial insult (infection) or hypermobility (22), but there is often no obvious trigger and vague recollections of the time of onset. The pain, as suggested, is generalized. There may be areas of allodynia, but there is often an absence of the autonomic changes that we see in more localized pain conditions (2). What is striking in the young people with diffuse pain is the fatigue, poor sleep pattern, and extremely low mood (48). It is widely believed, however, that the low moods in adolescents are reactive (to the pain-associated disability) rather than a primary depression. This is in contrast to adults with fibromyalga, where primary depression is frequently seen. This distinction is important when looking at rehabilitation and prognosis in these two populations (49). There are no DIP criteria for adolescents so the American College of Rheumatology criteria for adult fibromyalgia are still referred to. This has to be used with a little caution (48), not only because the outcome in adolescents is so much better but also there has been no definitive work looking specifically at tender points on children.

Localized Idiopathic Pain Syndrome, Including Complex
Regional Pain Syndromes

Localized idiopathic pain syndrome simply describes pain that remains in a localized area (such as a limb). Within this descriptive diagnostic group are the complex regional pain syndromes (CRPS 1 or reflex sympathetic dystrophy).

The diagnosis of CRPS 1 remains a clinical one. There is often a precipitating trauma (not always). The pain should be out of proportion to the inciting event and usually accompanied by allodynia. Autonomic changes are present; these include swelling, reduced cutaneous perfusion, and thermodynamic instability. There is also a marked reduction in range of movement and, in severe cases, trophic changes. In adolescents the legs are more commonly affected. The International Association for the Study of Pain (IASP) has diagnostic criteria for adults with CRPS (Table 1). Although these diagnostic criteria hold true for children and adolescents, it is widely believed that the dystrophic changes and long term disability are less common when compared with adults.

Occasionally more than one limb may be affected at presentation. It is not unusual for a hand or other leg to develop CRPS months after a leg has been affected. This may be due to the use of crutches and subsequent pain amplification but may also have no obvious trigger. Young people with CRPS may also develop low mood and overwhelming fatigue. This further complicates the clinical picture.

Table 1 International Association for the Study of Pain (IASP) Diagnostic
Criteria for Complex Regional Pain Syndrome

Presence of an initiating noxious event, or cause of immobilization
Continuing pain, allodynia, or hyperalgesia with which the pain is disproportionate
  to any inciting event
Evidence at some time of edema, changes in skin blood flow, or abnormal sudomotor
  activity in the region of the pain
This diagnosis is excluded by the existence of conditions that would otherwise
  account for the degree of pain and dysfunction
Type I: Without evidence of major nerve damage
Type II: With evidence of major nerve damage

Source: Adapted from Ref. 78.

Although the emphasis in this text is on pain syndromes, it must not be
forgotten that chronic pain can complicate any other musculoskeletal diseases, including JIA, muscular dystrophies, and dysplasias.

If the chronic pain condition is not recognized and treated, many of
these adolescents develop associated disabilities that continue into adult life.
They are unable to continue education; peer relationships fall away; family
life remains disrupted/dysfunctional; and physical and emotional well-being
is lost. Chronic fatigue and secondary depression become as disabling as
the pain.

THE IMPACT OF ADOLESCENT PAIN ON QUALITY OF LIFE

Recurring episodes of chronic pain often have a major impact on the daily
lives of adolescents and their families. Not only does the pain have a direct
affect on physical function but also on sleep, mood, appetite, social interaction, hobbies, and education. It is essential that that any planned rehabilitation takes these factors into account, concentrating solely on the pain is
often futile.

In the Roth-Isigkeit study, 54% of adolescents who reported pain also
had problems with sleep and appetite, 49% had long-term absences from
school and 47% were unable to meet friends (7). A separate outpatient
survey showed that 72% suffered impairment in sports activities, 51%
reported absence from school, 40% experienced limitations in social functioning, and 34% had problems with sleeping (77). Sleep disorders with
frequent nocturnal arousals or daytime somnolence are common in children
suffering juvenile rheumatoid arthritis (76); similar sleep disturbances
are seen in adolescents with chronic pain. In the German cohort study,
41% of the young people reported sleep disturbances attributable to pain.
This significantly increased with age. Restrictions at school, absenteeism,
and problems with school activities are widely reported in this population.

Key Areas Affected by Persistent Pain in Adolescents

As the pain continues the young person can quickly develop a pain-associated disability (Fig. 1) where there is deterioration in many aspects of quality of life.

Fatigue

Fatigue in any pain condition can be overwhelming. Continual pain, sleeplessness, and reduced fitness all contribute to an associated chronic fatigue problem.

Sleep

Sleep disturbances among adolescents affect many areas of their lives, including school attendance and performance, emotional state, and relationships with family members and friends. Initially, constant pain is the main factor in an adolescent's poor sleep pattern. Positioning in the bed is difficult and, with no distractions, the pain intensity increases. Over time the young person also has reduced physical activity in the day and a marked lowering of mood. These two elements are key in further deterioration of the sleep routine. The time getting to sleep gets later and there are frequent episodes of wakefulness throughout the night. It is not uncommon for a young person to fall asleep at 3 a.m. and to wake each hour following this. Catnapping in the day compounds this problem.

Activity

As pain continues the amount of physical activity that a young person can engage in reduces substantially. Previously fit, often competitive,

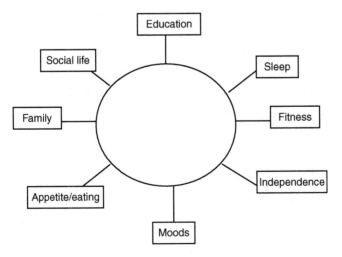

Figure 1   Pain-associated disability.

adolescents stop all sports and recreational activities, eventually becoming housebound.

Moods

The majority of young people with ongoing pain will develop a low mood. A small but important minority of these will go on to develop a secondary depression. This is not only due to the ongoing pain but also the deterioration in quality-of-life with an increasing dependence. Parents may report introversion, swinging moods, or outbursts of uncontrollable anger. Motivation for rehabilitation can reduce and communication difficult. Rarely, there is a "la belle indifference" where the young person is outwardly cheerful and unconcerned, despite a severe pain condition.

Education

Pain has considerable effect on concentration and memory. Adolescents find it difficult to retain facts and to remain attentive in lessons. Sitting for long periods increases discomfort and mobilizing around large secondary schools is often impossible. Multiple hospital appointments further reduce school attendance. In many cases the young person stops going to school. Home tuition may be instigated; this too depends on the young person's ability to participate.

Independence

Adolescence is a time of fierce independence. Chronic pain conditions markedly curtail this freedom as the young person relies totally on carers for tasks that were previously done with ease. Mobility, eating, toileting, and dressing may all need external help. This has an enormous impact on the emotional well-being of the young person.

Social Structure

As education and independence suffers so the peer relationships and social integration falls away. Previously popular young people become introverted and unwilling to communicate with friends and colleagues. Friendship groups can be challenging at this age for those who are well and at school full time—it is so much harder if you have a condition that is difficult to label and explain. Friends often stop making contact and move on.

Family

Chronic pain can cause enormous upheaval even in the most functional families. Initially there are the hospital visits and uncertainty about diagnosis. Parents lose time off work and it is not unusual for one parent to stop working completely. There have been a number of studies looking at parental stress and anxiety and affect on family function, perceived disability, and rehabilitation that show conclusively the importance of addressing these areas (70). Holidays, activities, socializing, and plans are all affected by adolescent pain. Siblings may feel neglected and anxious. Other relatives may become distant or overbearing.

There is a common misconception that chronic pain is only found in families that are, in some ways, dysfunctional. Most family units are, premorbidly, functioning normally. Ongoing pain has catastrophic effects on these families that can lead to overwhelming anxiety and breakdown of structure.

Future

Cruelly chronic pain often affects adolescents who are very able and highly functioning. Future goals become seemingly unattainable and motivation quickly disappears.

The pain increases beyond that expected from the original insult and the young person becomes gradually more disabled. Pain in adolescents and children creates understandable anxiety in families and medical arenas. This concern leads to frequent medical visits, investigations, and therapies.

ASSESSMENT OF AN ADOLESCENT WITH CHRONIC PAIN

As with all medical conditions, it is essential that a thorough history and examination is undertaken. Occasionally, what appears to be a chronic pain syndrome is part of another disease process that needs further investigation and directed medical therapy.

It is widely recognized that early assessment, targeted investigations, and multidisciplinary rehabilitation is key for returning these adolescents back to a more appropriate lifestyle.

The assessment should take place in a suitable environment and appropriate time set aside. Ideally a member of the multidisciplinary team should also be present. Several studies have shown that it is important to have key family members present during the assessment and periods of therapy. Parents' anxiety and perception of their child's disability has a direct effect on rehabilitation and the child's view of his/her condition.

Important Aspects of the History

1. Onset and characteristics of pain
2. Other symptoms
3. Effect of pain on quality of life (activities, sleep, etc.)
4. Past history—pain or other symptoms/illnesses
5. Family, emotional, and social circumstances

A thorough history is needed to ensure there is no other disease process occurring (Table 2). It is also important to gain insight into how the pain condition is affecting the young person's quality of life and the lives of family members (Fig. 1). The pain associated disability (from both young person and parent perspective) can be evaluated once the full medical evaluation has been completed.

Table 2   Assessment of the Adolescent with Chronic Pain: Important Aspects of the History

History
    Onset of pain
        When did the pain start?
        Was there a preceding infection, trauma or operation?
        Did it start gradually or suddenly?
        Where did it start?
    Characteristics of the pain
        Has the pain spread from original place?
        How would you describe the pain?
        How severe is the pain on a good day and on a bad day?
        Do you suffer pins and needles?
        Is the pain constant?
        Has the pain gotten any better or worse?
        Is there variation in the pain during the day?
        Does the pain alter at night? Does it wake you up?
        What makes it worse?
        What makes it better?
        Is it painful to lightly touch the area that is painful?
        Does that area look unusual?
    Other symptoms
        Is there a fever, rash, or weight loss?
        Has menstruation altered?
        Is there altered bowel habit?
        Do you have nausea?
        Do you suffer abdominal pain?
        Is there any muscle weakness?
        Do you have any areas that are numb?
        Do you suffer dizziness?
        Have you passed out or suddenly fallen to the floor?
        Is fatigue a problem?
        Do you suffer headaches/migraines?
        Do you feel colder/warmer than previously?
        Do you suffer from blurred vision?
        Has your mood been affected?

(*Continued*)

Table 2 Assessment of the Adolescent with Chronic Pain: Important Aspects of the History (*Continued*)

Effect of pain on daily living
    How is your sleep?
    Do you find it hard to get to sleep/stay asleep?
    Do you "catnap" in the day?
    What can you do on a "bad" day?
    What can you do on a "good" day?
    How much school have you managed over the past 6 months?
    How is your concentration/memory?
    On "bad days" how is your mood?
    On "good days" how is your mood?
    How has the pain affected your fitness?
    How has the pain affected your hobbies?
    Do you need help in areas where you were previously independent? Where?
    How has this affected your family?
    What do you think is causing this? Do you have fears about a particular illness?
    Do the parents have fears concerning the pain that they feel has not
    been addressed?
Past and family history of illness
    Have you suffered painful conditions previously?
    Have you suffered fatigue, sleeplessness, or anxiety previously?
    Any operations or illnesses as a younger child?
    Have any family members suffered illness?
    Is there a family history of painful conditions?
Family, emotional, and social circumstances
    Who currently lives at home?
    What are the occupations of the main carers?
    Have one or both carers changed/stopped their job since the pain
    condition started?
    Can you identify any stressors in school, family, or peer groups?

Important Aspects of Physical Examination

This should be thorough. It is important that the physician is confident with the diagnosis and is not concerned about other disease processes as a cause of the pain. Time spent at this stage may prevent repetition and unnecessary, distressing investigations at a later date. The list of differential diagnoses with any pain condition is long. An example of differential diagnoses of musculoskeletal pain is given in Table 3. A good history and examination will exclude most of these. If, however, there is concern, this is the time to order all investigations and ensure that these are followed up. Undue delay leads to catastrophization and often a worsening of pain symptoms and associated disability.

Table 3 Diagnostic Possibilities for Musculoskeletal Pain in Adolescents (Not Exhaustive!)

Lower limb
    Localized idiopathic pain syndrome
    Chronic regional pain syndrome type 1 (reflex sympathetic dystrophy)
    Chronic regional pain syndrome type 2
Hip
    Slipped femoral epiphysis
    Transient synovitis
    Spondyloarthropathy
Knee
    Arthritis (knee or radiating from hip)
    Osgood-Schlatter disease
    Chondromalacia
    Discoid meniscus
    Osteochondritis
Ankle and foot
    Enthesitis
    Arthritis
    Osteochondritis dissecans of talus
    Sever's disease
    Tarsal coalition
Upper limb
    Localized idiopathic pain syndrome
    Chronic regional pain syndrome type 1
    Chronic regional pain syndrome type 2
Shoulder
    Dislocation
    Transient synovitis
    Rotator cuff injury
Elbow
    "Pulled elbow"
    Arthritis
Wrist and hand
    Arthritis
    Raynaud's disease
    Erythromelalgia
Back
    Ankylosing spondylitis
    Spondylolysis
    Scheuermann's disease
    Osteomyelitis
    Hyperlordosis (with hypermobility)
Fractures, malignancies, and systemic illnesses can also present with localized
    musculoskeletal pain

Source: Adapted from Ref. 79.

Assessing the Impact of Pain

Pain has direct and indirect impact on a young person's life. It also impacts on the lives of those close to them. It is not easy to get a full picture of this pain- associated disability in a time-limited consultation.

The "pain spider" is a useful way to engage adolescents and gain insight into their lifestyle (Fig. 2). This is constructed with them during the assessment and they should be asked to highlight areas that are particularly difficult.

It is essential that there is also an understanding of the effect this situation has had on the family. Parental anxiety and their perception of their child's pain will have an effect on the rehabilitation plan.

Specific Pain Measures for Adolescents

Pain is a complex, subjective sensation that is influenced by many factors. Pain intensity has long been measured using the Visual Analogue Scale (50). This gives a subjective measure of the pain intensity according to the adolescent and/or that pain perceived by their carer. This is a 10-cm horizontal line anchored by "no pain" at the far left and "worst pain" at the right hand end. The young person marks where he or she feels the level of their pain is. While these are useful measures prospectively they give no indication of the impact of pain on the young person's life. For example, one adolescent with a pain score of 7 on the visual analogue scale (VAS) may

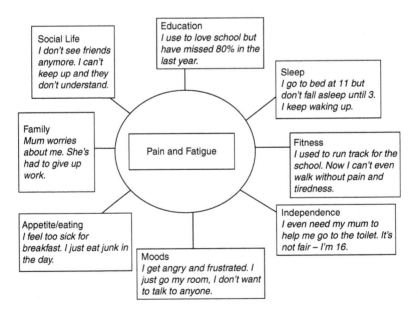

Figure 2   The pain spider.

still get to school where another adolescent with the same score may not be getting out of bed.

Multidimensional Pain Measures

The most frequently used multidimensional pain measure in pediatric rheumatology is the Varni/Thompson Pediatric Pain Questionnaire (51).

Recently, however, the Bath Adolescent Pain Questionnaire has been developed (52). This is a validated multidimensional measure that evaluates the impact of pain on a young person's life. It includes anxiety, disability, mood/ depression, somatomization, and sleep disorder. From this measure it is possible to specifically direct rehabilitation and prospectively monitor progress.

Physiological Measures of Pain

There is very little data on the role of physiological measures in assessing pain in adolescents. The role of thermography in CRPS has been studied (53), really evaluating its use in the early and late stages of this pain condition. Bone scintigraphy has also been looked at, the interest here is that in many adolescents with CRPS there is reduced uptake compared to the increased uptake that is seen in adult CRPS (54). Opinion is divided in the usefulness of both these measures in this condition.

Re-evaluation

It is important that a physician reevaluates the young person and family as soon as all the results of any investigations that have been undertaken have returned. During this second consultation any other differential diagnoses can be put to one side (assuming all appropriate investigations are normal) and other fears that the family may have had talked through (it is not uncommon for parents to worry about cancer or other life-threatening illnesses causing the ongoing pain). This in turn reduces catastrophization. At this stage the consultation can move onto pain education and begin to plan rehabilitation. If possible it is invaluable to share the consultation with an allied health professional that is part of the rehabilitation team.

PAIN EDUCATION

In order to move forward with rehabilitation it is essential that the adolescent and family have an understanding of chronic pain. This is a very difficult concept for many individuals to understand (including professionals) as there is a belief that pain is always a warning sign that a disease process or abnormality is present. There is a need for the young person and family to find a cause, and often skepticism from health professionals that the pains are present at all. During the consultation it is initially important to investigate what thoughts the family and the young person have about the cause of the pains. There are often fears that an undiagnosed condition such as cancer is triggering the discomfort. No family will move forward with pain education or future rehabilitation until these fears are allayed.

Essentially the team need to show and reinforce to the family the fact that many pains are not useful. It is helpful to give common examples of non-useful pain. Headaches are extremely common but very rarely due to conditions such as brain tumors or vascular events. Back pain is one of the most common presentations to general practitioners. But, again, very rarely does this signify malignancy or arthritis.

It is also useful to illustrate to families how complicated pain physiology is and how little is understood. Phantom limb pain is familiar to many—why, after a painful limb is amputated, do the pains remain, as severe as they were when the limb was present? Not only are the pains still present but they are in exactly the same place. This can lead onto an explanation of pain memory and amplification.

The young person will often be experiencing the pain-related symptoms and signs mentioned earlier in this chapter. By explaining that nausea, dizziness, blurred vision, sudden falls etc are all related to the pain effects the health professionals will not only educate but also alleviate some of the fears that other conditions are coexisting.

Analgesics are often unhelpful in chronic pain conditions. The adolescent may have tried a variety of nonsteroidals, codeine preparations, and/or opioids with no lasting effect. This can be confusing. An explanation that chronic pain conditions (whether directly related to disease, e.g., cancer or not) are notoriously difficult to treat should be given. For reasons that are unclear, the pains may be initially held but then breakthrough. This can be devastating both physically and emotionally.

From this point, one can move on to show how pain and the associated disability can amplify. An example is leg pain. If a young person has pain in an ankle then he/she is reluctant to move it. Over time this stiffens and the pain increases with smaller movements. The skin becomes hypersensitive. Weight bearing is difficult and the leg is held in an awkward position. This puts strain on the upper leg and hip. These in turn become painful and immobilized. The other leg takes more weight and becomes increasingly sore. Lower lumbar pain sets in as the pelvis is tilted. Sitting and standing become uncomfortable. By this stage sleeping is affected and fatigue increases. Other pain associated symptoms may develop. Activities drop off and mood lowers. The young person and their family will identify with this downward spiral.

It is important that they understand that slow, consistent physical and emotional rehabilitation is essential despite the pain—akin to re-educating the whole body. This approach has been shown to be successful. By introducing psychology in this way the family will hopefully understand the importance of emotional rehabilitation in chronic conditions.

In some cases of CRPS early, intensive physiotherapy may be appropriate (15) and this may be discussed.

At this stage, having answered as many questions as appropriate, one should be in a position to plan multidisciplinary rehabilitation.

REHABILITATING AN ADOLESCENT WITH CHRONIC PAIN

One of the most important aspects of rehabilitation is that of inclusion. A dedicated team that works consistently with the adolescent and the family will facilitate communication and enable goals to be reached earlier (47,55,56).

It is essential that the young person is worked up medically to ensure no ongoing disease process or trauma is present (57). If the pain is coexisting with a known illness, it is important that this is as stable as possible before rehabilitation. Once the attending physician has finished investigations then these should be explained fully to the family and young person. It is often difficult to show that investigations are normal when the pain is ongoing and a repeat consultation may be needed.

Medical Therapies

The number of analgesics and interventions used is a sign that there are no well controlled therapeutic trials in the arena of childhood chronic pain. It is becoming widely accepted, however, that any analgesic intervention should be alongside multidisciplinary therapy (58–61). It is unusual for analgesia to work alone.

Oral treatments that have been used, with variable success, include tricyclic antidepressants, nonsteroidals, opioids, anticonvulsants and glucocorticoids (62,63). Sympathetic blocks (64), TENS (23) and botulinum injections have been used in localized pain (62). In some centers spinal stimulation are also advocated. Complementary therapies are commonly utilized by patients with chronic pain (65). The evidence supporting many of these therapies in children and adolescents is poor (66) but many young adults find certain therapies such as acupuncture, massage and aromatherapy helpful.

Multidisciplinary Approach

The aim of treatment is to enable the young person to return to age appropriate activities and lifestyle. Ideally this would be pain free but, in many cases, this is initially with the pain. Physiotherapists, occupational therapists and psychologists (67–69) are key players in the team. They will be the primary professionals supporting the young person and the family. The physician is there to provide support if needed, occasional analgesic advice and very rarely, direct intervention. In some conditions, such as CRPS, intensive physiotherapy may be given for a set period of time (15).

The aim of this is accelerated mobilization (70). Many cases of diffuse pain will require a gentle, paced approach. In all cases the increase of activity should be consistent despite the pain. With musculoskeletal pains the more active the musculoskeletal system becomes, the more likely the muscle spasms and tightening are to reduce. Proprioception improves and autonomic changes subside. Where possible adolescents should work to devise their own "fitness plan." Fun games can be included with an aim to return gradually to activities the young person used to enjoy. Using a local gym rather than a hospital physiotherapy gym allows them to start to return to a more normal environment (71).

Working in this consistent, paced manner is extremely hard for the young person and their parents. The pain invariably continues at the beginning (if not throughout) and motivation is poor. Parental anxiety is high (72) and there is a fear that damage will be done. Psychological support during this time is key. The young person will need help setting goals, learning how to communicate pain to peers and family, keeping up motivation on "bad days," managing low mood, dealing with anger and frustration and overcoming fears. Often they have not been at school for a long period of time and need help in preparing again for this difficult environment. In some cases there may be other mental health needs that can be identified and appropriately treated. Relaxation, advice on sleep and eating and advice on how to pace other areas of life can all be given by members of the team.

In our experience it is essential that parents are included in this rehabilitation. We have shown that parental stress and anxiety can reduce the impact of any treatment plan. Parents often perceive their child as very disabled; there is a fear that any physical activity or intervention will lead to further pain and damage (72). It is important that they are able to see their child become functionally less disabled. They will need a great deal of emotional support but, as the rehabilitation plan continues, they will actually start to facilitate further improvement. An aim of treatment is to reduce the impact of pain on the whole family's life, not just that of the child.

Ideally most of the ongoing rehabilitation can be carried out by the young person and family and the input from the health care professionals gradually reduce.

OUTCOME

The natural history of chronic pain in children shows that, in many cases, outcome is improved compared to that in adults (73–75). It has been shown that early, multidisciplinary input (including cognitive behavioral therapy) has favorable outcome. In our outcome study we showed that the "back to school" rate significantly improved after an intensive, residential, multidisciplinary programme (71), as did functional ability, anxiety (parents and young person) and mood.

CRPSs in children have a favorable prognosis if early physiotherapy is initiated (with psychological support) (15). A prolonged time to treatment and the presence of marked autonomic changes are not good prognostic indicators. Relapses of pain are relatively common but, in our experience, if the young person and his/her family recognize the onset of similar pains and put into practice the physical and emotional strategies that have previously been taught, the impact of the pains can be significantly reduced. In some cases, despite a variety of interventions, the impact of pain remains disabling on the young person and family. We do not yet have prognostic indicators to show us, at initial assessment, how to identify this very small, but complex group.

REFERENCES

1. Sherry DD. Pain syndromes in children. Curr Rheumatol Rep 2000; 2(4): 337–42.
2. Malleson P, Clinch J. Pain syndromes in children. Curr Opin Rheumatol 2003; 15(5):572–80.
3. Sternbach RA. Pain and 'hassles' in the United States: findings of the Nuprin pain report. Pain 1986; 27(1):69–80.
4. Brattberg G. Do pain problems in young school children persist into early adulthood? A 13-year follow-up. Eur J Pain 2004; 8(3):187–99.
5. Jones GT, Silman AJ, MacFarlane GJ. Predicting the onset of widespread body pain in children. Arthritis Rheum 2003; 48:2615–21.
6. Perquin CW, Hazebroek-Kampschreur AA, Hunfeld JA, et al. Pain in children and adolescents: a common experience. Pain 2000; 87(1):51–8.
7. Roth-Isigkeit A, Thyen U, Stoven H, Schwarzenberger J, Schmucker P. Pain among children and adolescents: restrictions in daily living and triggering factors. Pediatrics 2005; 115:152–62.
8. Lamberg L. Girls' and boys' differing response to pain starts early in their lives. J Am Med Assoc 1998; 280(12):1035–6.
9. Groholt EK, Stigum H, Nordhagen R, Kohler L. Recurrent pain in children, socio-economic factors and accumulation in families. Eur J Epidemiol, 2003; 18 (10):965–75.
10. Brattberg G. The incidence of back pain and headache among Swedish school children. Qual Life Res 1994; 3(Suppl. 1):S27–31.
11. Smedbraten BK, Natvig B, Rutle O, Bruusgaard D. Self-reported bodily pain in schoolchildren. Scand J Rheumatol, 1998; 27(4):273–6.
12. Bates MS, Edwards WT. Ethnic variations in the chronic pain experience. Ethn Dis 1992; 2(1):63–83.
13. Bernstein BH, Singsen BH, Kent JT, et al. Reflex neurovascular dystrophy in childhood. J Pediatr 1978; 93(2):211–5.
14. Murray CS, Cohen A, Perkins T, Davison JE, Sills JA. Morbidity in reflex sympathetic dystrophy. Arch Dis Child 2000; 82(3):231–3.
15. Sherry DD, Wallace CA, Kelley C, Kidder M, Sapp L. Short- and long-term outcomes of children with complex regional pain syndrome type I treated with exercise therapy. Clin J Pain 1999; 15(3):218–23.

16. Varni JW, Walco GA. Chronic and recurrent pain associated with pediatric chronic diseases. Issues Compr Pediatr Nurs 1988; 11(2–3):145–58.

17. Buskila D, Odes LR, Neumann L, Odes HS. Fibromyalgia in inflammatory bowel disease. J Rheumatol 1999; 26(5):1167–71.

18. Jay SM, Elliott C, Varni JW. Acute and chronic pain in adults and children with cancer. J Consult Clin Psychol 1986; 54(5):601–7.

19. Stinson J, Naser B. Pain management in children with sickle cell disease. Paediatr Drugs 2003; 5(4):229–41.

20. Engel JM, Kartin D, Jaffe KM. Exploring chronic pain in youths with Duchenne Muscular Dystrophy: a model for pediatric neuromuscular disease. Phys Med Rehabil Clin N Am 2005; 16(4):1113–24, xii.

21. Ravilly S, Robinson W, Suresh S, Wohl ME, Berde CB. Chronic pain in cystic fibrosis. Pediatrics 1996; 98(4 Pt 1):741–7.

22. Gedalia A, Press J, Klein M, et al. Joint hypermobility and fibromyalgia in schoolchildren. Ann Rheum Dis 1993; 52(7):494–6.

23. Ashwal S, Tomasi L, Neumann M, Schenider S. Reflex sympathetic dystrophy syndrome in children. Pediatr Neurol 1988; 4(1):38–42.

24. Kristjansdottir G, Rhee H. Risk factors of back pain frequency in school-children: a search for explanations to a public health problem. Acta Paediatr 2002; 91(7):849–54.

25. Ciccone DS, Bandilla EB, Wu W. Psychological dysfunction in patients with reflex sympathetic dystrophy. Pain 1997; 71(3):323–33.

26. Sherry DD, Weisman R. Psychologic aspects of childhood reflex neurovascular dystrophy. Pediatrics 1988; 81(4):572–8.

27. Pillemer FG, Micheli LJ. Psychological considerations in youth sports. Clin Sports Med 1988; 7(3):679–89.

28. Aasland A, Flato B, Vandvik IH. Psychosocial factors in children with idiopathic musculoskeletal pain: a prospective, longitudinal study. Acta Paediatr 1997; 86(7):740–6.

29. Greene JW, Walker LS, Hickson G, Thompson J. Stressful life events and somatic complaints in adolescents. Pediatrics 1985; 75(1):19–22.

30. Mailis A, Wade J. Profile of Caucasian women with possible genetic predisposition to reflex sympathetic dystrophy: a pilot study. Clin J Pain 1994; 10(3):210–7.

31. Bruscas Izu, C, Beltran Audera CH, Jimenez Zorzo F. Polytopic and recurrent reflex sympathetic dystrophy in lower limbs in two siblings. Ann Med Int 2004; 21(4):183–4.

32. Postacchini F, Lami R, Pugliese O. Familial predisposition to discogenic low-back pain. An epidemiologic and immunogenetic study. Spine 1988; 13(12):1403–6.

33. Rush PJ, Wilmot D, Saunders N, et al. Severe reflex neurovascular dystrophy in childhood. Arthritis Rheum 1985; 28(8):952–6.

34. Buskila D, Neumann L, Hazanov I, Carmi R. Familial aggregation in the fibromyalgia syndrome. Semin Arthritis Rheum 1996; 26(3):605–11.

35. Imbierowicz K, Egle UT. Childhood adversities in patients with fibromyalgia and somatoform pain disorder. Eur J Pain 2003; 7(2):113–9.

36. Lampe A, Doering S, Rumpold G, et al. Chronic pain syndromes and their relation to childhood abuse and stressful life events. J Psychosom Res 2003; 54(4):361–7.
37. Ostensen M, Rugelsjoen A, Wigers SH. The effect of reproductive events and alterations of sex hormone levels on the symptoms of fibromyalgia. Scand J Rheumatol 1997; 26(5):355–60.
38. Seng JS, Graham-Bermann SA, Clark MK, et al. Posttraumatic stress disorder and physical comorbidity among female children and adolescents: results from service-use data. Pediatrics 2005; 116(6):e767–76.
39. Arnow BA, Hart S, Hayward C, et al. Severity of child maltreatment, pain complaints and medical utilization among women. J Psychiatr Res 2000; 34(6): 413–21.
40. Baraniuk JN, Casado B, Maibach H, et al. A Chronic Fatigue Syndrome-related proteome in human cerebrospinal fluid. BMC Neurol 2005; 5:22.
41. Diatchenko L, Slade GD, Nackley AG, et al. Genetic basis for individual variations in pain perception and the development of a chronic pain condition. Hum Mol Genet 2005; 14(1):135–43.
42. Buskila D, Neumann L, Zmora E, et al. Pain sensitivity in prematurely born adolescents. Arch Pediatr Adolesc Med 2003; 157(11):1079–82.
43. Buskila D, Neumann L. Musculoskeletal injury as a trigger for fibromyalgia/posttraumatic fibromyalgia. Curr Rheumatol Rep 2000; 2(2):104–8.
44. Gibson SJ, Littlejohn GO, Gorman MM, et al. Altered heat pain thresholds and cerebral event-related potentials following painful CO_2 laser stimulation in subjects with fibromyalgia syndrome. Pain 1994; 58(2):185–93.
45. Geisser ME, Casey KL, Brucksch CB, et al. Perception of noxious and innocuous heat stimulation among healthy women and women with fibromyalgia: association with mood, somatic focus, and catastrophizing. Pain 2003; 102(3):243–50.
46. Cohen H, Neumann L, Kotler M, Buskila D. Autonomic nervous system derangement in fibromyalgia syndrome and related disorders. Isr Med Assoc J 2001; 3(10):755–60.
47. Malleson PN, Connell H, Bennett SM, et al. Chronic musculoskeletal and other idiopathic pain syndromes. Arch Dis Child 2001; 84(3):189–92.
48. Buskila D. Fibromyalgia in children–lessons from assessing nonarticular tenderness. J Rheumatol 1996; 23(12):2017–9.
49. Buskila D, Neumann L, Hershman E, et al. Fibromyalgia syndrome in children–an outcome study. J Rheumatol 1995; 22(3):525–8.
50. Carlsson AM. Assessment of chronic pain. I. Aspects of the reliability and validity of the visual analogue scale. Pain 1983; 16(1):87–101.
51. Varni JW, Thompson KL, Hanson V. The Varni/Thompson Pediatric Pain Questionnaire. I. Chronic musculoskeletal pain in juvenile rheumatoid arthritis. Pain 1987; 28(1):27–38.
52. Eccleston C, Jordan A, McCracken LM, et al. The Bath Adolescent Pain Questionnaire (BAPQ): development and preliminary psychometric evaluation of an instrument to assess the impact of chronic pain on adolescents. Pain 2005; 118(1–2):263–70.

53. Lightman HI, Pochaczevsky R, Aprin H, Ilowite NT. Thermography in childhood reflex sympathetic dystrophy. J Pediatr 1987; 111(4):551–5.

54. Goldsmith DP, Vivino FB, Eichenfield AH, et al. Nuclear imaging and clinical features of childhood reflex neurovascular dystrophy: comparison with adults. Arthritis Rheum, 1989. 32(4):p. 480–5.

55. Christie D, Wilson C. CBT in paediatric and adolescent health settings: a review of practice-based evidence. Pediatr Rehabil 2005; 8(4):241–7.

56. Aitkenhead S. Managing chronic pain in children. Nurs Times 2001; 97(29): 34–5.

57. Kain ZN, Rimar S. Management of chronic pain in children. Pediatr Rev 1995; 16(6):218–22.

58. McGrath PA. An assessment of children's pain: a review of behavioral, physiological and direct scaling techniques. Pain 1987; 31(2):147–76.

59. Stanton-Hicks M, Baron R, Boas R, et al. Complex Regional Pain Syndromes: guidelines for therapy. Clin J Pain 1998; 14(2):155–66.

60. Shapiro BS. Treatment of chronic pain in children and adolescents. Pediatr Ann 1995; 24(3):148–50, 153–6.

61. Kashikar-Zuck S. Treatment of children with unexplained chronic pain. Lancet 2006; 367(9508):380–2.

62. Gordon N. Reflex sympathetic dystrophy. Brain Dev 1996; 18(4):257–62.

63. Eland JM. Pharmacologic management of acute and chronic pediatric pain. Issues Compr Pediatr Nurs 1988; 11(2–3):93–111.

64. Mailis A, Furlan A. Sympathectomy for neuropathic pain. Cochrane Database Syst Rev 2003(2):CD002918.

65. Carter B. Complementary therapies and management of chronic pain. Paediatr Nurs 1995; 7(3):18–22.

66. Tsao JC, Zeltzer LK. Complementary and Alternative Medicine Approaches for Pediatric Pain: A Review of the State-of-the-science. Evid Based Complement Alternat Med 2005; 2(2):149–59.

67. Eccleston C, Morley S, Williams A, et al. Systematic review of randomised controlled trials of psychological therapy for chronic pain in children and adolescents, with a subset meta-analysis of pain relief. Pain 2002; 99(1–2): 157–65.

68. Crombez G, Bijttebier P, Ecceleston C, et al. The child version of the pain catastrophizing scale (PCS-C): a preliminary validation. Pain 2003; 104(3): 639–46.

69. Walco GA, Ilowite NT. Cognitive-behavioral intervention for juvenile primary fibromyalgia syndrome. J Rheumatol 1992; 19(10):1617–9.

70. Littlejohn GO. Reflex sympathetic dystrophy in adolescents: lessons for adults. Arthritis Rheum 2004; 51(2):151–3.

71. Eccleston C, Malleson P, Clinch J, et al. Chronic pain in adolescents: evaluation of a programme of interdisciplinary cognitive behaviour therapy. Arch Dis Child 2003; 88(10):881–5.

72. Eccleston C, Crombez G, Scotford A, et al. Adolescent chronic pain: patterns and predictors of emotional distress in adolescents with chronic pain and their parents. Pain 2004; 108(3):221–9.

73. Ledingham J, Doherty S, Doherty M. Primary fibromyalgia syndrome–an outcome study. Br J Rheumatol 1993; 32(2):139–42.
74. Gedalia A, Garcia CO, Molina JF, et al. Fibromyalgia syndrome: experience in a pediatric rheumatology clinic. Clin Exp Rheumatol 2000; 18(3):415–9.
75. Krilov LR, Fisher M, Friedman SB, et al. Course and outcome of chronic fatigue in children and adolescents. Pediatrics 1998; 102(2 Pt 1):360–6.
76. Bloom BJ, Owens JA, McGuinn M, et al. Sleep and its relationship to pain, dysfunction, and disease activity in juvenile rheumatoid arthritis. J Rheumatol 2002; 29(1):169–73.
77. Konijnenberg AY, Uiterwaal CS, Kimpen JL, et al. Children with unexplained chronic pain: substantial impairment in everyday life. Arch Dis Child 2005; 90(7):680–6.
78. Merskey H, Bogduk N. Classification of Chronic Pain: Descriptions of Chronic Pain Syndromes and Definitions of Pain Terms. 2nd ed. Seattle: IASP Press, 1994.
79. Sherry DD, Malleson PN. Idiopathic Musculoskeletal Pain Syndromes Nonrheumatic Musculoskeletal Pain. In: Cassidy JT, Petty RE, eds. Textbook of Pediatric Rheumatology. 4th ed. Philadelphia, Pennsylvania: WB Saunders Co., p. 389.

10

The Young Person with Back Pain

Suzanne C. Li and Yukiko Kimura

*Section of Pediatric Rheumatology, Joseph M. Sanzari Children's Hospital,
Hackensack University Medical Center, Hackensack, and University of Medicine
and Dentistry of New Jersey (UMDNJ) Medical School, Newark, New Jersey, U.S.A.*

INTRODUCTION

Until recently, back pain was thought to be an uncommon pediatric problem that warranted significant investigation because it was almost always due to an underlying organic, often serious, cause (1–3). However, subsequent studies have shown that back pain is a relatively common complaint in children, and that the incidence increases with age. While less than 10% of children 10 years and younger report having had back pain, by mid to late adolescence over 50% will have had at least one episode of back pain [reviewed in (4,5)]. In the adolescent, back pain is equally likely to occur in either the mid back (thoracic) or low back (lumbosacral) region (6). In contrast, the younger child predominantly has mid back pain and the adult, low back pain (LBP) (6).

Compared to the younger child, mechanical and rheumatic etiologies are generally more common, and infectious etiologies less common in adolescents. Adolescents who participate in organized competitive sports are prone to back pain related to overuse and injury (7). Adolescents are less likely than adults to have disk herniation, spinal stenosis, or osteoarthritis as causes of back pain. Similar to adults, most adolescent back pain has no obvious etiology and is felt to represent nonspecific back pain (4,8–12). Although adult LBP accounts for as much as a third of workers' compensation costs, most adolescent back pain is felt to be mild, self-limited, and not associated with long-term disability (4,8,13).

CAUSES OF BACK PAIN

The main etiologies for adolescent back pain can be put into several general categories that are listed in Table 1.

Table 1 Etiologies of Adolescent Back Pain

Nonspecific back pain
  Mechanical
    Lumbar strain
    Spondylolysis, spondylolisthesis
    Scheuermann disease
    Disk herniation
    Scoliosis
    Osteoporosis
    Apophyseal ring fracture, sacral fracture
    Transitional vertebrae
    Spinal cord anomalies
    Nonaccidental trauma
Idiopathic pain syndromes
  Fibromyalgia
Rheumatic
  Enthesitis related arthritis
  Psoriatic arthritis
  Systemic lupus erythematosus, mixed connective tissue disease, dermatomyositis
Vascular
  Hemoglobinopathies (i.e., sickle cell disease, thalassemia)
  Arteriovenous malformation
  Spinal infarct
Infectious
  Osteomyelitis
  Discitis
  Epidural abscess
Tumor
  Benign bone tumors and tumor-like lesions
  Malignant bone tumors: primary and metastatic
  Spinal cord tumors
Psychological
  Psychogenic/conversion reaction
Referred pain
  Hip
  Abdominal (i.e., pyelonephritis, urinary tract infection, pancreatitis, appendicitis)
  Pelvic (i.e., ovarian cyst, perineural cyst, hematocolpos/imperforate hymen)
  Thoracic (i.e., pneumonia, pleuritis)

Nonspecific Back Pain

The majority of back pain found during adolescence does not have an identifiable etiology and falls into the category of nonspecific back pain. Most
studies have found that the prevalence of back pain rises during adolescence

(6,14–18), reaching adult levels in late adolescence. Generally, there is a 10% or lower lifetime prevalence of back pain in children 10 years or younger (4,15,16,19). The prevalence starts to rise in the next 1 to 2 years, with some studies reporting a lifetime prevalence of 7% to 30% (15,16,19,20). By 15 to 16 years, the reported lifetime prevalence is as high as 50–69% (15,19,21).

Many studies in several countries have been carried out to investigate the risk factors associated with the development of adolescent back pain and the relationship between back pain at this age versus adults (4,5,22). Most are cross-sectional studies, and are therefore unable to determine if the associated factor is a true marker or risk factor for back pain development (4). Most of the prospective studies involve small groups of subjects, which predispose them to potential subject selection bias. Conflicting results have been found when the same group of subjects is studied first by cross-sectional analysis and then prospectively. Comparison of the results of these different studies has been limited because of the multiple methodologies used. Inaccuracies also arise because of inconsistencies in the recall of back pain episodes by both children and adults.

In reviewing the factors that may be associated with adolescent back pain, we focused on the larger cross-sectional studies (6,14–19,21,23–28), and the six larger prospective studies (26,29–34). In these studies, the factors generally found to be associated with increased prevalence of back pain are older age, psychosocial factors, presence of other somatic symptoms and female gender. Less clear-cut factors include part-time work and smoking. Variable findings have been reported for sports activity. For example, a recent cross-sectional study of Danish adolescents found back pain to be associated with low isometric back extensor muscle endurance, with high isometric endurance being protective; no association was found with aerobic fitness, flexibility, functional strength, or physical activity (27). Factors not shown to be consistently associated with back pain include anthropomorphic factors (height, weight, body mass index), school bag use or weight, spinal or lower body flexibility, scoliosis, family history of back or other pain, and increased sedentary activities such as TV watching and computer use.

Mechanical/Traumatic

Mechanical problems are the most commonly diagnosed causes of back pain in adolescents. Some of these, such as Scheuermann's disease develop or progress during the adolescent growth spurt. Adolescent athletes are more likely to have back pain secondary to spondylolysis, spondylolisthesis, hyperlordotic mechanical back pain, or a herniated disk, especially in sports that require repetitive flexion, extension, or rotation of the spine (7) (see Chapter 11).

Although many mechanical etiologies of back pain are diagnosed on the basis of radiographs and other imaging, the significance of many of these "abnormal" findings have recently been called into question. Many studies have reported a significant frequency of abnormal radiographic spine findings in normal adults without back pain. In a review of 18 studies, for example, spondylolisthesis, spondylolysis, spina bifida occulta, transitional vertebrae, and Scheuermann-type changes were not found to be statistically associated with back pain in adults (35). There was only a weak association found between disk degeneration and nonspecific back pain, but, as most of these studies were cross-sectional, additional prospective studies are needed to better assess if there is a direct relationship (35).

Disk degeneration and herniation have also been found in asymptomatic adolescents (1,36), but some spinal changes may be more likely to be associated with back pain (37–39). A study of 439 Danish 13-year-olds found that upper lumbar disc and nucleus anomalies were associated with significant back pain in boys, while lower lumbar anomalies were associated with significant back pain in girls; endplate changes at L3 were associated with significant back pain irrespective of gender (38). In a 9-year prospective study comparing 40 adolescents with back pain to 40 without pain, disc degeneration at age 15 years was associated with a 16-fold relative risk of reporting recurrent LBP at age 23; disk protrusion and Scheuermann-type changes were also associated with an increased likelihood of recurrent back pain at 23 years (39). The frequency of spinal anomalies increases with age, and at 18 years, these spinal anomalies were less predictive of future back pain (39). Although a subset of adolescents with disc degeneration or other spinal anomalies may be more likely to have recurrent, significant back pain as adults, the majority of adolescents with these changes do not appear to be at risk for significant back pain later in life (39).

Lumbosacral Strain/Lordotic Mechanical Back Pain

Back pain may be caused by sprains or strains related to overuse. This problem is less common in adolescent athletes than in adult athletes (6% vs. 27%) (7). The activity or movement that triggered the injury aggravates pain, and there is often localized tenderness (7). There should be no associated neurological signs, although pain may be referred to the buttock or upper thigh (40). Patients improve with conservative measures over several weeks to 2 months (7,40).

Lordotic mechanical back pain has been found to be a common cause of back pain in adolescent athletes (7). Patients will have pain over the lumbar spine, and have an extension contracture of their lumbar spine that limits their ability to flex this area; there may be compensatory deformities of the thoracic spine (7). Pain is elicited by hyperextension or hyperflexion of the spine. These patients also usually improve with reduction in activities and conservative treatment.

Spondylolysis/Spondylolisthesis

Spondylolysis is a defect in the pars interarticularis of the L4 or L5 vertebra. If the vertebral body then slips forward, the condition is referred to as spondylolisthesis. Adolescent athletes with back pain often have the acquired traumatic form, where a fracture occurs through a normal pars interarticularis, usually at L5 (41). Sports that involve repeated lumbar hyperextension, such as gymnastics, dancing, figure skating, diving, soccer, football, hockey, and lacrosse, are particularly associated with traumatic spondylolysis and spondylolisthesis (3,36). In one study, 40% of pediatric soccer players with spondylolysis remembered maximum velocity kicking as a triggering event for their back pain (42). The high dysplastic developmental type of spondylolisthesis also often becomes symptomatic during adolescence and usually involves L5–S1 (41). This type of spondylolisthesis is more likely to be associated with bladder and bowel problems and L5 nerve radiculopathy (43).

The pain associated with spondylolisthesis and spondylolysis is typically a mild to moderate aching pain in the lower back, which is aggravated by extension and flexion, and relieved by rest. There may be paraspinal tenderness in the L5–S1 region, buttock pain, or pain radiating to the posterior thigh or buttocks (44). The onset is usually insidious unless it is precipitated by an acute fracture (1). Patients generally have tight hamstrings, which leads to a stiff legged gait with hip and knee flexion and a short stride length, also known as a "pelvic waddle" (43,44). The patient may have secondary postural changes, such as increased lumbar lordosis and a protruding abdomen. To test for this condition, the "one leg extension manoeuvre" is said to be best: the patient stands on one leg while the other hip and knee are flexed; the patient then hyperextends the lower back which elicits unilateral or bilateral LBP (1) (see Figure 11 in Chapter 11).

The oblique radiograph in a patient with spondylolysis usually shows the pars abnormality that is said to resemble a collar or broken neck of the "Scotty dog" in isthmic defects (Fig. 1), and the "greyhound sign" in dysplastic cases (44). Bone scan, single photon emission computed tomography (SPECT), and CT are all more sensitive, but bone scan and SPECT are unable to identify a chronic pars defect and cannot distinguish spondylolysis from other inflammatory problems (3,45). MRI offers the advantage of being able to detect impending spondylolysis before the actual pars breakage occurs (45). Earlier diagnosis improves the prognosis (45). Most patients respond to conservative treatment with analgesics, activity modification and/or bracing, and exercises to strengthen their abdominal and paraspinal muscles. (7,45); one study reported better results with cessation of sports activity for 3 months (42).

Scheuermann's Disease (Juvenile Kyphosis)

Scheuermann disease is a kyphotic deformity of the thoracic or thoracolumbar spine, which develops around 10–13 years of age and becomes more pronounced during the adolescent growth spurt (46). Adolescents may complain of aching back pain at the level of the deformity or in the lower

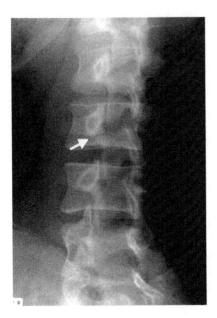

Figure 1 This 13-year-old girl heard a pop and had the acute onset of back pain while shoveling snow. AP view of her L spine did not show any defect, but an oblique view shows the "collar" or "broken neck" of the "Scotty dog" at L3 (*white arrow*), indicative of acute traumatic spondylolysis.

back, or may present with a painless thoracic kyphosis (1,47). The pain is often worse later in the day, and may be aggravated by prolonged sitting, standing or activity; those with lumbar involvement usually have more pain (3,44). About 1/3 of patients will have also have a mild to moderate scoliosis (36). AP and lateral X rays show narrowing of the intervertebral disk space, decreased vertebral height with anterior wedging of three adjacent vertebrae, irregular vertebral end plates, and sometimes Schmorl nodes (46). Patients with a mild degree of kyphosis can be monitored, treated with thoracic-extension and abdominal strengthening exercises, and will generally improve when their growth is finished (44). Patients with more severe kyphosis require bracing prior to skeletal maturity, and possibly surgery (44).

Lumbar Disk Herniation

Although disk herniation is commonly associated with adult back pain, only 1% to 4% of all documented cases of disk herniation occur during adolescence (36). Adolescent males, athletes, and those with a positive family history of lumbar disk herniation appear to be at increased risk (44,48). In contrast to the adult, where degenerative changes in the lumbar disk predispose the tissue to herniation, during adolescence herniation is usually secondary to a fracture (44).

Most herniations occur at L4–L5 or L5–S1 (36). As discussed above, the relationship between disc herniation and back pain is not clear, since herniation is a common finding in MRIs of asymptomatic adolescents and adults (1,36,38). Those that have significant, symptomatic disk herniation with actual disk protrusion and not just bulging, will have severe back pain and lumbar tenderness, and can have sciatica (3,49). If neurological signs are present, they rarely involve bladder or bowel changes; more common signs are gait abnormalities, abnormal reflexes, sensory deficits, and motor weakness (44,49,50). Most will have a positive straight leg raise sign (44).

Apophyseal Injury and Apophyseal Ring Fractures

Apophyseal ring injuries were found to be associated with back pain in a 3-year longitudinal study of adolescent athletes (37). The apophyseal ring fuses with the vertebral body between the ages of 17 and 20 years, and is subject to injury from traction or compression prior to fusion. Ring injuries are associated with figure skating and gymnastics, and can be detected by MRI (37).

Apophyseal ring fracture is an injury related problem that occurs in adolescent boys who participate in heavy weight lifting or similar activities. The onset of pain is usually acute; the pain is often described as constant and burning, and aggravated by activity and Valsalva maneuver. Pain is usually bilateral, and can be associated with sciatica and back stiffness (44). The posterior portion of the lumbar apophysis fractures, followed by partial disk herniation into the spinal canal, most commonly at L4. The condition may be visualized on a lateral X ray or by CT scan. If there are no neurological symptoms, patients can be treated conservatively with reduced activities, analgesics, and physical therapy. For those with neurological symptoms, excision of the bone fragment and lamina should be done (44).

Scoliosis

Scoliosis is relatively common during adolescence, but most cases are idiopathic and should not cause pain: the frequency of back pain in children with and without idiopathic scoliosis is similar (51). However, adolescents with idiopathic scoliosis need to have the magnitude of their curvature monitored as it can worsen during growth spurts, and those with rapidly progressive scoliosis or with 25 or more degrees of curvature may need bracing or surgery. Such patients should be referred to a pediatric orthopedist for further evaluation and management (52).

Scoliosis associated with severe pain should be regarded as a red flag, as it could represent pathologic osseous lesions such as a tumor (i.e., osteoid osteoma, osteoblastoma, eosinophilic granuloma, aneurysmal bone cyst) or infection (3). Other signs suggestive of intraspinal pathology include abnormal neurological findings, a left rather than right thoracic curve, very rigid scoliosis, rapid progression, and lack of compensatory curves above or below the lesion (3,51,53,54). Patients with these findings need a thorough evaluation.

Osteoporosis

Idiopathic juvenile osteoporosis is a rare cause of back pain in otherwise healthy adolescents. Patients will develop growth arrest, and some may present with an abnormal gait or progressive kyphosis (55). X rays show osteopenia, multiple growth arrest lines, progressive loss of height of the vertebrae, and often compression fractures of the long bones, especially around the joints. Other disorders that cause osteoporosis, such as leukemia, juvenile idiopathic arthritis (especially with chronic corticosteriod use), Cushing disease, thyroid disease, diabetes mellitus, growth hormone deficiency, homocystinuria, osteogenesis imperfecta, and dietary deficiencies (calcium, vitamin D, vitamin C) need to be excluded. Adolescent girls with behavioral eating disorders are also at increased risk for osteopenia (55) (see Chapter 12).

Transitional Vertebrae

Adolescents may have back pain associated with congenital anomalies of their L5 or S1 vertebrae. The L5 vertebrae can become sacralized or the S1 vertebrae can be lumbarized; these changes can be unilateral or bilateral. Pain is more likely with the unilateral asymmetrical form, and there may be sciatic pain down the leg opposite to the side of sacralization (56). Symptomatic transitional vertebrae may best be detected by SPECT scans. Adolescents with lumbar disk herniation are more likely to have transitional vertebrae, but again since transitional vertebrae can be found in many asymptomatic subjects, it is not clear if these radiographic findings are actually the cause of the back pain. (35).

Spinal Cord Anomalies

Adolescents with a tethered cord can present with painful scoliosis and neurological signs such as bladder dysfunction, motor weakness, atrophy of one limb, or a Babinski sign (40,44). Other associated physical findings include a cavovarus foot, lumbosacral hair patch, dermal cyst, or hemangioma. Radiographs can show spina bifida occulta or diastematomyelia (44); MRI will define this problem, which will require neurosurgical intervention.

About 25% of patients with syringomyelia, or spinal cord cysts, will present with painful scoliosis. Other associated symptoms include headache, neck pain, pes cavus, and neurological signs such as abnormal gait, loss of abdominal reflexes, and change in sensation for pain or temperature (44). When syringomyelia is present, it is recommended that the entire spine of these patients be examined by MRI to look for other anomalies (44).

Nonaccidental Injury

The child that has back pain who has had unusual or suspicious trauma should be evaluated for signs of nonaccidental injury. These signs could include multiple fractures, bruises, skin scars suggestive of burns or other unusual traumas, frequent school absences, and signs of neglect. This problem is more likely to be found in the younger child than in the adolescent.

Rheumatic

Juvenile Idiopathic Arthritis (JIA)

Adolescents with back pain related to JIA are most likely to have either enthesitis-related arthritis (ERA) or psoriatic arthritis. Back pain in these disorders results from inflammation of the spine and/or sacroiliac (SI) joints. In contrast to the pattern seen with mechanical back pain, inflammatory back pain is worsened by rest (i.e., morning stiffness), and improved by activity. ERA is more common in adolescent Caucasian boys and in those with a family history of HLA-B27–associated diseases (57,58,84,85). These adolescents often present with enthesitis of the heel or knee, peripheral arthritis, and less commonly acute anterior uveitis (57,83,84). Although adults with ankylosing spondylitis (AS) frequently have inflammatory spinal pain at onset, only a minority of children with ERA (12.8–24%) has been reported to have pain, stiffness, or limitation of movement of the lumbosacral or SI region during the first year of disease (57,83). Instead, most develop back symptoms after 5–10 years of disease (58). A minority of adolescents with inflammatory bowel disease (IBD) may develop spine and SI arthritis in a pattern similar to ERA. This can occur months to years before or after the onset of the gastrointestinal symptoms (82,83), and the arthritis in these patients appears to be independent of the bowel disease activity. Patients with psoriatic arthritis can have varying patterns of joint involvement, such as dactylitis, oligoarthritis or polyarthritis, and 11–47% will develop back pain due to sacroiliitis, again in a pattern similar to ERA (58). The majority of children with psoriatic arthritis will develop joint inflammation before the onset of skin disease, often making the diagnosis a challenge (58,83). Typical skin findings include psoriasis vulgaris, nail pitting, and less commonly, onycholysis (58,85). Most children with psoriatic arthritis have a family history of psoriasis (58,85).

Direct palpation over the SI joint, compression of the pelvis, or distraction of the SI joint may elicit pain in the SI joint. (58). The development of sacroiliitis in ERA seems to be associated with disease duration and intensity (59). Radiographs may show diffuse pelvic osteoporosis as well as changes in the bones surrounding the SI joint, such as blurring of the subchondral margins, erosions, joint space narrowing, reactive sclerosis, and fusion (57) (Fig. 2). Arthritis of the spine may be detected as a flattening of the lumbar curve on forward flexion, decreased lumbar expansion as measured by the Schober test, decrease in hyperextension, or restriction of chest wall expansion (58). Late radiographic changes of the spine include anterior vertebral squaring and anterior ligament calcification (57). MRI with gadolinium can detect signs of inflammation much earlier than radiographs (57,59), so should be done if suspected. Laboratory studies may show mild anemia, elevated inflammatory markers, thrombocytosis, and occasionally leukocytosis; the ANA and rheumatoid factor will be negative, while the HLA-B27 can be positive in 70% to 90% of patients (57,83,84). Patients presenting with back pain who have IBD may have anemia, high ESR, low albumin, a positive peripheral staining anti-neutrophil cytoplasmic antibody (P-ANCA), or anti-Saccharomyces cerevisiae antibody (ASCA), and/or occult or frank hematochezia (57). (For further discussion of JIA, see Chapter 7.)

Other Autoimmune Disorders

Adolescents with systemic lupus erythematosus (SLE), mixed connective tissue disease, chronic vasculitis, or dermatomyositis may also develop back pain. SLE and MCTD are most common in the adolescent female, while dermatomyositis is more common from mid childhood through early adolescence (86–89). Back pain in these patients may be secondary to arthritis, infection, osteoporosis, osteonecrosis, referred from pathology in the chest or abdomen, or transverse myelitis, but these patients can also develop other more common causes of back pain in adolescents such as mechanical problems, nonspecific back pain, or fibromyalgia. Arthritis as a cause of back pain is unusual in these patients who are more likely to have peripheral small joint arthritis rather than axial arthritis (86–89).

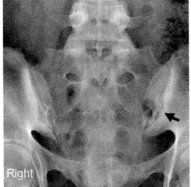 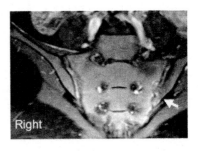

(A)   **(B)**

Figure 2 This 16-year-old girl had a 3-week history of progressive daily arthralgias involving her knees, neck, back, and upper extremity joints. She had morning stiffness, fatigue, and limping. Her laboratory studies showed a Hg of 11.2 gm/dl, platelet count of 414K/mcl, ESR 82, negative ANA, and a positive HLA-B27. (A) An X-ray of her SI joints shows bilateral sclerosis on both sides of her SI joint, with widening of the left side (*arrow*) suggestive of erosion, and irregularity on the right side. (B) An MRI at this time (T1 TSE coronal with fat saturation after gadolinium) shows moderate erosive changes bilaterally, with large erosion on the left side (*arrow*), and enhancement along both the sacral and iliac sides.

Vascular

Hemoglobinopathies

Patients with sickle cell anemia may develop vaso-occlusive crises in their spine, especially in the lumbosacral region (60). Onset of pain is usually acute, severe, and may be accompanied by localized spine tenderness, fever, and tachycardia. Most patients will have worsening hemolytic anemia, elevated leukocyte counts, and have evidence of sickling on their smear; such patients should be treated with hydration and analgesics (60,61). Radiographs can show osteopenia, sclerosis, fractures, and cuplike depressions in the vertebral bodies (61). Patients with sickle cell disease are at risk for osteomyelitis and bony infarcts of the spine. Thalassemia intermedia or thalassemia major can lead to growth failure, osteoporosis, spinal deformities, and back pain (62).

Infectious

Vertebral Osteomyelitis

About 1% to 2% of children and adolescents with osteomyelitis have the infection localized to their spine. Within the spine, the lumbosacral area is the most common followed by the thoracolumbar region. There is a peak incidence in adolescence. Common presenting symptoms include back pain which can be severe, muscle spasm, vertebral tenderness, and fever (1). Patients may limp or refuse to walk, and usually appear quite ill, but may have had insidious symptoms for several weeks to months (63). Most will have an elevated ESR and white blood count. Blood cultures are positive in only slightly more than half of the patients. When an organism is detected, the most common organism is *Staphylococcus aureus*. Rare causes include *Bartonella henselae* and Salmonella species, and in patients from developing countries, tuberculosis is a major cause. Radiographs can often be normal in early vertebral osteomyelitis; therefore, if suspicion is high, bone scintigraphy and/or MRI should be done (1,63). Treatment with antibiotics is usually successful, especially if a bone aspiration or biopsy identifies the causative organism, although there may be permanent bony defects.

Discitis

Discitis can present with many of the same features found with vertebral osteomyelitis but is more common in younger children (<5 years of age). However, a history of intravenous drug abuse in the adolescent increases the risk in this age group (63,64). Over 80% of cases involve the lumbar spine, generally L3/4 or L4/5 (1,64). The patient may refuse to walk, bend forward, or sit, and may present with back stiffness, malaise, poor appetite, muscle weakness, or hyporeflexia. Teenagers often have localized back pain that radiates to the buttocks and legs (44). Patients tend to have symptoms for several weeks, and most do not have fever or appear ill. The ESR, and often the white blood count, is elevated; the CRP is normal in the majority of patients (63,64). Varying frequencies of positive cultures from direct biopsy samples have been reported (0–88%) but only a minority of blood cultures have been positive (63,64). *S. aureus* is the most common etiologic agent when an organism is isolated (1,65). As it may take 2–3 weeks for radiographs to show disc space narrowing and vertebral end plate irregularity, MRI is considered the preferred imaging method (1,44). MRI also allows discitis to be distinguished from osteomyelitis and epidural abscess, both of which need to be treated more emergently (44). Treatment with intravenous antibiotics has been reported to lead to a faster and more complete recovery, but since many patients recover without antibiotic treatment, this is controversial unless there is a history of intravenous drug abuse (64).

Epidural Abscess

Although an epidural abscess can cause back pain, fever, and symptoms similar to those seen in patients with discitis or osteomyelitis, it is rare in the pediatric patient. Even in adults, there is usually an associated risk factor such as diabetes mellitus, intravenous drug abuse, alcoholism, skin infections, or spinal trauma (66). About 12% of the cases are pediatric patients, with males older than 10 years the most likely to be affected (66). About one-third of cases occur in the lumbar or lumbosacral region, another third in the thoracic region. Irritability, back pain, localized tenderness, and neurological signs such as muscle weakness, incontinence, or paraparesis/paraplegia are common symptoms (66). These symptoms can be acute or chronic, making diagnosis difficult (1). Most patients will have fever and an elevated ESR and white blood count. Epidural abscess is a medical and surgical emergency, since delay in treatment often leads to irreversible neurological residua or even death (1). MRI is the best imaging method (44). Surgical drainage and antibiotics are required, and again *S. aureus* is the most common pathogen (66).

Tumors

Back pain and stiffness is a common symptom in patients with both benign and malignant spinal tumors, but malignant tumors are more likely to be associated with neurological symptoms (44,53). Other symptoms suspicious for malignancy include bone pain, night sweats, fever, anorexia, weight loss, and fatigue (67). Fortunately, in adolescence, most spinal tumors are benign. Primary benign tumor and tumor-like lesions of the vertebrae, except for those of the sacrum, are more common during childhood and adolescence than later in life (53). Sacral lesions in children and adolescents are more likely to be malignant than in adults (53). Children with either benign or malignant lesions can have symptoms for months to several years before diagnosis (11,53,68), and may develop a painful scoliosis and rigid spine secondary to bony destruction or muscle spasm; the lesion is usually located on the concave aspect of the curve, with the scoliosis convex to the side opposite the lesion (3,53).

Benign bone tumors and lesions include osteochondroma, osteoid osteoma, osteoblastoma, aneurysmal bone cysts, eosinophilic granulomas, and osteoclastomas (53). Osteoid osteoma and osteoblastoma are classically associated with nocturnal pain that is readily relieved by NSAIDs, but many patients do not have this pattern (53). Osteoblastomas are often located in the lumbar spine and associated with a radicular type of pain (53). Although larger than osteoid osteomas, osteoblastomas are usually less painful (1,3). Aneurysmal bone cysts are also often found in the lumbar spine, and can be associated with pathological fractures and neurological symptoms as these lesions tend to extend into the vertebral body and adjacent vertebrae (3,53). Osteoclastoma is more commonly seen after skeletal maturity is attained and in the spine, is most common in the sacrum (53). Although eosinophilic granuloma is a benign lesion, it is often associated with fever and weight loss. Patients with these lesions need a skeletal survey and bone scan to look for other lesions (1,44). All of these benign lesions should be surgically removed, except for eosinophilic granuloma, which can often be treated conservatively with bracing as needed (1,44,53).

Malignant tumors of the spine include primary osseous tumors, neural spinal cord tumors, and skeletal metastases. In the adolescent patient, Ewing's sarcoma, osteosarcoma, and lymphoma are the most common spinal malignancies, while in the younger patient, leukemia, neuroblastoma, and astrocytoma are more common (44). It can be difficult to diagnose these benign and malignant lesions on plain radiographs, since less than half show the typical radiographic features (53). Bone scintigraphy is helpful when radiographs are normal usually have increased uptake. Osteosarcoma, Ewing sarcoma, osteoid osteoma, osteoblastoma, and aneurysmal bone cysts (53). MRI allows better definition of the extent of the lesion and evaluation of spinal cord and adjacent soft tissue involvement; CT allows better evaluation of the extent of bony destruction (3).

Psychogenic

Conversion reactions are predominantly found in late childhood to early adolescent girls, and may begin after a minor illness or trauma (1). Patients may report diffuse spinal tenderness, with marked allodynia, numbness, paralysis, or a bizarre gait. These are often inconsistent with organic pathology (1,57). Despite their reports of pain and limitation, the patient is often smiling or cheerful ("la belle indifference"). Physical examination does not reveal any neurological or organic pathology. Treatment consists of psychological and graded physical therapy (1).

Idiopathic Pain

Fibromyalgia and other forms of idiopathic pain are a relatively common diagnosis in new patients presenting with back pain to North American pediatric rheumatology centers (90,91). Fibromyalgia generally develops during late childhood and adolescence, with girls much more commonly

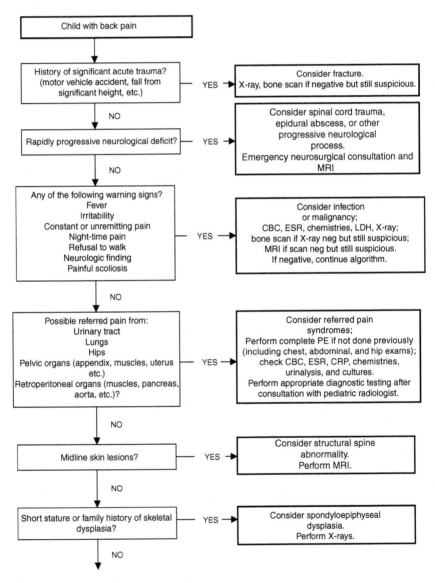

Figure 3   *(Continued on next page)*

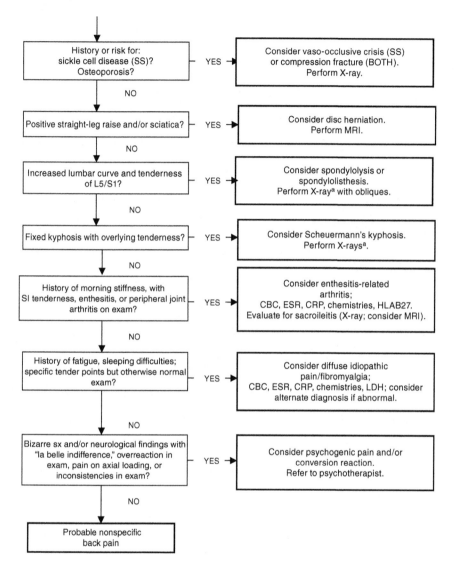

Figure 3 An algorithmic approach to diagnosis of causes of back pain. [a]These are common X-ray findings that may not be causative; therefore continue algorithm to look for other causes. *Abbreviations*: PE, physical exam; SI, sacroiliac; Sx, symptoms. *Source*: Reprinted with permission from Ref. 92.

affected than boys (90,91). In addition to back pain, these patients usually complain of widespread musculoskeletal pain, and on examination have significant tenderness at specific soft tissue locations called tender points. The symptoms often have a gradual onset, and patients frequently have associated symptoms such as fatigue, difficulty sleeping, non-restorative sleep, headaches, abdominal pain, dizziness, and mood disturbances (90,91). No evidence for inflammatory, mechanical musculoskeletal, or neurological problems are found on exam, and blood tests should be normal (90,91).

GENERAL DIAGNOSTIC APPROACH TO ADOLESCENT WITH BACK PAIN

Back pain in the adolescent is less likely to represent a serious problem compared to the younger child, and less likely compared to adults to represent spinal pathology compared to adults. Therefore, the majority of adolescents with back pain will have a mild, self-limited problem and will not need an extensive work-up. A careful history and physical exam should distinguish nonspecific back pain from more serious etiologies. Figure 3 is one algorithmic approach to back pain diagnosis. In general, an urgent evaluation is required in an adolescent with neurological signs and symptoms suspicious of a possible or impending spinal cord compression as can occur with tumor, epidural abscess, or fracture. Plain radiographs are indicated in those assessed to be likely to have a problem associated with radiographic changes or with a history of significant trauma prior to back pain onset. MRI is best for further investigation of a significant plain radiographic abnormality, or in those who have serious or persistent symptoms. Laboratory studies, such as CBC, comprehensive serum chemistry screening, urinalysis, ESR, CRP, should be done in those suspected of having a systemic problem. If a rheumatic condition is suspected, then depending on what is suspected, tests such as HLA-B27 (in ERA), ANA (lupus), ANCA, and/or ASCA (IBD) may be helpful.

Patterns of Clinical Presentation

Symptom Patterns

Symptom pattern recognition is the key to diagnosis in any age group. Tumors are characterized by nocturnal, constant, and severe pain that often limits activities (Fig. 4). While the pain associated with the benign tumors of osteoid osteoma and osteoblastoma are often dramatically relieved by NSAIDs, pain associated with other tumors is generally not relieved by analgesics. Some mechanical causes such as disk herniation and spinal or sacral fracture usually present acutely or following a significant trauma, while others such as spondylolysis and Scheuermanns disease have a more insidious and chronic onset. Mechanical causes of back pain are typically worse later in the day but not at night, and are aggravated by activities and relieved by rest; spondylolysis and spondylolisthesis are usually worsened by hyperextension and flexion. Some conditions such as spondylolysis, disk herniation, apophyseal ring injuries and fractures often present with very localized pain, others such as Scheuermann present with a broader area of

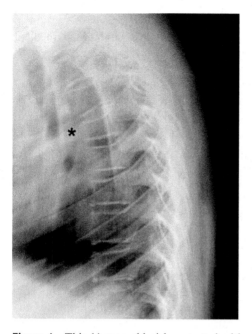

Figure 4 This 11-year-old girl presented with complaints of severe neck, shoulder, and back pain. On examination, she was found to have significant limitation in movement and diffuse severe tenderness around her shoulder and upper back. X-rays showed generalized osteoporosis of her thoracic spine with collapse of upper thoracic vertebra (*asterisk*). She had a white blood count of 2.6 K cells/mcl with a normal differential hemoglobin of 9.6 gm/dl; platelet count of 117,000/mcl; ESR of 49; and CRP of 1.8 (normal to 0.8). She was found to have acute lymphoblastic leukemia on her bone marrow aspirate.

pain, and still others such as disk herniation with pain that radiates into the buttock or down a leg. In contrast, inflammatory spine pain is usually characterized by stiffness that is improved by moderate activity and worsened by rest and lying supine. The pain is usually relieved by NSAIDs to some degree. Infectious causes can be either acute or insidious in onset, but the pain tends to be constant.

Systemic symptoms such as fever, weight loss, malaise, or night sweats are more likely to be associated with serious conditions such as infection, tumor (usually malignant), IBD, or a major rheumatic disease. Patients that have a history of significant trauma to their back prior to the onset of their pain should be carefully examined for possible spinal fracture or disk herniation. A change in the bladder or bowel pattern is suspicious for tumor, infection, or a major spinal cord injury. Severe or progressive limitation of activities or limping is also suggestive of infection or tumor, although a severe mechanical or rheumatic disease can also cause these problems.

Adolescents should also be asked about their level of participation in sports to assess their risk for mechanical problems. Underlying medical problems in the patient or the family such as psoriasis, IBD, intravenous drug use, frequent infections, or use of immunosuppressive medications, may indicate potential disease risks. A poor sleep pattern, fatigue, and mood changes are suggestive of fibromyalgia. Excessive school absences might be suggestive of psychogenic pain or school avoidance. These patients will generally have poorly characterized, diffuse, and variable patterns of pain.

Physical Examination Patterns

The spine should be examined for painful scoliosis and a left curve, findings that are often associated with a tumor. Paravertebral muscle spasms, a rigid spine, and spinal point tenderness are seen with tumor and infection, but can also be associated with mechanical etiologies (spondylolysis and disk herniation). A waddling gait with flexed knees indicates spinal nerve root irritation, which can occur with tumors, disk herniation, spondylolisthesis, or intervertebral disk disease. In contrast, a bizarre gait, with prancing steps or other non-organic pattern of walking, is suggestive of a psychogenic problem. If a spinal cord problem is suspected, reflexes, including of the abdomen and anus, and strength and sensory testing should be done. Tenderness of the sacroiliac joints, spine tenderness in a broad area, and decreased lumbar flexibility are findings associated with JIA; patients are also likely to have peripheral joint arthritis and enthesitis or other findings such as dactylitis or nail pitting (psoriatic arthritis), or skin findings (erythema nodosum or oral ulcers in IBD). Occult spinal or sacral anomalies such as a dimple, hair patch, or vascular markings are suggestive of a tethered cord or other congenital spinal canal malformation of spinal canal.

MANAGEMENT

Adolescents with specific causes of back pain should be treated according to the diagnosis. For example, if a mechanical etiology is suspected, patients should be managed with conservative treatment such as short-term restriction of activity or modification of activity, followed by flexibility and strengthening exercises. Bracing can be helpful for some mechanical problems such as posterior verterbral arch stress fracture, spondylolysis, spondylolisthesis, or Scheuermann's disease (7,45,69). Only rarely is surgery required for adolescent mechanical back problems. Back pain due to arthritis and inflammation should be treated initially with NSAIDs, and if there is little or no response, other anti-rheumatic medications can be considered.

The appropriate treatment for nonspecific back pain is less clear, and only a limited number of studies have been carried out in adolescents. Most adolescent back pain is mild and self-limited, and does not require more than conservative treatment (8,70). Treatment recommendations are based on studies in adults, which are also controversial. Many studies have contradictory findings, and comparison between studies is difficult because of differences in methodology, study quality, and populations (13,71,72).

Although many medications have been used to treat adult LBP, only limited evidence supports their use. NSAIDs and acetaminophen may be beneficial for acute LBP, but their benefit for chronic LBP is less clear (13,71). Opioids and muscle relaxants have not been shown to be more effective than NSAIDs or acetaminophen (13). Tricyclic antidepressants have been shown to cause a small reduction in pain in patients with chronic LBP, but no consistent functional improvement has been found in those who are not depressed (73).

A recent review of 61 randomized controlled trials of exercise therapy found that exercise had no clear benefit for adult acute LBP, but was mildly helpful at decreasing pain and improving function in adults with chronic LBP (74). Bed rest is not advised for patients with LBP, and only has limited benefit for patients with sciatica (13). Conflicting results have been reported for other treatments such as physical therapy, spinal manipulation, TENS, acupuncture, biofeedback, and behavioral therapy (71,73). Although some treatments, such as spinal manipulation, can improve acute symptoms, no clear long-term benefit has been found (13). The combination of medical care with PT or manipulation may be slightly more effective than a single type of treatment in reducing pain and perceived disability (73). Multidisciplinary approaches combining physical rehabilitation with educational, psychological, and behavioral treatment have been reported to lead to improved outcome that is sustained over many months, but success varies depending upon the program and the patient population (13,71).

PROGNOSIS

Adolescent back pain generally has a better prognosis than adult back pain. Mechanical causes usually respond to conservative treatment, as they are only rarely caused by degenerative or progressive conditions such as spinal stenosis or disk herniation. Nonspecific back pain in adolescents is also thought to have a better outcome than adult nonspecific back pain. Few adolescents (7–11%) seek medical treatment for their back pain, and only rare cases are hospitalized or become disabled (4,6,15,19,20,5,70,75). In contrast, back pain in adults is the fifth most common reason for physician visits (76), and although most adults with acute LBP will improve within three months, 6% to 20% will develop chronic back pain, and 25% to 75% still have back pain one year later (13,72,73,77). In adults, preexisting psychological distress, work compensation issues, other chronic pain issues and job dissatisfaction are all associated with an increased risk of developing chronic LBP (73). Other associated factors include poor self-rated health, low level of physical activity, and smoking (78).

A few prospective studies have been done that followed adolescents into adulthood to evaluate long-term prognosis and risk factors for incident or persistent back pain, and they have shown that having had back pain during adolescence was associated with a somewhat higher likelihood of having LBP later in adulthood (33,47,79). Other risk factors for developing adult back pain appear to include a family history of LBP (47), emotional or behavioral disorders during childhood, and lower parental education in childhood (32), but one large prospective study did not find a significant association between childhood emotional problems and onset of LBP in the preceding year (80). A dose-response relationship between smoking and adult LBP was reported in another large prospective study of adolescents, but no association was found for alcohol consumption or being overweight as an adolescent (34). Exercise may be beneficial: adolescents who continued to exercise 3 hours/week or more into adulthood were found to have a lower prevalence of LBP as adults in a small study (81). However, being physically active was also associated with a lower frequency of smoking, being sick, being unemployed, being in a low socioeconomic class, and a shorter school education, so other factors may be important for the observed reduction in back pain prevalence (81). Additional long-term prospective studies in adolescents are needed to better understand the factors that determine the development of LBP as adults.

WEB RESOURCES

www.espalda.org/english/divulgativa/su_espalda/escolares.asp. The Kovacs Foundation, a Spanish organization interested in promoting medical work, runs this site. This site reviews anatomy, etiologies, diagnosis, and exercises. It also provides the information in Spanish.

www.spine-health.com/topics/cd/kids/kids01.html. This site has a medical advisory board from different areas related to spine care, which provide peer-reviewed patient information. Topics covered included spondylolysis, Scheuermann disease, scoliosis, and sports related back problems in children and teens. Calcium requirements during growth are also reviewed. Adult topics include back exercise, chronic pain, osteoporosis, surgical treatment, office furniture selection, and sleep advice.

www.painconnection.org/MyTreatment/articles/BackAndNeck_Part_1.asp. This web site of the National Pain Foundation reviews common causes of adult and pediatric back pain, and discusses psychological factors related to chronic pain in pediatric patients and their treatment.

www.nlm.nih.gov/medlineplus/backpain.html. This is the site of the National Institutes of Health, with links to other sites. Many topics are covered including anatomy, etiologies, treatment strategies, exercises, and there are links to the American Academy of Orthopedics's website on childhood causes of back pain., backpack use (Nemours), and pediatric pain management (National Pain Foundation site). The website also provides explanations in Spanish.

www.allaboutbackandneckpain.com/html/articles.asp. This site is managed by DePuy Spine Inc, a subsidiary of Johnson & Johnson. There are articles about spinal anatomy, back pain in athletes, scoliosis, and other etiologies. They describe the different radiographic imaging techniques used to evaluate back pain and provide information about medications and surgical treatment. The site states that it is intended for the U.S. audience.

REFERENCES

1. Hollingworth P. Back pain in children. Br J Rheumatol 1996; 35:1022.
2. Grattan-Smith P, Ryan M, Procopis P. Persistent or severe back pain and stiffness are ominous symptoms requiring prompt attention. J Paediatr Child Health 2000; 36:208.
3. Afshani E, Kuhn J. Common causes of low back pain in children. RadioGraphics 1991; 11:269.
4. Jones G, Macfarlane G. Epidemiology of low back pain in children and adolescents. Arch Dis Child 2005; 90:312.
5. Balagué F, Troussier, B, Salminen, JJ. Nonspecific low back pain in children and adolescents: risk factors. Eur Spine J 1999; 8:429.
6. Wedderkopp N, Leboeuf-Yde C, Andersen L, Froberg K, Hansen H. Back pain reporting pattern in a Danish population-based sample of children and adolescents. Spine 2001; 26:1879.
7. Micheli L, Wood R. Back pain in young athletes. Arch Pediatr Adolesc Med 1995; 149:15.
8. Burton A, Clarke R, McClune T, Tillotson K. The natural history of low back pain in adolescents. Spine 1996; 21:2323.
9. Turner P, Green J, Galasko C. Back pain in childhood. Spine 1989; 14:812.
10. Combs J, Caskey P. Back pain in children and adolescents: a retrospective review of 648 patients. South Med J 1997; 80:789.
11. Feldman D, Hedden D, Wright J. The use of bone scan to investigate back pain in children and adolescents. J Pediat Orthop 2000; 20:790.
12. Mirovsky Y, Jakim I, Halperin N, Lev L. Nonspecific back pain in children and adolescents: a prospective study until maturity. J Pediat Orthop 2002; 11:275.
13. Atlas S, Nardin R. Evaluation and treatment of low back pain: an evidence-based approach to clinical care. Muscle Nerve 2003; 27:265.
14. Kristjansdottir G, Rhee H. Risk factors of back pain frequency in school-children: a search for explanations to a public health problem. Acta Paediatr 2002; 91:849.
15. Balagué F, Dutoit G, Waldburger M. Low back pain in schoolchildren. Scand J Rehab Med 1988; 20:175.

16. Leboeuf-Yde C, Kyvik K. At what age does low back pain become a common problem? A study of 29,424 individuals aged 12–41 years. Spine 1998; 23:228.

17. Taimela S, Kujala U, Salminen J, Viljanen T. The prevalence of low back pain among children and adolescents: a nationwide, cohort-based questionnaire survey in Finland. Spine 1997; 22:1132.

18. Watson K, Papageorgiou A, Jones G, et al. Low back pain in schoolchildren: the role of mechanical and psychosocial factors. Arch Dis Child 2003; 88:12.

19. Balagué F, Nordin M, Skovron M, Dutoit G, Yee A, Waldburger M. Nonspecific low-back pain among schoolchildren: a field survey with analysis of some associated factors. J Spinal Disorders 1994; 7:374.

20. Olsen T, Anderson R, Dearwater S, et al. The epidemiology of low back pain in an adolescent population. Am J Public Health 1992; 82:606.

21. Kovacs F, Gestoso M, Real Md, López J, Mufraggi N, Méndez J. Risk factors for nonspecific low back pain in schoolchildren and their parents: a population based study. Pain 2003; 103:259.

22. Leboeuf-Yde C. Back pain-individual and genetic factors. J Electromyogr Kinesiol 2004; 14:129.

23. Siambanes D, Martinez J, Butler E, Haider T. Influence of school backpacks on adolescent back pain. J Pediatr Orthop 2004; 24:211.

24. Korovessis P, Koureas G, Papazisis Z. Correlation between backpack weight and way of carrying, sagittal and frontal spinal curvatures, athletic activity, and dorsal and low back pain in schoolchildren and adolescents. J Spinal Disord Tech 2004; 17:33.

25. Harreby M, Nygaard B, Jessen T, et al. Risk factors for low back pain in a cohort of 1389 Danish school children: an epidemiologic study. Eur Spine J 1999; 8:444.

26. Jones G, Watson K, Silman A, Symmons D, Macfarlane G. Predictors of low back pain in British schoolchildren: a population-based prospective cohort study. Pediatrics 2003; 111:822.

27. Andersen L, Wedderkopp N, Leboeuf-Yde C. Association between back pain and physical fitness in adolescents. Spine 2006; 31:1740.

28. Skaggs D, Early S, D'Ambra P, Tolo V, Kay R. Back pain and backpacks in school children. J Pediatr Orthop 2006; 26:358.

29. Feldman D, Shrier I, Rossignol M, Abenhaim L. Risk factors for the development of low back pain in adolescence. Am J Epidemiol 2001; 154:30.

30. Brattberg G. The incidence of back pain and headache among Swedish school children. Qual Life Res 1994; 3:527.

31. Szpalski M, Gunzburg, R, Balagué, F, Nordin, M, Mélot, C. A 2-year prospective longitudinal study on low back pain in primary school children. Eur Spine J 2002; 11:459.

32. Mustard C, Kalcevich C, Frank J, Boyle M. Childhood and early adult predictors of risk of incident back pain: Ontario Child Health Study 2001 Follow-up. Am J Epidemiol 2005; 162:779.

33. Hestbaek L, Leboeuf-Yde C, Kyvik K. Is comorbidity in adolescence a predictor for adult low back pain? A prospective study of a young population. BMC Musculoskelet Disord 2006; 7:29.

34. Hestbaek L, Leboeuf-Yde C, Kyvik K. Are lifestyle-factors in adolescence predictors for adult low back pain? A cross-sectional and prospective study of young twins. BMC Musculoskelet Disord 2006; 7:27.
35. Tulder Mv, Assendelft W, Koes B, Bouter L. Spinal radiographic findings and nonspecific low back pain. A systematic review of observational studies. Spine 1997; 22:427.
36. King H. Back pain in children. Orthop Clin North Am 1999; 30:467.
37. Kujala U, Taimela S, Erkintalo M, Salminen J, Kaprio J. Low-back pain in adolescent athletes. Med Science Sports Exercise 1996; 28:165.
38. Kjaer P, Leboeuf-Yde C, Sorensen J, Bendix T. An epidemiologic study of MRI and low back pain in 13-year-old children. Spine 2005; 30:798.
39. Salminen S, Erkintalo M, Pentti J, Oksanen A, Kormano M. Recurrent low back pain and early disc degeneration in the young. Spine 1999; 24:1316.
40. Sponseller P. Evaluating the child with back pain. Am Fam Physician 1996; 54: 1933.
41. Hammerberg K. New concepts on the pathogenesis and classification of spondylolisthesis. Spine 2005; 65:S4.
42. El Rassi G, Takemitsu M, Woratanarat P, Shah S. Lumbar spondylolysis in pediatric and adolescent soccer players. Am J Sports Med 2005; 33:1688.
43. Cavalier R, Herman M, Cheung E, Pizzutillo P. Spondylolysis and spondylolisthesis in children and adolescents: 1. Diagnosis, natural history, and nonsurgical management. J Am Acad Orthop Surg 2006; 14:417.
44. Ginsburg G, Bassett G. Back pain in children and adolescents: evaluation and differential diagnosis. J Am Acad Orthop Surg 1997; 5:67.
45. Cohen E, Stuecker R. Magnetic resonance imaging in diagnosis and follow-up of impending spondylolysis in children and adolescents: early treatment may prevent pars defects. J Pediatr Orthop B 2005; 14:63.
46. Ali R, Green D, Patel T. Scheuermann's kyphosis. Curr Opin Pediatr 1999; 11:70.
47. Harreby M, Neergaard K, Hesselsøe G, Kjer J. Are radiologic changes in the thoracic and lumbar spine of adolescents risk factors for low back pain in adults? A 25-year prospective cohort study of 640 school children. Spine 1995; 20:2298.
48. Varlotta G, Brown M, Kelsey J, Golden A. Familial predisposition for herniation of a lumbar disc in patients who are less than twenty-one years old. J Bone Joint Surg 1991; 73-A:124.
49. Kurth A, Rau S, Wang C, Schmitt E. Treatment of lumbar disc herniation in the second decade of life. Eur Spine J 1996; 5:220.
50. Atalay A, Akbay A, Atalay B, Akalan N. Lumbar disc herniation and tight hamstrings syndrome in adolescence. Childs Nerv Syst 2003; 19:82.
51. Ramirez N, Johnston C, Browne R. The prevalence of back pain in children who have idiopathic scoliosis. J Bone Joint Surg 1997; 79-A:364.
52. Roach J. Adolescent idiopathic scoliosis. Orthop Clin North Am 1999; 30: 353–65.
53. Knoeller S, Uhl M, Adler C, Herget G. Differential diagnosis of benign tumors and tumor-like lesions in the spine. Own cases and review of the literature. Neoplasma 2004; 51:117.

54. Schwend R, Hennrikus W, Hall J, Emans J. Childhood scoliosis: clinical indications for magnetic resonance imaging. J Bone Joint Surg 1995; 77–A:46.
55. Kauffman R, Overton T, Shiflett M, Jennings J. Osteoporosis in children and adolescent girls: case report of idiopathic juvenile osteoporosis and review of the literature. Obstet Gynecol Sur 2001; 56:492.
56. Keim H. The Adolescent Spine. 2nd ed. New York: Springer-Verlag; 1982.
57. Cassidy JT, Petty RE. Juvenile Ankylosing Spondylitis. In: Cassidy JT, Petty R, Laxer RM, Lindsley CB, eds. Textbook of Pediatric Rheumatology. 5th ed. Philadelphia: WB Saunders Co., 2005; Chapter 13, pp. 304–323.
58. Petty RE, Southwood TR. Psoriatic Arthritis. In: Cassidy JT, Petty R, Laxer RM, Lindsley CB, eds. Textbook of Pediatric Rheumatology. 5th ed. Philadelphia: WB Saunders Co., 2005; Chapter 14, pp. 324–333.
59. Bollow M, Biedermann T, Kannenberg J, et al. Use of dynamic magnetic resonance imaging to detect sacroilitis in HLA-B27 positive and negative children with juvenile arthritides. J Rheumatol 1998; 25:556.
60. Roger E, Letts M. Sickle cell disease of the spine in children. Can J Surg 1999; 42:289.
61. Borenstein D, Wiesel S, Boden S. Low Back and Neck Pain. Comprehensive Diagnosis and Management. 3rd ed. Philadephia: Saunders; 2004.
62. Vichinsky E. The Morbidity of Bone Disease in Thalassemia. Ann NY Acad Sci 1998; 850:344.
63. Fernandez M, Carrol C, Baker C. Discitis and vertebral osteomyelitis in children: An 18-Year Review. Pediatrics 2000; 105:1299.
64. Ring D, Johnston C, Wenger D. Pyogenic infectious spondylitis in children: The convergence of discitis and vertebral osteomyelitis. J Pediatr Orthop 1995; 15:652.
65. Brown R, Hussain M, McHugh K, Novelli V, Jones D. Discitis in young children. J Bone Joint Surg (Br) 2001; 83-B:106.
66. Reihsaus E, Waldbaur H, Seeling W. Spinal epidural abscess: a meta-analysis of 915 patients. Neurosurg Rev 2000; 232:175.
67. Cabral D, Tucker L. Malignancies in children who initially present with rheumatic complaints. J Pediatr 1999; 134:53.
68. Parker A, RObinson R, Bullock P. Difficulties in diagnosing intrinsic spinal cord tumours. Arch Dis Child 1996; 75:204.
69. Kujala U, Kinnunen J, Helenius P, Orava S, Taavitsainen M, Karaharju E. Prolonged low-back pain in young athletes: a prospective case series study of findings and prognosis. Eur Spine J 1999; 8:480.
70. Watson K, Papageorgiou A, Jones G, et al. Low back pain in schoolchildren: occurence and characteristics. Pain 2002; 97:87.
71. Grabois M. Management of chronic low back pain. Am J Phys Med Rehabil 2005; 84(Suppl.):S29.
72. Furlan A, Clarke J, Esmail R, Sinclair S, Irvin E, Bombardier C. A critical review of reviews on the treatment of chronic low back pain. Spine 2001; 26:E155.
73. Carragee E. Persistent Low Back Pain. N Engl J Med 2005; 352:1891.
74. Hayden J, Tulder Mv, Malmivaara A, Koes B. Meta-analysis: exercise therapy for nonspecific low back pain. Ann Intern Med 2005; 142:765.

75. Jones M, Stratton G, Reilly T, Unnithan V. A school-based survey of recurrent nonspecific low-back pain prevalence and consequences in children. Health Educ Res 2004; 19:284.

76. Hart L, Deyo R, Cherkin D. Physician office visits for low back pain. Frequency, clinical evaluation, and treatment patterns from US national survey. Spine 1995; 20:11.

77. Croft P, Macfarlane G, Papageorgiou A, Thomas E, Silman A. Outcome of low back pain in general practice: a prospective study. Br Med J 1998; 316:1356.

78. Thomas E, Silman A, Croft P, Papageorgiou A, Jayson M, Macfarlane G. Predicting who develops chronic low back pain in primary care: a prospective study. Br Med J 1999; 318:1662.

79. Brattberg G. Do pain problems in young school children persist into early adulthood? A 13-year follow-up. Eur J Pain 2004; 8:187.

80. Power C, Frank J, Hertmzan C, Schierhout G, Li L. Predictors of low back pain onset in a prospective British study. Am J Public Health 2001; 91: 1671.

81. Harreby M, Hesselsøe G, Kjer J, Neergaard K. Low back pain and physical exercise in leisure time in 38-year-old men and women: a 25-year prospective cohort study of 640 school children. Eur Spine J 1997; 6:181.

82. Lindsley GB, Laxer RM. Arthropathies of Inflammatory Bowel Disease. In: Cassidy JT, Petty R, Laxer RM, Lindsley CB, eds. Textbook of Pediatric Rheumatology. 5th ed. Philadelphia: WB Saunders Co., 2005; Chapter 15, pp. 334–339.

83. Southwood TR, Passo MH. Spondyloarthropathies in childhood. In: Maddison P, Isenberg D, Woo P, Glass D, eds. Oxford Textbook of, Rheumatology. 2nd ed, Oxford: Oxford University Press, 1998; Chapter 5.5.2, p. 1049–58.

84. Petty RE. Enthesitis Related Arthritis. In: Szer IS, Kimura Y, Malleson PN, Southwood TR, eds. Arthritis in Children and Adolescents. Oxford: Oxford University Press, 2006; Chapter 2.7, pp. 259–264.

85. Cabral DA. Psoriatic Arthritis. In: Szer IS, Kimura Y, Malleson PN, Southwood TR, eds. Arthritis in Children and Adol scents. Oxford: Oxford University Press, 2006; Chapter 2.6, pp. 252–258.

86. Petty RE, Laxer RM. Systemic Lupus Erythematosus. In: Cassidy JT, Petty R, Laxer RM, Lindsley CB, eds. Textbook of Fediatric. Rheumatology. 5th ed, Philadelphia: WB Saunders Co., 2005; Chapter 16, pp. 342–391.

87. Cassidy JT, Petty R. Overlap Syndromes. In: Cassidy JT, Petty R, Laxer RM, Lindsley CB, eds. Textbook of Pediatric Rheumatology. 5th ed, Philadelphia: WB Saunders Co., 2005; Chapter 21, pp. 482–491.

88. Cassidy JT, Lindsley CB. Juvenile Demiatomyositis. In: Cassidy JT, Petty R, Laxer RM, Lindsley CB, eds. Textbook of Pediatric Rheumatology, 5th ed, Philadelphia: WB Saunders Co., 2005; Chapter 18, pp. 407–441.

89. Li SC, Imundo LF. Major rheumatic diseases. In: Szer IS, Kimura Y, Malleson PN, Southwood TR, eds. Arthritis in Children and Adolescents, Oxford: Oxford University Press, 2006; Chapter 1.6, pp. 86–115.

90. Sherry DD, Malleson PN. Pain and the Pain Amplification Syndromes. In: Cassidy JT, Petty R.Laxer RM, Lindsley CB, eds. Textbook of Pediatric

Rheumatology. 5th ed. Philadelphia: WB Saunders Co., 2005; Chapter 37, pp. 697–715.

91. Imundo LF. Idiopathic pain syndromes. In: Szer IS, Kimura Y, Malleson PN, Southwood TR, eds. Arthritis in Children and Adolescents. Oxford: Oxford University Press, 2006; Chapter 1.9, pp. 147–154.

92. Kimura Y. Common presenting problems. In: Szer IS, Kimura Y, Malleson PN, Southwood TR, eds. Arthritis in Children and Adolescents. Oxford: Oxford University Press; 2006, Chapter 1.3, pp. 24–48.

11

Adolescents with Joint Pain: A Sports Medicine Perspective

Rebecca A. Demorest

Department of Orthopedics and Sports Medicine, Children's National Medical Center, and The George Washington University School of Medicine and Health Sciences, Washington, D.C., U.S.A.

It is estimated that more than 30 million children in the United States participate in organized sports each year, with more than 7.5 million high school students playing competitive sports during the 2005/2006 school year. With the advent of year round recreational and competitive teams along with travel teams there are more and more opportunities for adolescents to participate in sports. Through Title IX, the first comprehensive federal law in the United States to prohibit sex discrimination against students and employees of educational institutions, girls have had an explosion in the number and variety of sports opportunities available to them. Along with this increase in sports participation has come the recognition that injuries do occur. In 2000–2001, there were more than 4.3 million visits to the ER for sports and recreation injuries with a majority of these injuries occurring in the 5- to 24-year-old age group. There are more than 10 million annual injury visits to pediatricians' offices with the number one reason being sports injuries and overexertion. More than 25% of adolescent injury visits are attributable to knee injuries. Overuse injuries have become more prevalent in this age of sports participation. This chapter will review some of the most common musculoskeletal injuries seen in this active adolescent age group.

Adolescent sport injuries are unique in that due to rapid growth, teenagers are more likely to injure a growth plate rather than the surrounding muscle-tendon unit. Apophyses (secondary centers of ossification where tendons attach) are frequently injured both acutely and chronically in adolescents. As these growth plates fuse at different ages, knowing the general patterns of ossification can help distinguish theses injuries.

Adolescents are sometimes hesitant to report injuries or pain because of peer pressure and their desire to participate in their sport. Close attention to the psychological impact injuries impart on adolescents is important in helping them fully recover and return to activity.

THE KNEE

The knee is one of the most common joints injured during sports activity (Fig. 1). Common sports knee injuries are listed in Table 1. Careful evaluation of the hip is required in anyone presenting with knee pain as hip pain is frequently referred to the knee in children and adolescents. Signs of a more serious knee injury include a knee effusion, knee catching or locking, instability, inability to bear weight, and a concerning history. Knee radiographs should include an anteroposterior (AP), lateral, tunnel, and sunrise view for all acute injuries (Fig. 2). Oblique radiographs can be useful to visualize fractures but are not a standard view. Secondary imaging should not be ordered without initial plain films. Immobilization is necessary for fractures, patellar tendon ruptures, and medial collateral ligament (MCL) injuries with most other injuries responding to early range of motion. Rest, ice for 20 minutes at a time, compression, and elevation of the joint above the heart (RICE) should be implemented after an acute injury.

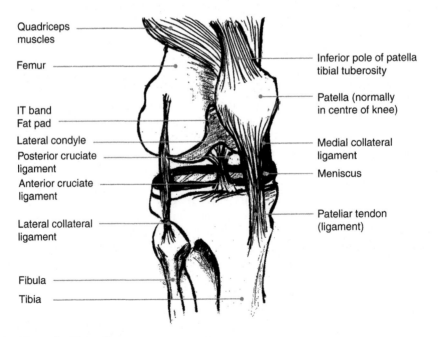

Figure 1 Knee diagram.

Table 1 Common Sports Knee Injuries

Injury	Acute/chronic	Mechanism of injury/symptoms	Physical examination
Anterior cruciate ligament	Acute	Usually noncontact; the planted leg is twisted; hear or feel a pop; instability; swelling within a few hours	Large effusion; positive Lachman's; may have concomitant ligament or meniscus injury
Fat pad impingement	Chronic	Pain with running/jumping; pain under or next to the patellar tendon	Pain medial or lateral to patellar tendon; no effusion; pain with repetitive knee extension
IT band syndrome	Chronic	Lateral knee pain with running; clicking sensation of lateral knee	Lateral knee pain over IT band; positive Ober's test
Medial collateral ligament	Acute	Valgus stress to the knee; swelling, instability	Moderate effusion; pain along MCL; pain or instability noted with valgus stress test at $0°$ or $30°$
Meniscus	Acute	Twisting mechanism; may have catching or locking; may lack full extension	Small effusion; posterior-medial, or posterior-lateral jointline tenderness; pain with full flexion of the knee
Osgood Schlatter	Chronic	Pain with running, jumping, kneeling	Pain over tibial tuberosity; tight hamstrings
Osteochondritis dessicans	Chronic	Intermittent pain and/or swelling with running, jumping, walking	$+/-$ effusion; $+/-$ pain at medial femoral condyle
Patellofemoral stress syndrome	Chronic	Retropatellar or peripatellar tenderness with running, stair climbing, prolonged sitting, giving way sensation	$+/-$ medial or lateral facet tenderness, positive compression and apprehension test, no effusion

(Continued)

Table 1 Common Sports Knee Injuries (*Continued*)

Injury	Acute/chronic	Mechanism of injury/symptoms	Physical examination
Patellar dislocation	Acute or chronic	Twisting mechanism or fall; pain and immediate swelling around patella	Large effusion; pain around patella and facets, medial retinacular pain, positive compression and apprehension test
Patellar tendonitis	Chronic	Pain with running and jumping	Pain over patellar tendon; tight hamstrings
Posterior cruciate ligament	Acute	Fall or hit with knee in flexed position; swelling	Effusion; positive sag sign and posterior drawer test
Salter Harris I fracture of distal tibia or proximal femur	Acute	Valgus stress to the knee with swelling; may have decreased range of motion	Effusion; pain at distal femoral or proximal tibial physis, pain with valgus stress
Sinding Larsen-Johansson syndrome	Chronic	Pain with running, jumping, kneeling	Pain at inferior pole of patella; tight hamstrings

Abbreviations: IT, iliotibial; MCL, medical collateral ligament.

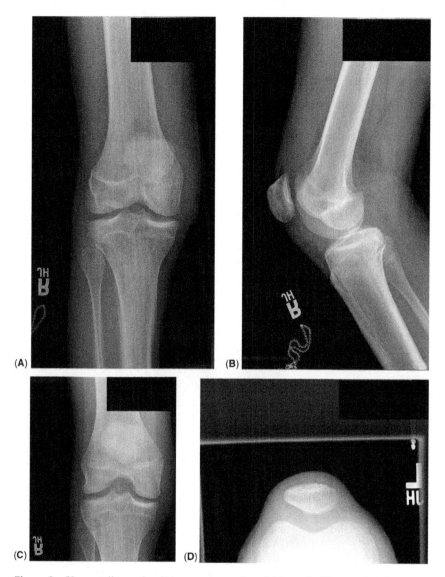

Figure 2   Knee radiographs: (**A**) anteroposterior; (**B**) lateral; (**C**) tunnel; (**D**) sunrise.

Case 1: A 16-year-old field hockey player has had four months of bilateral knee pain that worsened in the last week since field hockey started. She denies any injury or trauma that began her symptoms. She says the pain began during lacrosse season last spring and is worse with running, stair climbing, and prolonged sitting. She denies swelling but says the knee does occasionally buckle on her. She has used pain medications and some occasional ice along with an over the counter knee brace without much relief. She took most of the summer off from sports and noticed pain when she began running three miles a day for lacrosse tryouts last week.

Patellofemoral Stress Syndrome

Patellofemoral stress syndrome (PFSS) is a broad, nondescript term used in sports medicine to describe anterior knee pain when the true etiology is multifactorial or unknown. Multiple factors such as an increased Q angle, femoral anteversion, foot hyperpronation, gluteal/hip weakness, tight hamstrings, and patellar malalignment are suggested contributors to anterior knee pain. PFSS is commonly seen in adolescent females but occurs in males and females of all ages. Pain can be unilateral or bilateral and is not usually associated with trauma or injury. Pain occurs with prolonged walking, running, stair climbing, jumping, or prolonged sitting (theater sign), but not usually at rest or at night. Many adolescents experience an increase in pain when they return to sports activity, especially if they do not condition in the preseason. Pain may occur in athletes, nonathletes, or overweight adolescents.

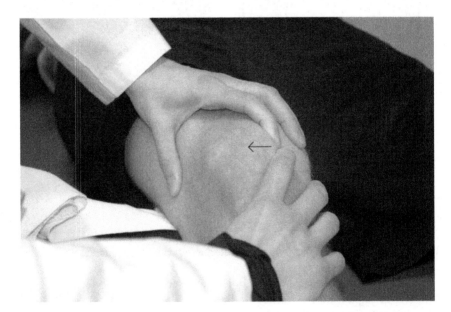

Figure 3 Apprehension test for patellar instability. Placing your knee underneath the patient's knee to allow 30° of relaxed flexion, gently try to laterally sublux the patella. A look of apprehension or pain is a positive finding. Instability/laxity may be noted. Be careful not to displace too aggressively as one could dislocate the patella.

Physical examination may show hyperpronation upon gait evaluation. There is typically no knee effusion and a normal ligament examination. There is frequently patellar hypermobility, medial and lateral patellar facet tenderness, and pain with patellar compression and apprehension testing (Fig. 3). There may also be patellar malalignment or maltracking. The vastus medialis, the medial quadriceps muscle, may be mildly atrophied. The athlete may experience pain with tightening of the quadriceps muscles. Hamstrings are typically tight (Fig. 4). Core strength is usually weak and single leg squats may reveal knee valgus (Fig. 5). Knee radiographs are usually normal but may reveal a laterally displaced patella or a shallow femoral groove on sunrise view.

Rehabilitation consists of daily physical therapy to increase flexibility of the hamstrings and hip flexors along with strengthening of the lower extremity and especially the core body. Pilates is an excellent way to strengthen the core body muscles. Icing for 15 to 20 minutes after activity and use of nonsteroidal anti-inflammatories (NSAIDs) after activity on an as needed basis provide some pain relief. McConnell taping or a patellar stabilizing brace helps provide central patellar alignment if tracking or subluxation is a problem. Avoiding running for conditioning and cross

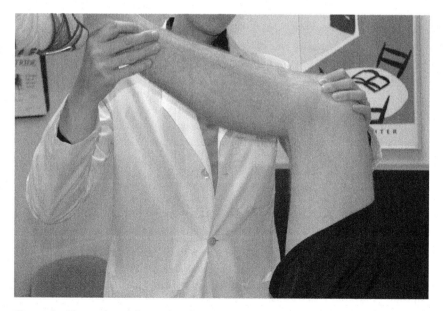

Figure 4 Hamstring tightness/popliteal angle. With the patient relaxed and the hip and knee flexed to 90° gently try to extend the lower leg to gauge hamstring flexibility. Do not have the patient help push. Less than 160° (90° = lower leg horizontal) is considered tight.

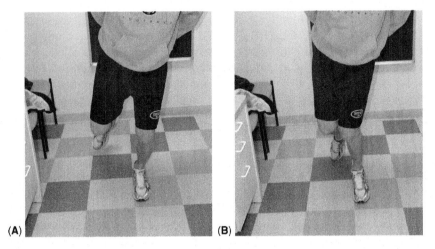

Figure 5 Single leg squat for core body strength. Have the patient stand on one leg, and without holding on perform a single leg squat to 90° of knee flexion. If core body strength is good, the hip, knee, and ankle will remain in a straight vertical line as shown in (**A**). If core body strength is poor the knee will buckle into valgus as shown (**B**).

training on the bike, elliptical machine or in the pool helps to decrease symptoms while allowing the athlete to remain active. Orthotics to correct hyperpronation along with supportive, new running shoes can also be recommended.

Case 2: A 14-year-old soccer player has a 3-month history of left knee pain without a mechanism of injury. Pain occurs at the tibial tuberosity with running and jumping and any time the area is hit. There is no knee effusion but the tibial tuberosity is prominent on the left side. Three years ago he had similar pain along the inferior patella. He has been growing a lot lately and has very tight hamstrings.

Osgood Schlatter and Sinding-Larsen-Johansson Syndrome

Osgood Schlatter (OS) is a traction apophysitis of the tibial tuberosity that is seen in children ages 11 to 17. This growing part of the bone is more vulnerable to injury that the surrounding patellar tendon. Insidious onset of pain, which may be unilateral or bilateral, occurs at the tibial tuberosity with running, jumping, or kneeling. Physical examination may reveal an enlarged, tender, swollen tibial tuberosity. Many athletes will have tight hamstrings and feel an anterior knee stretch with full flexion of the knee. Lateral radiographs may show fragmentation of the tibial tuberosity but are not necessary for diagnosis (Fig. 6). Treatment consists of daily physical

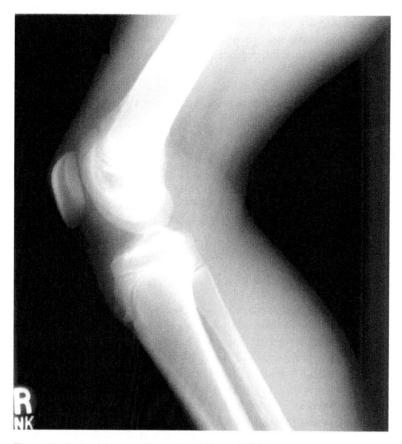

Figure 6 Lateral knee radiograph of Osgood Schlatter.

therapy to increase flexibility of the hamstring, quadriceps, and hip flexors along with core body strengthening. Icing after activity for 15 to 20 minutes and NSAIDs on an as needed basis after activity can help control pain. A patellar tendon strap (a Velcro strap placed across the patellar tendon to decrease tension on the tibial tuberosity) may also decrease pain. Athletes may continue to participate in sports as long as they are not limping or having a significant increase in pain. The enlarged tibial tuberosity is a permanent feature of OS that lasts into adulthood. Beware of an athlete presenting with "acute OS" as he/she must be evaluated for a Salter Harris type III fracture of the proximal tibia or tibial avulsion. If an athlete can not perform a straight leg raise concern for a more serious injury such as those listed above or a patellar tendon rupture should be addressed. Rarely, if conservative methods fail, casting in extension or surgical excision of ossicles may be recommended.

Sinding-Larsen-Johansson (SLJ) syndrome is a similar traction apophysitis that occurs at the inferior pole of the patella in 9- to 14-year-olds. Fragmentation of the inferior pole of the patella may be seen on lateral radiographs. It causes discomfort with the same activities as OS and is treated similarly. Beware the acute SLJ as one may have a patellar sleeve fracture that requires surgical management. Straight leg raise testing can evaluate this extensor mechanism.

LIGAMENT AND MENISCUS

The four stabilizing ligaments of the knee and meniscus can be injured with acute twisting or traumatic injuries. Knowing the mechanism of injury is paramount in helping to distinguish which structure may be damaged. Injuries to the MCL and posterior cruciate ligament (PCL) can usually be treated conservatively whereas injuries to the anterior cruciate ligament (ACL), lateral collateral ligament, and meniscus typically require surgical fixation.

Anterior Cruciate Ligament

Case 3: A 16-year-old lacrosse player injured her right knee after she planted her right leg to take a shot on goal during a game. As she twisted her knee she felt a pop and had immediate pain. She had significant swelling within a few hours and has a hard time putting full weight on her knee. She has a large knee effusion and a positive Lachman test.

The ACL is the stabilizing ligament of the knee that prevents the tibia from moving forward off of the femur. The ACL is injured 2–8 × more frequently in adolescent females than males. Improper landing mechanisms are thought to be one of the reasons for this female predominance. ACL prevention programs are popular in sports such as soccer, basketball, and volleyball. The goal of these programs is to teach proper landing techniques to help prevent ACL injury.

The mechanism of injury is usually noncontact, with the foot planted when a twisting injury occurs at the knee. Athletes usually hear or feel a pop and have immediate pain and swelling within 24 hours. Contact injuries may also damage the ACL. On examination they can usually weight bear but have a large effusion. They have a positive Lachman test suggesting that the ACL is torn (Fig. 7). Radiographs are usually normal although a Segund Fracture is pathognomonic for an ACL tear (Fig. 8). An MRI may be useful in equivocal cases or in those with a soft endpoint on Lachman testing. Athletes with a torn ACL need surgical repair if they wish to return to cutting and pivoting sports as without an ACL, cutting and pivoting will damage the meniscus and may lead to early arthritis. Adolescents may also sustain a tibial spine fracture with the same mechanism that tears the ACL. Mechanisms that injure the ACL can also cause damage to the MCL or meniscus.

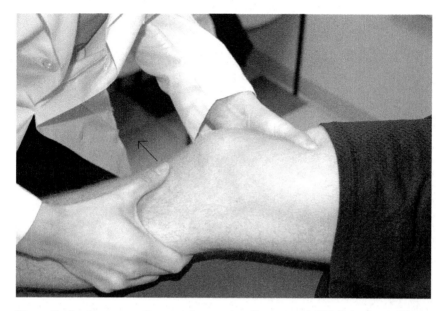

Figure 7 Lachman test for anterior cruciate ligament (ACL) integrity. With the patient's hip relaxed and slightly externally rotated, place your hands on the femur and tibia. You should be able to move the leg up and down with the hand supporting the distal femur. Place the tibia hand with the thumb just medial to the tibial tuberosity and the rest of the hand supporting the calf musculature. Hold the relaxed knee at 20–30° of flexion. While stabilizing the femur quickly pull upwards toward your shoulder (*without rotating the leg*) with the hand holding the tibia. If the ACL is intact, an endpoint (*taught rubberband ending*) will be appreciated. If the ACL is torn, no endpoint or a soft stoppage will be felt.

Medial Collateral Ligament

Case 4: A 17-year-old football running back injured his knee in Friday's football game. An opponent came from the side and fell into his knee as he was being tackled. He had immediate pain on the inside of the knee and was unable to continue playing. He has pain with full knee extension and flexion and has a knee effusion. He has discomfort and instability noted with valgus stress testing of the knee at 30°.

The MCL, a medial stabilizer of the knee, is injured after a valgus stress is placed to the knee, such as being tackled during football. There is usually a moderate effusion, pain, and decreased knee range of motion. Tenderness to palpation is present over the MCL and pain or instability is present with a valgus stress to the knee at 0 or 30°. In skeletally immature adolescents, the tibial or femoral physis may be damaged by the same mechanism that damages the MCL. These adolescents will have pain with palpation over the physis as opposed to the ligament. Stress radiographs can

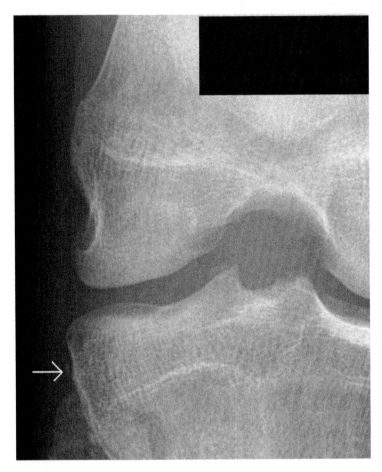

Figure 8   Segond fracture of anterior cruciate ligament tear.

be helpful in determining a physeal injury. MCL injuries are usually treated with immobilization in a straight leg brace for 2–3 weeks to allow the ligament to heal, followed by aggressive physical therapy to return them to their sport.

Meniscus

Case 5: A 15-year-old wrestler injured his knee in practice. He was taking someone down, and as his knee pad got stuck on the mat, he twisted his right knee. He can not fully extend the knee and has pain along the posteriorlateral joint line along with a small knee effusion.

The meniscus are the shock absorbers that cushion the knee and protect the femur and tibia from being bone on bone. They are C shaped structures that absorb shock with weight bearing activity. Meniscal injuries are not very common in adolescents although may occur after a traumatic twisting injury that may cause other ligament damage. Meniscal injuries cause pain along the posterior joint lines and athletes will have significant discomfort with full flexion or McMurray's testing of the knee. They may be unable to full straighten their knee and have a flexion contracture. Locked knees are orthopedic emergencies and anyone unable to full extend the knee should remain non-weightbearing on crutches. Radiographs are normal. MRIs usually show meniscal damage. Surgical repair or excision is necessary depending on the injury.

Some people are born with a congenital malformation where the meniscus are shaped like discs. Those with a discoid meniscus are predisposed to injuring or tearing the meniscus secondary to increased forces across the meniscus. These athletes may present with recurrent catching, locking, or swelling of the knee after activity or twisting. An MRI can help define a discoid meniscus. Recurrent mechanical symptoms or tears require surgical evaluation.

Patellar Tendonitis and Fat Pad Impingement

Case 6: A 16-year-old basketball player has had intermittent anterior knee pain for the last six months that gets worse during basketball. He has pain with prolonged running and jumping. He denies an injury that began his symptoms. He points to the patellar tendon as to where he gets his pain. He has pain with resisted knee extension. He has tight hamstrings and difficulty with single leg squats as he goes into a valgus maneuver.

Patellar tendonitis (PT) or "jumper's knee" is a tendonitis (acute inflammation) or a tendonosis (chronic scarring and changes of the tendon) of the patellar tendon. It is a common overuse injury in sports that require jumping such as basketball. Pain occurs along the patellar tendon with knee flexion/extension, running and jumping. There is no knee effusion or instability. Athletes typically have very tight hamstrings and a weak core body. Treatment consists of daily rehabilitation focusing on core body strengthening and flexibility of the hamstrings and quadriceps. Iontophoresis (electrical delivery of a steroid) can be helpful in decreasing pain. Icing after activity for 15 to 20 minutes along with use of a patellar tendon strap as coutertraction can help decrease pain. Athletes may participate as long as they are not limping or having a significant increase in pain.

Fat pad impingement occurs with the same overuse mechanism as PT. A medial and lateral fat pad lie beneath the patellar tendon and may become inflamed with activity. Treatment is the same as PT although sometimes a steroid injection into the fat pad can decrease exquisite pain. Patellar tendons are never injected with steroids as they may cause tendon rupture or atrophy.

Patellar Dislocations

Case 7: A 17-year-old ice hockey goalie injured her right knee during a game. She was trying to block a shot and felt her patella move out of place. She had immediate pain and swelling and was unable to continue playing. She has a large effusion and pain around the patella. She has discomfort along the medial retinaculum and a positive apprehension test. Ligament testing in stable although she can only flex to 60°. She has had one previous patellar dislocation and has a hypermobile patella on the left side.

Lateral patellar subluxations and dislocations are a frequent sports injury. Subluxations occur when the patella moves partially out of joint with instant relocation as opposed to dislocations where the patella comes fully out of joint and needs to be relocated. The mechanism of injury is usually a twisting/cutting maneuver or fall. Athletes may hear or feel a pop as their patella slides out of place and may remember this sensation of patellar movement. Immediate swelling of the knee along with pain surrounding the patella and the medial retinaculum (the tissue just medial to the patella that gets torn during dislocation) occurs. Athletes with hypermobile patellas or lateral tilt may be predisposed to patellar dislocations. Those with recurrent dislocations may have a positive apprehension test and may have subluxation or dislocation of their patella with range of motion of the knee. Radiographs may show a subluxation/dislocation or lateral tilt on sunrise views. Small fragments of the patella may be fractured with a dislocation.

Treatment consists of initial RICE for the first 48 hours followed by range of motion exercises to help decrease swelling. The key to long-term treatment is an aggressive daily rehabilitation program consisting of core body strengthening especially the hip abductors, along with hamstring and quadriceps flexibility. Icing for 15 to 20 minutes after activity and use of a patellar stabilizing brace can be helpful. McConnell taping can also help guide proper patellar movement during activity. Athletes usually can return to activity in 4 to 12 weeks depending on their motivation regarding rehabilitation.

Once a patella dislocates it becomes easier for the same mechanism to cause further dislocations. For this reason continued rehabilitation exercises for as long as the athlete plays sports is required. If no improvement after 6 months of physical therapy or continued patellar dislocations, surgical evaluation may be necessary.

Osteochondritis Dissecans Lesion

Case 8: An 11-year-old dancer states she has had random right knee pain and swelling over the past 6 months but does not remember injuring the knee. Sometimes after dancing she gets swelling and pain that dissipates over

3 to 4 days with a decrease in activity. She denies any mechanical symptoms. She has no pain in between episodes. Her examination shows a small effusion of the knee and some minimal tenderness with palpation over the medial femoral condyle.

Osteochondritis dissecans lesions (OCD), an injury to the subchondral bone, can develop in almost any joint but are commonly found in the knee along the posterior portions of the femoral condyles or behind the patella. The most common area is the lateral portion of the posteriormedial femoral condyle. Osteochondral fragments may happen with acute trauma however OCD lesions are more chronic in nature. The exact mechanism is unknown but most believe that repetitive trauma or poor blood flow contributes to these lesions. Unilateral or bilateral, OCD lesions occur in both active and inactive adolescents.

Adolescents typically present with months of intermittent knee swelling and pain that lasts for a few days and then dissipates. If the lesion becomes unstable the adolescent may experience mechanical symptoms including catching or locking of the knee. Examination of the knee may reveal a small effusion with vague knee discomfort, a locked knee, or may be normal. The history of intermittent swelling gives more information than the examination typically provides. Four radiographic views of the knee should be obtained however; a tunnel view is the best view to visualize the posterior condyles and may show the lesion (Fig. 9). MRIs are useful in assessing the stability of the lesion. Skeletally immature adolescents with small stable lesions may heal on their own over time.

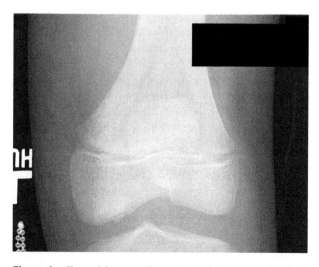

Figure 9 Tunnel knee radiograph depicting an osteochondritis dessicans lesion of the lateral portion of the medial femoral condyle.

Conservative therapy consists of restriction of impact activity and radiographs every 3 months to assess progress. In this author's experience most OCD lesions take a minimum of 6 to 12 months to heal. Skeletally mature adolescents, those with large or unstable lesions, or those with significant pain require surgical evaluation. Many suggest an aggressive surgical approach for most lesions as conservative therapy interferes with lifestyle activity choices during a vulnerable age. Untreated OCD lesions raise the concern for early onset arthritis.

BACK

Back pain in adolescents is a frequent concern as they become more involved in sports. The most common reason for an adolescent to present with back pain is a stress fracture of the pars interarticularis (spondylolysis). Adolescents may also experience muscular pain or spasms, disc disease, or sacroiliac (SI) dysfunction. Typical lumbar spine views include an AP, lateral and occasionally obliques if a spondylolysis is suspected.

Spondylolysis

Case 9: A 16-year-old level 9 gymnast has had right sided low back pain for the past three weeks. She denies a specific injury but notes pain with bending backwards or backwards tumbling. She has no radiation of pain and notes no improvement with ibuprofen or ice. She has pain with palpation just lateral to the right L5 spinous process and has pain with hyperextension and one legged hyperextension (Stork test) on the right.

Spondylolysis is the most common cause of low back pain in adolescents seeking medical evaluation; most commonly seen in the lower lumbar spine at L4 or L5. A spondylolysis is a stress fracture of the pars interarticularis. Athletes who perform repetitive hyperextension, such as dancers, gymnasts, divers, wrestlers, rowers, soccer players, and football lineman, are at increased risk to develop spondylolysis. Low back pain may be unilateral or bilateral, of acute or insidious onset, or worsen after an inciting event. Some may experience radiation of pain into the buttocks. Pain with lumbar spine hyperextension or one-legged hyperextension (the stork test) is sensitive but not specific for spondylolysis (Fig. 10). Examination may also reveal hyperlordosis and tight hamstrings. Radiographs of the lumbar spine should include an AP, lateral, and left and right oblique to evaluate for a stress fracture. On oblique radiographs, the "broken neck" on the Scottie dog represents the pars defect (Fig. 11). Fractures visible on radiographs are usually older and may not have the capacity to heal further. As many acute stress fractures are not visualized on radiographs, if clinical suspicion is high, either a bone scan with single photon emission computed tomography (SPECT) or thin cut CT are recommended for further evaluation.

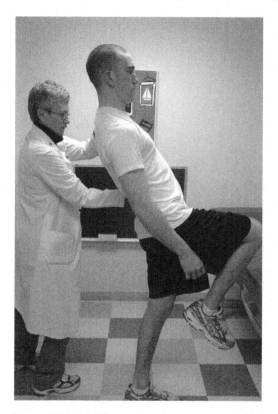

Figure 10 Stork/hyperextension test.

Treatment consists of rest from ALL activity (sports, running, jumping, riding, lifting etc.) until the athlete is pain free. Controversy surrounds the need for a thoricolumbarsacral orthotic or a lumbar sacral orthotic to stabilize the back, prevent movement, and promote healing. If an athlete is deemed reliable to follow treatment guidelines and has no pain with activities of daily living, this author does not always use a brace. When the athlete is pain free at rest and with hyperextension, a monitored daily physical therapy program focusing on core stability and lumbar strengthening in neutral or flexion (avoiding extension) is recommended. Most athletes can return to play within 3 to 8 months of their stress fracture.

Most young athletes with spondylolysis report excellent functional outcomes after diagnosis, with poorer outcomes seen in those with bilateral defects. Complications of a pars interarticularis fracture include nonunion, chronic pain, and a spondylolisthesis. A spondolisthesis or "slip" occurs if there are bilateral pars defects with forward slippage of the anterior vertebral body. A spondylolisthesis can be seen and measured on a lateral

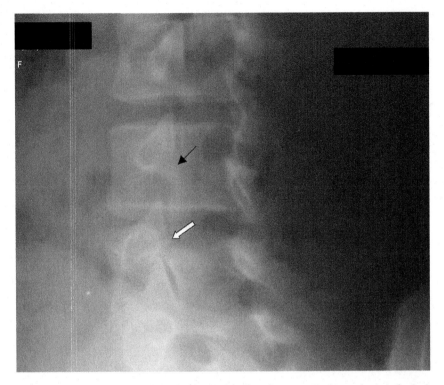

Figure 11 Oblique view of the lumbar spine showing a normal pars interarticularis (*black arrow*). The pars interarticularis shows a lucency along the Scottie dog's neck (*white arrow*) representing a spondylolysis.

lumbar spine radiograph. A large slip (> 50% of the body width) can cause spinal cord compression symptoms and may require surgical management. As slips may worsen during growth periods, adolescents with bilateral spondylolysis should be radiographed every 6 months until maturity to evaluate for a slip or any progression of a slip.

MUSCULAR/HYPERLORDOSIS

Case 10: A 17-year-old overweight male presents with 6 months of intermittent low back pain. Most of his pain occurs with prolonged sitting or standing. He does not remember an injury but has pain when he does his homework on his bed. He has hyperlordosis along with tenderness to palpation of his lower lumbar paraspinal muscles. He has a normal neurologic exam but does go into a valgus maneuver with single leg squats.

Muscular low back pain during adolescence may be acute secondary to a muscle pull or more chronic due to rapid growth, poor posture, and core body weakness. Muscular pain usually occurs with prolonged sitting or standing especially in those with poor posture. Pain may also be elicited during or after sports activity or with overuse. Adolescents with hyperlordosis may experience pain as they grow secondary to pulling along the apophyses of the lumbar spine. Pain occurs along the low back paraspinal muscles or spinous processes and is usually bilateral. There is no radiation of pain, neurologic symptoms, night pain, or bowel/bladder dysfunction.

On examination adolescents may have hyperlordosis or hyperpronatin. They have full range of motion of the back but may have difficulty with full forward flexion secondary to tight hamstrings. They may have discomfort with extremes of motion, side bending or twisting. They have a normal neurologic exam. Many have poor core body strength and go into a valgus maneuver with a single leg squat.

Treatment consists of daily physical therapy focusing on core body strengthening and hamstring flexibility. Weight control measures are important to discuss with overweight adolescents. Heating before activity may help to increase stretch of muscles. Pilates and yoga are excellent activities for this group. Pain medications may be used but are not particularly helpful for relieving discomfort. Proper posture, workspace/computer ergonomics, use of a lumbar support pillow for sitting and shoewear with good arch supports during prolonged walking may benefit adolescents with muscular low back pain.

Disc Disease

Case 11: A 16-year-old football lineman presents with 3 weeks of low back pain in the off-season. He has been doing team conditioning and weight training and remembers his back hurting after squatting 350 pounds. He has right sided low back pain that goes into his buttocks region. He denies weakness into his legs. He has pain when he drives in the car or sits for a long time.

Disc disease, a bulging of the intervertebral disc with or without nerve root impingement, is more frequently an adult back disorder but does occur in adolescents. Athletes lifting weights are particularly prone to disc problems due to improper positioning or lifting excessively heavy weight especially with squatting. Athletes present with low back pain that may radiate into the buttocks or leg or cause parasthesis into the lower extremities. Pain worsens with forward flexion, sitting, or driving. Straight leg raises may be positive however, some adolescent disc bulging may be more central without nerve root impingement resulting in a negative straight leg test. Lower extremity strength and sensation is usually normal but may be compromised with nerve root impingement. Atrophy, weakness, or neurologic symptoms signal more serious disease and should be evaluated appropriately. Radiographs (AP and lateral) are normal although may show some narrowing of the joint spaces on lateral view. An MRI may show disc bulging or nerve root impingement.

Treatment is typically conservative and consists of a daily core body/ lumbar stabilization rehabilitation program in the neutral or extension biased position along with hamstring and hip rotator flexibility. Use of a lumbar support pillow can decrease stress on the disc while sitting. Avoiding prolonged sitting or stationary positions may help circumvent significant discomfort. In acute cases, steroids may be used to help decrease inflammation but are not a mainstay of treatment in adolescents. Rarely, surgery is necessary for disc decompression. Proper weight training technique and discussion regarding weight training is suggested.

SI Dysfunction

Case 12: A 16-year-old tennis player has had 3 weeks of worsening low back pain. She thinks it may have started after twisting to hit a forehand out of her reach. She isolates the pain to the right low back and has pain with sudden movements and twisting. She has some radiation of pain into the buttocks. She has extreme tenderness when she tries to get out of bed, a chair, or the car. She is tender over the right SI joint and has decreased mobility and pain on this side with forward flexion. She has a positive Patrick/FABER test.

The sacroiliac (SI) joint has limited movement (2–4°) but can be a source of pain in adolescent athletes, especially females. Twisting or loading of the joint with activity may cause acute pain. Symptoms are similar to those with muscular low back pain but are directed at the SI joint. Tenderness to palpation at the SI joint along with a positive Patrick's/ FABER test (*f*lexion, *ab*duction, *e*xternal *r*otation of the hip) are typical. Mobility of the SI joint may be excessive or limited on the affected side with forward flexion. Radiographs of the SI joint are normal.

Treatment is conservative. Physical therapy consists of daily flexibility and core body strengthening. Mobilization or manipulation of the joint by a physical therapist may help relive acute symptoms. Attention to equal weight loading of the legs especially when changing positions can help to decrease acute increases in pain. Heat, ice, and nonsteroidal antinflammatories are used but do not typically relieve all pain. Occasionally injections (steroids or prolotherapy) are used to relieve discomfort. (For further discussion of back pain during adolescence, see Chapter 10.)

HIP/GROIN

Case 13: A 15-year-old basketball player has intermittent left hip/back pain for 4 months. She denies an injury but notes pain with twisting activities and prolonged running. She denies radiation of pain or pain at night. She has tenderness to palpation along the iliac crest.

Pelvic Apophyseal Injuries

Case 14: A 15-year-old hurdler injured his right hip when jumping over a hurdle during a track event. He felt a pop and had immediate pain and could not bear weight. He has tenderness over his anterior superior iliac spine and limited range of motion of his hip.

Common pelvic apophyseal injuries occurring during adolescence are listed in Table 2. These injuries are unique to growing adolescents because the growth plate is weaker than the surrounding muscle tendon unit making it more prone to injury. Acute apophyseal avulsion injuries commonly occur during sprinting, hurdling, or jumping after a sudden forceful muscular contraction. Radiographs (AP pelvis) reveal an apophyseal avulsion (Fig. 12). Pain at the apophysis occurs with activity and at rest with restricted range of motion and muscle weakness. Chronic apophyseal injuries can occur with running, skating, soccer, or other endurance sports yet radiographs do not always reveal abnormalities. Chronic traction apophyseal injuries may present with tenderness at the apophysis along with some limitation of motion or weakness. Most apophyseal injuries heal with conservative treatment although large displaced avulsion fragments, especially of the ischial tuberosity, may require surgical fixation. Conservative treatment, over 4 to 16 weeks, consists of rest and protection of the area to limit muscle spasm with acute injuries, ice, and NSAIDs. Progressive resistance exercises begin once full range of motion is achieved. Daily therapy focuses on hip, back and lower extremity flexibility along with a structured core body strengthening program. Noncontact proprioceptive and pliometric drills specific to the athlete's sport complement the strengthening program. Practice and competition may begin when the athlete is pain free and has full motion and strength of the affected area.

Slipped Capital Femoral Epiphysis

Case 15: A 12-year-old overweight male presents with four weeks of an intermittent left leg limp. He denies an injury but remembers landing from catching a ball and having some pain. He points to the groin and thigh area and says he has pain with prolonged running and walking but no pain at rest or at night. He walks with a slight limp and has pain and mild limitation with internal rotation and abduction of the hip.

A slipped capital femoral epiphysis (SCFE) is an orthopedic emergency. Typically seen in overweight adolescents ages 11 to 15, SCFEs present with hip, thigh, or knee pain and a limp that may be unilateral or bilateral. Pain may be acute or more chronic in nature. Adolescents may

Table 2 Common Adolescent Pelvic Apophyseal Injuries

Apophysis	Age at apophyseal ossification	Muscle attachments	Mechanism	Physical exam findings	Sports
Iliac crest	18–21	Abdominals, gluteus maximus	Abdominal contraction with contraction of gluteals; sudden change of direction while running	Pain with abdominal contraction and resisted hip abduction	Running Hockey Football
Anterior superior iliac spine	21–25	Sartorius	Contraction of sartorius with hip extended and knee flexed	Pain with passive hip extension; active hip flexion	Hurdlers Jumpers Sprinters
Ischial tuberosity	18–21	Hamstrings	Hamstring contraction with hip flexed and knee extended	Pain with resisted hip extension or passive hip flexion; difficulty sitting	Hurdlers Jumpers Sprinters
Anterior inferior iliac spine	16–18	Rectus femoris	Contraction of rectus femoris with kicking	Pain with passive hip extension; active hip flexion	Sprinting Kicking

Source: Adapted from Ref. 13.

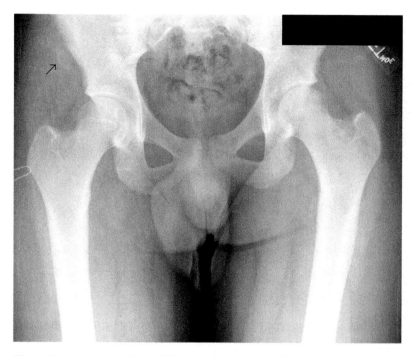

Figure 12 Avulsion injury of the anterior superior iliac spine.

walk with a limp with the affected leg in an externally rotated position. They may have limited internal rotation or abduction and have pain with hip movement. Some will have obligatory external rotation of the hip with flexion of the knee. AP and frog view of the hips show slippage of the epiphysis (Fig. 13). SCFEs need immediate surgical management to prevent further slippage and damage of the hip joint. Adolescents should be made non-weightbearing on crutches and sent for immediate orthopedic evaluation.

Stress Fractures

Case 16: A 16-year-old year-round runner has had left groin pain for two weeks. The pain initially started after an 8-mile run and has gradually progressed to occur during running and occasionally with walking. Menses began at age 14 but have never been regular as she has cessation of her periods during her heavy running. She has adequate calcium intake but a history of a tibial and metatarsal stress fracture last year. She sticks to a 2200 calorie/day diet to maintain her weight. She has painfully limited internal rotation of the hip and has pain with femoral loading.

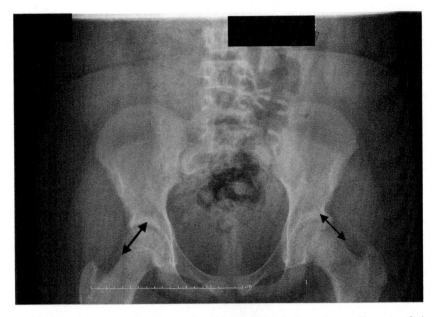

Figure 13 Slipped capital femoral epiphysis. Klein's line shows slippage of the epiphysis on the left with a normal epiphysis on the right.

Stress fractures of the femoral shaft and neck are not common but do occur in adolescents, especially female athletes. Females with the female athlete triad (disordered eating, amenorrhea, and osteopenia/osteoporosis) are at significant risk for stress fractures secondary to poor bone density. Runners, dancers, gymnasts, and those in aesthetic sports are at high risk for this injury. Athletes present with hip, groin, or leg pain with or without a limp. Weight bearing activities increase pain. Pain initially occurs after activity and progresses to happen during activity, with walking, at rest, and then at night.

Physical examination may show a limp and pain or limited rotation of the hip especially internal rotation. Femoral loading may also increase pain. AP and cross table lateral or frog view may show a periosteal reaction or lucency suggestive of a stress fracture. A high index of suspicion is necessary as some stress fractures do not show up on radiographs for weeks. If suspected, the patient should be made non-weight bearing, evaluated with an MRI and sent for orthopedic care. Some stress fractures are stable and will heal with rest and others are unstable and require surgery. Discussion of training patterns, nutrition, menses, shoewear, and other stress injuries is necessary before considering return to sports activity. Proper calcium intake of 1500 mg a day for females/1200 mg a day for males should also be discussed.

THE SHOULDER

Shoulder pain in adolescents occurs after acute trauma or secondary to sports overuse (Fig. 14). A differential diagnosis of acute and chronic shoulder pain is listed in Table 3. Typical shoulder radiographs include an AP, axillary, and scapular Y view. The key to most shoulder injuries is early range of motion and daily physical therapy focusing on scapular stabilization, rotator cuff, and core body muscles along with scrutiny of proper technique.

Multidirectional Instability of the Shoulder Causing Impingement

Case 17: A 14-year-old year round right handed swimmer has three months of intermittent right shoulder pain. The pain usually occurs with butterfly stroke. She feels as though the shoulder clicks and slips with certain movements. She denies paresthies or an injury. She has limited internal rotation of her shoulder and weakness with resisted external rotation and supraspinatous testing. She has a positive sulcus sign along with a positive apprehension and relocation test. She has scapulothoracic dysfunction and weak scapular muscles. She goes into a valgus maneuver with single leg squats.

Throwers, swimmers, wrestlers, tennis players, and athletes participating in overhead activities commonly present with shoulder pain.

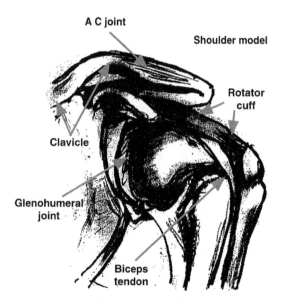

Figure 14 Shoulder diagram.

Table 3 Sports Shoulder Injuries

Injury	Mechanism/history	Physical exam	Treatment
AC sprain (shoulder separation)	Fall on an outstretched hand or lateral blow to shoulder	Pain at AC joint; limited shoulder ROM; positive crossover test	Rest, ice, rehabilitation for grades I–III; surgery for grades IV–VI
Biceps tendonitis	Overuse injury from repetitive throwing/overhead activity	Pain at insertion of long head of biceps; weakness of rotator cuff muscles; positive Speed's test	Rest, ice, rehabilitation of scapular/shoulder muscles; review of technique; iontophoresis prn
Burner/stinger	Compression or traction injury to the neck resulting in stretch of brachial plexus	Limited shoulder ROM/weakness; occasional weakness of upper extremity/numbness or tingling; negative axial load/Spulring's maneuver	Rehabilitation, including ROM and strengthening, ice
Clavicle fracture	Fall or hit to area (usually mid-clavicle)	Pain/deformity at clavicle, limited shoulder ROM	Ice, pain medications, sling for support; use of arm as tolerated; 6–8 weeks for healing
Rotator cuff tendonitis	Overuse injury from repetitive throwing or overhead activity	Limited/painful ROM, weakness of rotator cuff especially external rotators and supraspinatous	Rest, ice, rehabilitation of scapular muscles and rotator cuff; review of technique
Chronic Salter Harris I fracture of proximal humerus	Overuse injury from repetitive throwing/overhead activity	Pain at proximal humeral physis, limited ROM especially internal rotation, weakness of rotator cuff, scapular stabilizers and core body, poor throwing technique (throwing with arm not the body)	Rest from throwing activity, rehabilitation of core body and scapular stabilizers, throwing program once pain free, review of proper pitching mechanics, avoid overuse in future
Shoulder dislocation	Hit to shoulder in an abducted/externally rotated position as with throwing a football; traumatic hit or fall	Swelling, pain with shoulder palpation, limited ROM especially internal rotation, weakness of rotator cuff, decreased sensation along deltoid if axillary nerve injury	Rest, ice, sling for support for 2–5 days, early rehabilitation, debate over need for surgery with first time dislocators

Abbreviations: AC, acromioclavicular; ROM, range of motion.

Shoulder instability from repetitive overload causing impingement combined with muscular imbalance and scapulothoracic dysfunction has been implicated in overuse shoulder injuries in overhead athletes. The shoulder joint is a ball and socket joint likened to a golf ball (humeral head) on a golf tee (glenoid rim). As the bony stability of the shoulder is not structurally sound (i.e., the golf ball is not stable on the small golf tee on which it sits), the shoulder relies on the strength of the surrounding labral capsule, musculature of the shoulder, scapula and neck along with ligamentous integrity to provide support and maintain dynamic stability. When participating in repetitive overhead activities, adolescents may experience pain and impingement if there is increased laxity in the shoulder joint. As many adolescent athletes have natural ligamentous laxity, this instability can cause subsequent impingement of the soft tissues of the subacromial space and act like rotator cuff impingement or tendonitis, seen more often in adults. During swimming, the initial pull through and recovery portions of both freestyle and butterfly stroke cause excessive shoulder impingement as does the overhand tennis serve.

History often reveals an overuse picture with repetitive overhead movements causing shoulder pain. Pain along the anterior shoulder or along the lateral deltoid region may occur with activity, rest, and at night. Pain can be elicited along the long head of the biceps tendon in many athletes. Adolescents with multidirectional instability have increased laxity with anterior, posterior, and inferior shoulder movements. Many symptomatic athletes have scapulothoracic and scaplohumeral dysfunction. This scapulothoracic dysfunction can be visualized by standing behind the patient and watching scapular movement with slow active shoulder abduction. Athletes will have weakness of the rotator cuff, specifically with resisted external rotation and supraspinatous testing (empty can test) (Fig. 15). Anterior and posterior apprehension and relocation testing may be positive and patients may have a sulcus sign, suggesting inferior instability. Impingement testing is commonly positive. AP, axillary, and scapular Y radiographic views of the shoulder are usually normal.

Rehabilitation consists of rest from overuse in the overhead position. Yearlong swimmers or throwers may need a complete break (minimum of 3 months) from the sport to allow for rest and rehabilitation. Rehabilitation focuses on daily scapular stabilization, internal rotation flexibility, rotator cuff strengthening and core strengthening. Icing the shoulder for 15 to 20 minutes after activity and occasional NSAID use after activity is used for pain control. Technique should be reviewed and intensity decreased until symptom free. Decreasing activity by at least 50% in terms of time/yardage and intensity is essential as this is an overuse injury. Avoiding specific activities, such as the butterfly or freestyle stroke, throwing or tennis serves, may help decrease symptoms.

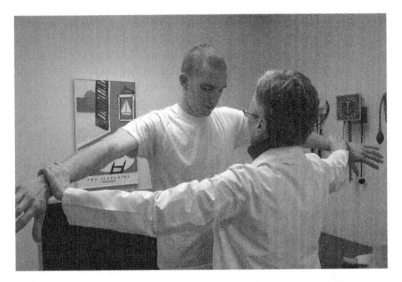

Figure 15 Supraspinatous/empty can test. The examiner places his or her hands on the patient's wrists. With the patient's arm abducted to 90°/forward flexed to 30°/ thumbs pointed downward, have them resist downward displacement of their wrists. Weakness or inability to resist downward displacement suggests injury to the supraspinatous rotator cuff muscle.

Very rarely are subacromial bursal cortisone injections recommended for overuse injury in adolescents. Shoulder stabilization surgery is occasionally necessary for those that fail conservative therapy or have frank dislocations of the shoulder.

THE HEEL

Case 18: A 10-year-old soccer player presents with left heel pain for the last three weeks. The pain began two weeks into soccer practice. She denies an injury but has pain with running and prolonged walking causing her to limp. She has more pain when she goes barefoot or wears her cleats. She has pain along the calcaneal physis and a positive calcaneal squeeze test. She has tight heel cords.

Calcaneal Apophysitis

Sever's disease is a traction apophysitis of the calcaneous seen in children ages 7 to 13. Some studies suggest that the etiology of Sever's disease may be more stress related as opposed to a true traction apophysitis. Insidious onset of heel pain with running is the hallmark symptom. Pain can be elicited with the calcaneal squeeze test (squeezing the medial and lateral portions of the calcaneous together) and palpation of the Achilles insertion onto the calcaneous. As long bone growth may precede tendon and ligamentous growth, many children with calcaneal apophysitis have tight heel cords on examination. Radiographs show a normal appearing apophysis and are not clinically necessary. Soccer players seem to be particularly plagued with this "growing pain" as soccer shoes provide very little cushioning or support. Daily physical therapy to increase flexibility of the gastrocnemius/Achilles complex along with heel cups is helpful in alleviating symptoms. Ice massage for 15 to 20 minutes after activity also controls pain. All conditioning and running should be done in proper running shoes as opposed to cleats when possible. Athletes may participate in sports as long as they are not limping or having a significant increase in pain. Pain usually resolves completely when the apophysis ossifies, around ages 13 or 14.

ELBOW

Elbow injures may occur acutely after a fall or more chronically with overuse activity. Acute injuries after a fall may result in a supracondylar or epicondylar fracture or elbow dislocation visible on radiographs. Typically patients have deformity, pain, swelling, and limited range of motion. Inflammation of the olecranon bursa may occur after a direct fall causing pain and swelling. Chronic injuries to the elbow are seen in overhead athletes, gymnasts, and wrestlers. Insidious elbow pain may suggest an overuse injury to the growth plate, osteochondritis dissecans, or Panner's disease of the elbow. Panner's disease is an avascualar necrosis to the capitellum and usually occurs insidiously in 5- to 12-year-olds. Radiographs usually show the lesion but MRI may be necessary. Ligament injuries are uncommon but may occur especially in baseball pitchers.

Medial Epicondyle Apophysitis (Little League Elbow)

Little league elbow, seen in throwers aged 8 to 14 years, especially pitchers and catchers, is an overuse injury to the fusing medial epicondyle apophysis from repetitive throwing. During the acceleration phase of pitching or the pull through during swimming a large valgus stress is placed on the medial elbow. Athletes typically present with medial elbow pain during throwing and sometimes at rest. Weakness and pain are present with resisted wrist flexion and pronation. The athlete has pain with valgus stress to the elbow and may lack full elbow extension. Occasionally, ulnar nerve irritation causes parasthesias in the ulnar distribution. Comparison radiographs may be necessary to appreciate widening or sclerosis of the medial epicondyle

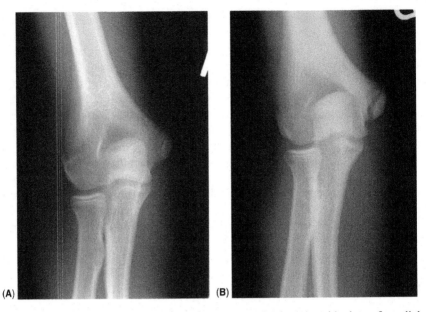

(A)   (B)

Figure 16 Normal open medial epicondyle apophysis (**A**); widening of medial epicondyle apophysis (**B**) consistent with little league elbow.

apophysis (Fig. 16). Acute avulsion injuries may present with acute mechanical symptoms of catching and locking.

Rehabilitation focuses initially on rest from throwing, pitching, and overhead activity for six weeks to six months. This restriction includes no upper extremity weight bearing or lifting activities, which may continue to injure the affected area. The daily rehabilitation program focuses on flexibility and strengthening of the scapular stabilizers, rotator cuff, and wrist flexors. Core body strengthening is another important focus of rehabilitation as power and control during pitching comes from these muscles and deficits can contribute to injury and reinjury. Occasionally, surgical fixation of the avulsed fragment is necessary. Attention to proper throwing form is imperative when the athlete returns to throwing and pitching. Athletes must complete a throwing program before returning to overhead throwing activity. Prevention of little league elbow should be a primary focus of baseball organizations, coaches, parents, and athletes. Recent studies suggest that some degree of conditioning is necessary to avoid injury; however, excessive pitching or overhead activity may lead to further injury. Players younger that 14 years of age should not throw curve balls or sliders. Pitch counts should be followed to prevent excessive throwing and the likelihood for injury.

WRIST

Chronic Salter Harris I Fracture of the Distal Radius in Gymnasts

Case 19: A 12-year-old level 8 gymnast has had right wrist pain for the past three months. The pain began with tumbling activity and now occurs with all weight bearing activity including conditioning. He says the wrist occasionally swells. He has pain along the distal radial physis and discomfort with forced dorsiflexion. He has a normal neurologic examination.

Gymnasts are unique in that they bear up to four times their body weight on their arms when they tumble and perform their sport. Many will experience wrist pain and swelling with repetitive weight bearing activity. A differential diagnosis of wrist pain in this group consists of a chronic Salter Harris I fracture of the distal radius, wrist tendonitis, stress injury or fracture, ganglion cyst, compartment syndrome, or nerve entrapment.

Chronic Salter Harris I fractures are common in both elite and non-elite gymnasts with open physes. Pain at the distal radius occurs with weight bearing dorsiflexion. Athletes may lack full wrist extension or have pain with passive and active extension or radial and ulnar deviation. These athletes typically have weak scapular stabilizers which may be partly to blame for this injury. Radiographs (AP, lateral, and oblique) show widening, sclerosis and cystic changes of the distal radius (Fig. 17). Contralateral views may be necessary to appreciate all changes.

Treatment consists of rest and ice along with daily rehabilitation focused on the scapular stabilizers, upper back muscles, and core body. A wrist splint may be useful for relief of symptoms during the day and while

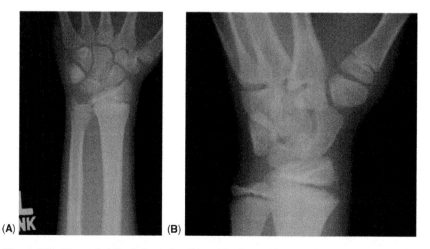

(A)   (B)

Figure 17 Normal AP of the wrist (**A**); widening and sclerosis of the distal radial and ulnar physes on oblique view (**B**) consistent with Salter Harris I fractures.

sleeping. Upon return to sports activity which can be 6 weeks to 6 months, tiger paws (specialized gymnast wrist splints that prevent excessive dorsi-flexion) can be used while performing their sport. Not all athletes with radiographic changes have pain. Not all athletes with pain have radiographic changes. Chronic changes in the wrist could lead to arthritis or chronic pain. Damage to the radial growth plate may cause early cessation of radius growth or an ulnar variance.

CONCLUSION

Sports foster many lifelong essential skills and qualities including independence, teamwork, socialization, coordination, determination, self-worth, and a healthy lifestyle and should be enjoyed by all. Unfortunately, injury has become a common problem due to overuse and intense sport participation in many adolescent athletes. Recognition and education regarding youth injuries are important to prevent further and future injury. The National Institutes of Health web site carries multiple patient handouts for sports injury prevention (www.nlm.nih.gov/medlineplus/sportsinjuries.html) Prevention strategies focusing on rules, proper technique, education, and societal awareness of injury need to be implemented so that sports can continue to be a fun and integral part of every adolescent's life.

ACKNOWLEDGMENTS

Special thanks to Officer Tommy Gold and Susan Gold, RN.

SUGGESTED READING

1. Burt CW, Overpeck MD. Emergency visits for sports related injuries Ann Emerg Med 2001; 37:301–8.
2. Christopher NC, Congeni J. Overuse injures in the pediatric athlete: evaluation, initial management and strategies for prevention. Clin Pediatr Emerg Med 2002; 3(2):118–20.
3. Coady CM, Micheli LJ. Stress fractures in the pediatric athlete. Clin Sports Med 1997; 16(2):225–38.
4. DiFiori JP, Puffer JC, Aish B, Dorey F. Wrist Pain, distal radial physical injury and ulnar variance in young gymnasts: does a relationship exist? Am J Sports Med 2002; 30(6):879–85.
5. Hambridge SJ, Davidson AJ, Gonzales R, Steiner JF. Epidemiology of pediatric injury related primary care office visits in the US. Pediatrics 2002; 109 (4):559–65.
6. Lyman SL, Fleisig GS, Waterbor JW, et al. Longitudinal study of elbow and shoulder pain in youth baseball pitchers. Med Sci Sports Exerc 2001; 33(11): 1803–10.

7. Lyman SL, Fleisig GS, Anderws AR, Osinski ED. Effect of pitch type, pitch count, and pitching mechanics on risk of elbow and shoulder pain in youth baseball pitchers. Am J Sports Med 2002; 30(4):463–8.
8. Martin TJ, Martin JS. Special Issues and concerns for the high school and college-aged athlete. Pediatr Clin N Am 2002; 49(3):533–52.
9. Mahaffey BL, Smith PA. Shoulder instability in young athletes. Am Fam Phys 59(10): 1999; 2773–82, 2787.
10. Nattiv A, Armesy TD. Stress injury to bone in the female athlete. Clin Sports Med 1997; 16(2):197–224.
11. Naughton G, Farpour-Lambert N, Carlson J, et al. Physiological issues surrounding the performance of adolescent athletes. Sports Med 2000; 30(5): 309–25.
12. Nonfatal Sports and Recreation Related Injuries Treated in Emergency Departments—US July 2000–July 2001. MMWR 2002; 51(33):736–40.
13. Paletta GA Jr, Andrish JT. Injuries about the hip and pelvis in the young athlete. Clin Sports Med 1995; 14(3):591–628.
14. Patel DP, Nelson TL. Sports injuries in adolescents. Med Clin N Am 2000; 84(4): 983–1007.
15. Saperstein AL, Nicholas SJ. Pediatric and adolescent sports medicine. Pediatr Clin N Am 1996; 43(5):1013–33.
16. Shea KG, Apel PJ, Pfeiffer RP. Anterior cruciate ligament injury in paediatric and adolescent patients: a review of basic science and clinical research. Sports Med 33(6):455–71.
17. Stricker PR. Sports Training Issues for the pediatric athletes. Pediatr Clin N Am 2002; 49(4):793–802.
18. Waicus KM, Smith BW. Back injuries in the pediatric athletes. Curr Sports Med Rep 2000:1–7.

12

The Young Person with Low Bone Mineral Density

Rolando Cimaz

Department of Pediatrics, Meyer Children's Hospital, Firenze, Italy

Maria Luisa Bianchi

Bone Metabolism Unit, Istituto Auxologico Italiano, IRCCS, Milano, Italy

Osteoporosis is characterized by loss of bone mass and microarchitectural integrity, and its awareness is increasing in the pediatric age as well. Peak bone mass is a key determinant of the lifetime risk of osteoporosis; therefore its prevention begins by optimizing gains in bone mineral throughout childhood and adolescence.

LOW BONE MINERAL DENSITY DEFINITION AND RELEVANCE

Low bone mineral density (BMD) can be defined as "a reduction of bone mineral mass per volume unit of bone tissue, in the absence of mineralization defects." The last point is particularly important regarding infants and children, to avoid confusion with rickets. Clinically significant low BMD is increasingly observed in younger patients. While this condition in adults is normally referred to as osteoporosis (1), there is no consensus about the definition of osteoporosis in children before the appearance of fragility fractures, and there are not widely accepted cut-off densitometric values, such as those proposed by WHO for adult women (2). This is due to two main reasons.

The first is the problematic interpretation of densitometric values in a growing skeleton. Bone size, shape, and mineral density are rapidly changing, and some regions can be affected by low mineral density more than others (e.g., the trunk more than lower limbs). Moreover, the growing process itself—including the onset and progression of puberty—can be influenced by the primary disease. Therefore, it is often difficult to identify an appropriate control group to define normal densitometric values. The usual comparison with sex- and age-matched controls can be inadequate in the presence of chronic diseases affecting skeletal growth and maturation, and can lead to inaccurate evaluations in terms of actual bone mass loss. The second reason is that, while BMD is a strong predictor of the fracture risk in adults (3–5), there are no comparable evidences on this point in the young, although some recent findings may support it (6,7). Presently, most researchers would consider a diagnosis of osteoporosis in the young only after at least one fracture with minimal trauma (8).

Regarding the different forms of osteoporosis, the primary forms of osteoporosis are relatively rare, while a growing number of causes of secondary osteoporosis are now known, mainly as a consequence of the improved long-term outcome of chronic diseases in the young.

Some basic information on the growth, development, and consolidation of bones are desirable as an introduction to the bone problems of adolescents affected by chronic rheumatic diseases.

Skeletal Growth and Development

Growth and physical development depend on a multitude of genetic, nutritional, and environmental factors, and may be optimal only in the presence of optimal health. The skeletal apparatus is no exception. From birth to the end of the pubertal phase, the skeleton of a healthy child increases almost three times in length. The faster skeletal growth occurs from birth to about three years of age, although at a rapidly decelerating yearly rate. From age three to the onset of puberty, there is a relatively slower growth in both sexes, with a small spurt at around eight years. Then, during puberty, a rapid acceleration occurs and the skeleton has another phase of rapid growth. After that, another deceleration phase follows, until full resorption of the growth cartilages occurs. This means the complete cessation of bone lengthening, while the bone mineral content (BMC) continues to increase for several more years. During puberty, the differences between genders become evident. Both the starting age of the pubertal spurt and the growth process are earlier in girls, but the duration of the growth spurt and the maximal peak of growth are greater in boys (see Chapter 3).

Bone Growth Factors

Bone growth is mainly determined by the hypothalamic-pituitary, gonadal, and pituitary-thyroid axes. The balance between cell proliferation and maturation is controlled by several hormones and local factors.

The best known action is that of growth hormone (GH). GH acts on a variety of target cells, including those of growth plates, inducing the release of insulin-like growth factor 1 (IGF-1). The GH/IGF-1 system and the androgens are the main stimulants of cell proliferation in the growth plate cartilages, and are thus the main factors in the linear growth of long bones. Less known is the role of thyroid hormones, thyroxine (T4), and the active metabolite triiodothyronine (T3). Children with hypothyroidism have a reduced linear growth of bones. T3 is known to have direct effects on the growth plate chondrocytes, starting both their proliferation and their maturation process (9).

Gonadal hormones (mainly testosterone and estradiol) are secreted only in minimal quantities in infancy. After puberty, they are secreted in large quantities and are obviously involved both in the appearance of the pubertal growth spurt and in the subsequent disappearance of the growth plate and permanent cessation of growth. They are thought to promote both the proliferation and the maturation of growth plate cells, even though their specific actions at this level are not fully understood.

Bone Mass Acquisition

The fetal skeleton at term contains about 21 g of calcium, the adult skeleton about 1000 g. Many studies evaluated the factors controlling calcium accumulation in the skeleton during growth and development. Maximal accumulation occurs during puberty. Ninety percent of adult bone mass is accumulated by age 18 years, while the remaining 10% will be added in the subsequent skeletal consolidation phase. It is important to know that bone mass acquisition has different characteristics in cortical and trabecular bone. Trabecular bone density is strongly influenced by the hormonal and metabolic factors associated with sexual development during adolescence. On average, spine bone mass (mostly trabecular bone) increases by 13% during puberty, in both sexes. Beyond their direct action, sex hormones act also indirectly, through the modifications that they induce on protein and calcium metabolism, and through the sequence of events triggered by the higher production of GH and IGF-1. Consolidation of cortical bone is slower. So, the "peak of bone mass" is reached at the end of the second decade in the axial skeleton, while in the appendicular skeleton it is reached much later, somewhere between age 30 and 35 years (10).

Effect of Puberty on Bone Mass

Puberty is a complex maturational process involving genetic, environmental, endocrine, and nutritional factors, and has a profound impact on bone mass accrual (11). Longitudinal studies have demonstrated that bone mass accrual is extremely rapid during adolescence, and that about 25% of the peak bone mass is accumulated during the two years of peak height gain. Sabatier et al. (12) have followed with dual energy X-ray absorptiometry (DXA) a large group of healthy females, showing that the four perimenarcheal years, beginning with the first pubertal clinical signs, are essential for bone acquisition. A recent study has confirmed that the age of the onset of menstruation is a predictor of BMD in the lumbar spine (13).

Specific Determinants of Bone Density in Adolescents

Many factors influence bone mass accrual during growth and development: heredity, nutrition, mechanical forces (physical activity and body weight), endocrine factors, and presence of other risk factors. The influence of all these factors on bone mass as well as their interrelationships are very complex and only some key points can be presented here.

Heredity: Genetic factors are considered the most important determinants of the variability of bone mass gain during pubertal maturation. Several genes are involved in bone modeling and remodeling, and influence bone mass determining also its peak value. The polymorphisms of more than 20 candidate genes have been studied (14).

Physical activity: The response of bone to mechanical strain is greater during the growing age than in adult life. Several studies demonstrated that intense physical exercise is associated with an increase in bone mass acquisition at weight-bearing skeletal sites during childhood and especially during adolescence (15). Some studies have observed a positive association also between bone mass and mild physical activity, even if some other studies reported controversial data (16,17). In young girls excessive physical activity, such as that of adolescents female athletes, may lead to hypogonadism with amenorrhea, and a secondary low bone mass.

Nutrition: Increasing dietary calcium intake during childhood and adolescence is associated with a greater bone mass gain and a higher peak of bone mass. The skeleton seems to be more responsive to an increase in calcium intake before the onset of pubertal maturation (18). Benefits are more marked in the appendicular than the axial skeleton. Among other nutrients, protein intake is especially important (19). During the period of growth, inadequate energy and protein intake can affect bone development. Low protein intake also reduces the production of IGF-1. During adolescence, a relative deficiency in IGF-1 may result not only in a reduction of bone longitudinal growth but also of cross-sectional growth. Young people affected by anorexia nervosa or other forms of eating disorders are at high risk of osteoporosis, also because they may have severe calcium, protein or energy (caloric) deficits.

PRIMARY FORMS OF OSTEOPOROSIS: IDIOPATHIC JUVENILE OSTEOPOROSIS

Idiopathic juvenile osteoporosis (IJO) is a rare, self-limited disease, first described in 1965 by Dent and Friedman (20). IJO reveals itself in otherwise healthy children, more often 2 to 3 years before puberty, even if more precocious cases are observed (21). It does not appear to be hereditary and is equally distributed among genders. Affected children have pain in the back, pelvis, knees, feet, and sometimes have difficulties in walking. Compression vertebral fractures are frequent and may reduce the trunk's length. Long bone fractures, more commonly at metaphyses, are also observed. Clinical examination may reveal kyphosis, scoliosis, pigeon chest, long bone deformities and the already mentioned difficulties in walking.

The pathognomonic feature of IJO is the radiological evidence of impaction-type fractures, typically located at weight-bearing metaphyses (e.g. distal tibiae), and characterized by abnormal newly formed bone (*neoosseous osteoporosis*). Long bones have no alteration in dimensions, while vertebral bodies may present height reductions because of biconcave or wedge deformities. There are no relevant laboratory anomalies, except possible nonspecific alterations of bone turnover markers. The diagnosis of IJO is based on the exclusion of other forms of osteoporosis. The differential diagnosis between IJO and the mild forms of Osteogenesis imperfecta may be difficult. The most characteristic clinical feature of IJO is its spontaneous resolution within 2 to 5 years, more frequently occurring at puberty. In some cases, however, the disease persists in adult age (22).

Pathogenesis is not known. Recent histomorphometric studies on bone biopsies of children affected by IJO show alterations in osteoblast activity, with reduced bone formation limited to the trabecular bone, and more specifically to the zones in contact with bone marrow (23). Such data seem to indicate that the skeleton of patients affected by IJO is unable to respond to the greater mechanical requirements of growth and development. Its association with the onset of puberty might also point to a role—not proved until now—of sexual hormones.

The spontaneous resolution of the disease makes it difficult to evaluate treatment efficacy. Positive effects with calcitriol, sodium fluoride or pamidronate have been reported. Presently, the best choice seems to optimize calcium and vitamin D intake according to the recommended daily allowance, recommend regular physical activity (with low risk of trauma), and avoid excessive loads on spine. Bisphosphonate use should be limited to selected cases with significant pain following repeated vertebral or limb fractures.

CHRONIC RHEUMATIC DISEASES AND THEIR EFFECT ON BONE DENSITY DURING ADOLESCENCE AND ON PEAK BONE MASS

The effects of chronic illnesses such as the rheumatic disorders on bone density are well known. Failure to develop adequate bone mineralization is common in children with chronic arthritis. (For a comprehensive review, see Reference 24). Juxta-articular osteopenia can be evident in plain radiographs even in early disease, whereas diffuse osteopenia or osteoporosis can develop later and lead to the risk of vertebral collapse and long-bone fractures after minimal trauma. Multiple risk factors are known to be associated with decreased bone mass, and active arthritis has an osteopenic effect both around affected joints and systemically, by means of a complex and still partly unknown network of proinflammatory cytokines. For example, Henderson and coworkers have studied predictors of BMD in prepubertal patients never treated with glucocorticoids. Almost 30% of mild to moderately ill patients had low total body BMD; parameters of disease severity (number of swollen joints, articular severity score, ESR) exerted a negative effect on bone mineralization. In another study from the same group, approximately 30% of postpubertal females who had never received systemic glucocorticoids demonstrated low bone mass (25,26).

Of particular importance when dealing with adolescents is the fact that chronic disorders are frequently accompanied by pubertal delay. A complex network of endocrine (i.e., the GH-IGF1-IGFBP system) and nutritional factors is usually responsible for this complication. In recent years, several studies have demonstrated that adult subjects with a past history of juvenile arthritis had a lower bone mass than matched controls (27–29). Zak et al. (27) have assessed BMD of the hip and spine in 65 young adults with a history of juvenile chronic arthritis (JCA). They found that BMD was significantly lower (and the frequency of osteopenia and osteoporosis was higher) in patients than in age-, sex-, height- and weight-matched healthy controls. Factors associated with a lower BMD included active disease at the time of the study, baseline erosions, higher Steinbrocker functional class, polyarticular course and chronic corticosteroid treatment. The presence of JCA by itself explained about 20% of BMD variation. The persistence of active inflammation in adulthood—estimated to occur in a third of the patients—is accompanied by a lower BMD than in healthy controls of the same sex and age. In another recent study (28) the impact of disease activity on peak bone mass was assessed in 229 young adults with juvenile arthritis in their mid-twenties, 15 years on average after disease onset. Patients with persistent disease had a significantly lower BMD than did healthy subjects, while patients whose disease was in remission had a normal bone mass overall. However, even in women with only a history of arthritis, BMD was significantly lower in the total body (but not in the lumbar spine or the radius). Moreover, almost half of the patients who were in remission had a history of oligoarthritis. This subtype of disease is more frequent and more benign than the other childhood arthritides and could partly explain the discrepancies between the results of this study and that by Zak et al. where the percentage of patients with oligoarticular disease was lower. Therefore, according to these authors, even the full remission of the disease is not able to completely normalize bone mass at all skeletal sites. Finally, French et al. (29) found osteopenia at spine or femoral neck in 41% of a cohort of adults with a history of juvenile rheumatoid arthritis. This observation is particularly striking given the predominance of patients with pauciarticular JRA in their population based group. Several variables present during adolescence were associated with later low bone density, the most important being a higher Steinbrocker functional class, reduced physical activity, tobacco use and lower calcium intake. These observations, if confirmed by larger studies, are extremely important, since they indicate that there is an increased risk of osteoporosis and fragility fractures in the adult population who suffered from a chronic inflammatory disease many decades before, during childhood and adolescence.

OTHER SECONDARY FORMS OF OSTEOPOROSIS IN ADOLESCENTS

Secondary forms of osteoporosis can be found in a variety of other illnesses (Table 1).

Secondary osteoporoses are constantly increasing in the young for several reasons, such as the longer survival in many severe chronic diseases, the greater pediatric use of potentially bone-damaging drugs, and—last but not least—the greater attention now paid to the alterations of bone and mineral metabolism.

In all forms of secondary osteoporosis in addition to the direct bone derangements caused by the primary disease malnutrition, reduced dietary intake of calcium, protein and vitamin D, limited physical activity, reduced exposure to sunlight, all contribute to alter the skeletal growth and development and the acquisition of bone mass.

Among the most frequent causes of osteoporosis also in pediatric age, we must remember long-term glucocorticosteroid (GC) treatment. Many studies have demonstrated that GCs induce osteoporosis, compromise the attainment of a normal peak of bone mass, and increase the fracture risk even in the young (30). A negative correlation between cumulative steroid dose and bone mass has been demonstrated, particularly in children (31,32). Much discussed are the possible effects on bone mass of inhaled corticosteroids (33), a significant problem considering the increasing incidence of asthma in the young.

DIAGNOSTIC METHODS

Bone densitometry can be performed with three different techniques, each with its own advantages and drawbacks. Among them, DXA has emerged as the preferred—and more widely used—technique in pediatric bone mass evaluation.

Dual-Energy X-Ray Absorptiometry

DXA is the most widely used technique even in children, adolescent, and young people, because of the availability of instruments, accuracy, and precision (reproducibility). It has been much studied both in vivo and

Table 1   Primary and Secondary Osteoporoses in Children and Adolescents

Primary osteoporosis
Idiopatic juvenile osteoporosis
Heritable disorders of connective tissue

Secondary osteoporosis
Neuromuscolar disorders
  Cerebral palsy
  Duchenne muscular dystrophy
  Prolonged immobilization

Chronic diseases
  Leukemia
  Systemic connective tissue diseases
  Cystic fibrosis
  Inflammatory bowel diseases
  Malabsorption syndromes (celiac disease)
  Thalassemia
  Primary biliary cirrhosis
  Nephropathies (nephrotic syndrome)
  Anorexia nervosa
  Organ transplants
  HIV infection

Endocrine diseases
  Delayed puberty
  Hypogonadism
  Turner syndrome
  Growth hormone deficiency
  Hyperthyroidism
  Juvenile diabetes mellitus
  Hyperprolactinemia
  Cushing syndrome

Inborn errors of metabolism
  Protein intolerance
  Glycogen storage diseases
  Galactosemia
  Gaucher disease

Iatrogenic causes
  Glucocorticoids
  Methotrexate
  Cyclosporine
  Heparin
  Radiotherapy
  Anticonvulsant drugs

in vitro, also in younger subjects (34). The radiation dose is low and there have been pediatric dose studies (35). The main advantage of DXA in pediatrics is the possibility to perform a separate analysis of the different skeletal regions, and of the whole skeleton, because the dual-energy X-rays overcome the problem of soft tissues surrounding bone. This also allows an evaluation of the body fat and lean mass, a particularly important aspect in pediatric patients. DXA bone mass measurement is the sum of the cortical and trabecular bone components of the studied skeletal segment. The limit of DXA is that it uses a two-dimension projection of the examined area, so that the calculated "density" is actually the mineral density per unit of bone projection area rather than per unit of bone volume.

Interpretation of DXA During Adolescence in Chronic Rheumatic Diseases

The DXA instruments have obtained ample scientific validation and have been approved by the Food and Drug Administration in the United States of America. The manufacturers have significantly improved their software, and have developed sensitive and specific algorithms for pediatric age and for the recognition of bone and soft tissues, so that even very reduced bone masses can be measured (36). However there are intrinsic limits in the use of DXA for studying a growing skeleton. BMD as calculated by DXA is the ratio of the bone mineral content to the area of the projection of the examined bone, instead of the bone volume. This introduces an error in the presence of different bone volumes. To overcome this problem, some mathematical corrections have been proposed, both for the vertebrae and for the femur. For example, assuming that a vertebral body is a cylinder, its volume has been calculated on the basis of the height and width of the anteroposterior projection of vertebrae. The BMD corrected for this "apparent" vertebral volume has been called "apparent BMD" (BMAD, g/cm^3) and can be calculated with a simple mathematical expression: BMAD = BMD * 4/(3.14 * width of the vertebral body) (37). Other corrections assume that the vertebral body is a cube, or a cylinder with an ellyptic base.

Quantitative Computed Tomography

The main advantage of quantitative computed tomography (QCT) is that of actually measuring the volume (and, consequently, mineral density) of the studied bone. Normally, QCT instruments—endowed with a specific software and calibration phantom—can measure BMD only at the level of lumbar spine. More recently, specific peripheral QCT (pQCT) instruments have been developed to measure BMD at appendicular sites (forearm and femur). Both QCT and pQCT can measure cortical and trabecular bone density separately. The limits are however in the much higher X-ray dose with respect to DXA. Moreover, in the evaluation of vertebral BMD (mainly trabecular bone), the precision can be reduced because trabecular thickness can be lower than the diameter of the "pixel." In evaluating long bone metaphyses, particularly the radius, the measurement of trabecular bone is influenced by cortical bone thickness, a source of error (38). In order to obtain precise measurements in children, a special pediatric phantom must be available for instrument calibration. Moreover—a crucial aspect in longitudinal studies—the used phantom must always be the same, as different phantoms give significantly different results.

Quantitative Ultrasonography

Quantitative ultrasonography (QUS) gives a global evaluation of both the cortical and the trabecular components of examined bones. QUS measurements can only be done at peripheral sites (calcaneus, fingers, tibia, etc.), and each instrument is designed to measure one specific site only. Only some instruments have been adapted for pediatric use, but still may lack the specific devices for smaller children. The main advantages of QUS in pediatrics are essentially two: absence of ionizing radiations and transportability (very important for mass screenings). However, what is exactly measured by QUS is still an open question.

QUS provides two main values: the "speed of sound" (SOS) and the "broadband ultrasonic attenuation" (BUA). While SOS is essentially determined by bone density, BUA depends on several structural parameters of the examined bone. BUA is often considered an index of the bone structure. QUS measurements appear to depend on bone size. So, changes of QUS values with age could possibly reflect bone size changes during growth, rather than actual changes in bone density. A crucial point, for example, for calcaneus-measuring instruments, is the difficulty of a precise repositioning, which might undermine reproducibility and longitudinal studies.

Clinical Problems with Bone Mass Measurement in Pediatrics

The use of densitometry is not only a matter of instruments, but is strongly related to the availability of normative data. The reference databases supplied by the manufacturers are generally not adequate for serious studies. It is essential that the normal reference sample be of adequate size and stratified by sex, age and ethnicity. In studying pediatric patients, the pubertal status must also be considered. Weight and height should also be included in the normal sample (and actually measured in the examined subject) in order to normalize densitometric data for body size. From birth to about 25 years of age (i.e., until the achievement of peak bone mass), the normal reference population must be that of healthy subjects of the same sex and age. BMD comparisons are made in terms of the number of standard deviation (SD) below the average value of the reference population. This index is called the Z-score, and is calculated with the formula: Z-score = Examined subject's

BMD – Average BMD of the reference population/SD of the reference population (39).

In pediatric studies, much more than in adult subjects, the adoption of rigorous protocols for scanning and data analysis is necessary. Regular calibration of the instruments is necessary. The correct positioning (and repositioning) of a patient is a particularly delicate point in order to obtain comparable serial data.

As the skeletal changes in a growing subject are much faster than in adults, and are particularly sensitive to the influence of chronic diseases, the interval between two successive DXA measurements must be adapted to the individual situation, and may be as short as 6 to 12 months.

The simple finding of low bone mass in a child or an adolescent should always be considered a serious warning, but by itself does not allow any diagnosis. Clinical examination, X-rays, biochemical tests, and sometimes also bone biopsy, are needed. Table 2 illustrates the key points in the

Table 2   Initial Diagnostic Workup for Young Patients with Low Bone Mass

History
    Evaluation of primary disease (if any)
    History of fractures (familiar and personal)
    History of drug use (including inhalatory steroids)
    History of gastrointestinal disorders (diarrhea)
Evaluation of lifestyle
    Dietary intake of calcium and protein
    Physical activity (frequency, duration, intensity)
    Exposure to sunlight (or not)
    Smoking
Examination
    Auxological parameters (height, weight, BMI, growth velocity)
    Pubertal stage
    Spine abnormalities (kyphosis, scoliosis)
    Deformities, trunk/limbs proportion
    Joint laxity
    Color of sclerae
    Pain
    Deambulation
Basic blood tests
    Calcium, phosphate
    Alkaline phosphatase
    25-hydroxyvitamin D
    Parathyroid hormone
Basic tests
    Bone density
    Wrist X-ray for bone age

Table 3   Most Common Available Bone Biochemical Markers

Formation
Serum
  Bone specific alkaline phosphatase (BSAP)
  Osteocalcin (OC)
  Carboxyterminal propeptide of type I collagen (PICP)
  Aminoterminal propeptide of type I collagen (PINP)

Resorption
Urine
  Hydroxyproline (rarely used now, due to determination problems)
  Free and total pyridinolines (Pyd)
  Free and total deoxypyridinolines (Dyd)
  N-telopeptide of collagen cross-links (NTx)
  C-telopeptide of collagen cross-links (CTx)

Serum
  Tartrate-resistant acid phosphatase (TRACP)
  Cross-linked C-telopeptide of type I collagen (ICTP)
  NTx
  CTx

---

diagnostic workup. Of note, a recent large study has shown that a low BMD in adolescence is associated with a history of fracture occurrence (40).

Markers of Bone Metabolism During Adolescence

Table 3 lists the most common available markers of bone formation and bone resorption. Changes in bone biochemical markers during growth, and especially during adolescence, are more complex to interpret than in adults. In the growing skeleton, and particularly during puberty, all the mechanisms contributing to bone turnover (longitudinal growth, modeling, and remodeling) are accelerated (41). In girls, the peak of bone markers is earlier but lower than in boys, reflecting gender differences in pubertal development. The plasma levels of bone formation markers are highest when the velocity of bone mineral accrual is maximal. Plasma and urinary concentrations of bone resorption markers progressively decrease after the growth spurt, reaching adult levels at the end of pubertal maturation (on average, 15 to 16 years for girls and 17 to 18 years for boys). These changes are an expression of the reduction in resorption rate associated with the reduction and arrest in longitudinal bone growth.

In adolescents affected by chronic rheumatic diseases the evaluation of bone markers requires special caution. Age, sex, pubertal stage, disease activity, and therapy must all be taken into account in order to evaluate the actual bone damage (reduced bone formation or increased bone resorption). As in many chronic diseases, growth can be affected, determining low levels of bone markers. An apparently paradoxical increase in bone markers is observed during the successful treatment of rheumatic diseases: it reflects the acceleration of growth and pubertal maturation. Moreover, the bone turnover changes linked to pubertal maturation overlap with the changes due to the effects on bone of chronic inflammation (increased osteoclastogenesis and bone resorption), and to the effects of therapy, mainly corticosteroids.

BONE HEALTH PROMOTION

As a general measure, in order to create the most favorable environment for bone growth and development, the correct intake of nutrients, especially calcium, according to the patient's age, sex, and physical characteristics should be actively promoted. Physical activity has also a major role in the full attainment of an individual's genetically determined potential peak of bone mass. This is extremely important, since it has been estimated that a 10% increase of peak bone mass reduces by 50% the risk of one osteoporotic fracture during adult life. Diet should be varied and correctly balanced. For example, fruit and vegetable consumption is positively linked with BMD in girls (42).

Adolescents should be encouraged not only to acquire healthy habits (balanced diet, regular exercise), but also to avoid bone-damaging behaviors such as smoking or excessive alcohol consumption (43,44).

Special attention must of course be paid to disease-specific needs. For example, protein-energy malnutrition has been reported in 10% to 50% of adolescents with JIA (45).

Calcium

Many studies have demonstrated the positive effect of high calcium intake on bone mass, especially in pre-pubertal children (19,46). On the basis of longitudinal data, during the two years of peak bone accretion, the estimated calcium need increases to 1500 mg daily for girls and 1700 mg daily for boys (47). However, in many countries, even healthy adolescents of both sexes consume only 60% to 70% of the recommended amount of calcium, as the so-called "soft drinks" rapidly substitute traditional milk beverages (48).

Chronically ill children require at least the same amount of calcium as healthy subjects of the same sex and age. Low-calcium intake in childhood is associated with increased risk of fracture not only in later life but even in adolescence. Adult women with low milk intake during childhood and adolescence have a lesser bone mass and a greater risk of fracture, an effect independent of current milk or calcium intake (49).

Calcium-rich foods should be preferred, but when they cannot be taken, calcium supplements can be considered. However the long-term compliance with calcium salts in adolescents is low, mostly because of gastrointestinal side effects such as mild abdominal pain, meteorism and constipation.

Vitamin D

Vitamin D is essential for bone health, being necessary for both the intestinal absorption of calcium and a correct skeletal mineralization. Vitamin D is normally synthesized in the skin upon exposure to ultraviolet rays (UVB). If there is insufficient exposure to natural sunlight, the serum 25-hydroxyvitamin D level—the best clinical indicator of the vitamin D status—drops down. In such cases, vitamin D supplements are indicated to avoid insufficient bone mineralization. In some countries, vitamin D fortified foods are available and such additional dietary intake is normally recommended. For example, the recommended dietary intake of vitamin D is 280 IU/day for children aged 3 years or more in the United Kingdom, and 200 IU/day for those aged 0 to 18 years in the United States.

There are no recommendations for supplementation during adolescence in many countries, in spite of serious evidence of vitamin D deficiency in those with dark skin who wear concealing clothing and live at latitudes where solar UVB is inadequate for cutaneous vitamin D synthesis during the winter months (50).

Young people with chronic illness may be at high risk of vitamin D deficiency because of reduced outdoor activities or the necessity to avoid sunlight exposure (e.g., in systemic lupus erythematosus or dermatomyositis). Liver, kidney, and intestinal dysfunction linked to many diseases can affect the metabolism and function of vitamin D. Finally, some drugs (e.g., corticosteroids, anticonvulsants, heparin, cyclosporine A, tacrolimus) can interfere with vitamin D metabolism. All these conditions can increase the risk of a true vitamin D deficiency, or of inappropriately low levels of circulating vitamin D metabolites.

Low serum vitamin D levels can induce an increase in parathyroid hormone secretion (secondary hyperparathyroidism), which can in turn influence bone health.

Protein Intake

Protein (mainly collagen) constitutes one-half of the volume of the extracellular material of bone. In bone remodeling, many constituent such as aminoacids cannot be recycled, thus bone turnover requires a continuous input of fresh dietary proteins. Proteins are now recognized as an important co-factor for bone health along with calcium. On the contrary, an excess of dietary protein may lead to an increased urinary loss of calcium.

Physical Activity

Physical activity and weight-bearing exercises have been shown to increase BMD in different pathological conditions, as well as in health (51,52). Of course the type, quantity and quality of physical activity must be tailored on the basis of sex, age, and primary disease. Children physically active at a younger age show a higher periosteal bone formation, resulting in a greater diameter of the long bones, with an increased BMC. On the contrary, those who started regular activity after puberty tend to have bone mass increases as the result of endocortical formation. The periosteal growth of the former potentially results in a lifelong larger skeleton, providing greater resistance to fractures and periosteal remodeling.

MEDICAL TREATMENT

A correct approach to low bone mass in adolescents with rheumatic diseases should always start with the simplest measures, that is, correct calcium intake and a physical activity program. Whenever serum vitamin D levels are inappropriately low, active metabolites of vitamin D should be initially used. Among more specific drugs, only bisphosphonates have been consistently used, especially in the presence of a high fracture risk, even if only a few studies have been carried out in young patients.

Of course, after a therapy for bone loss has been started, accurate periodical evaluation is required. This should include clinical history and examination (growth, presence of pain, kyphosis, fractures) as well as a thorough study of bone mass and bone turnover, which are essential instruments to evaluate treatment efficacy.

Vitamin D

Vitamin D (400 IU/day) and 25-hydroxy-vitamin D (0.5 mcg/kg/day) have been studied in pediatric patients with various rheumatic diseases, with or without steroid treatment (53–55).

These studies treated small numbers of patients with different characteristics (age, type, duration, and severity of the disease), so comparing their results is impossible. Data on the efficacy of vitamin D treatment in reducing or preventing bone loss are not conclusive, even if an increase in bone mass has been reported.

Bisphosphonates

Bisphosphonates have been extensively used in adult osteoporosis with positive effects on bone fracture risk. Their use in younger patients has been limited by fear of adverse effects on a growing skeleton and their long-term permanence in bone tissue. However, after more than 10 years of use in severe conditions such as osteogenesis imperfecta, bisphosphonates have been shown to be quite safe. No adverse effects on growth, pubertal spurt and healing of fractures have been reported, even after a long follow-up. Bone biopsies of treated patients show normal bone structure and no mineralization defects (56). Typical radiological alterations in pre-pubertal patients are radiolucent sclerotic bands (57), but they do not appear to have clinical relevance. Bisphosphonate use is now growing also in young patients (58–60), even if careful selection of cases and strict monitoring is required.

Regarding the studies on low bone mass in rheumatic diseases, different compounds and dosages have been used. Intravenous alendronate, oral olpandronate, IV pamidronate, oral clodronate, or oral alendronate have been used in children/adolescents affected by rheumatic diseases (mainly JIA), in most cases treated with steroids. Some studies are limited to single patients or small series, while other studies considered slightly larger samples (61–63). All these studies demonstrated an increase in BMD and a positive effect on pain related to vertebral fractures, without significant untoward side effects. The largest published study available is still that on the use of oral alendronate in 38 children (64,65), which showed a BMD increase of $+14.9 \pm 9.8\%$ on average (13 patients having attained normal range) and no new fractures after 12 months of therapy. The highest BMD increase was observed in the patients who had the pubertal spurt during the year of alendronate therapy. A significant decrease in bone resorption and bone formation markers was also observed in these patients.

Adverse effects of bisphosphonates have not been reported in greater frequency in adolescents than in adults. A mild flu-like syndrome may occur after IV administration, usually the first one only. Transient hypocalcemia and mild abdominal discomfort or dyspepsia are also occasional complaints. According to present knowledge, the use of bisphosphonates in pregnancy cannot be considered safe, since they are known to cross the placenta and could have effects on the fetal bones. If bisphosphonates are needed in a sexually active girl, contraceptive methods must be adopted.

In conclusion, all the published studies so far have consistently showed that bisphosphonates are effective in counteracting bone loss induced by rheumatic diseases and/or corticosteroid therapy in young patients. However, larger studies, particularly controlled with placebo, are needed.

The previous observations apply only to the correct, prudent use of appropriate drug doses on the basis of age and body weight. Whyte reported a case of frank misuse, with very high biophosphonate doses for a very long time, without adequate clinical, biochemical and densitometrical monitoring, which led to severe untoward effects (66). New administration schedules (e.g., once-a-week pills, once-a-month injections) may be appealing in order to improve the compliance and the quality of life, especially in adolescents.

Growth Hormone

The effects of growth hormone (GH) on bone mass are still controversial. Simon et al. observed that in 14 children treated for 1 year with GH and followed for two more years after stopping it, height velocity and height as well as lean mass increased significantly during the year on GH, but fell to pre-treatment values after withdrawal (67). A significant increase in bone turnover was also observed in 14 children with systemic JIA on long-tem steroid therapy, treated with GH for one year (68). Bone turnover returned to the pre-GH velocity after discontinuation of the growth hormone. A not significant increase in bone mass was observed.

Bechtold and colleagues followed 11 children with JIA treated with GH for 4 years, and did not find statistically significant improvement of vBMD (BMD corrected for vertebral size) (69).

On the contrary, an increase of bone mineral content, correlated with increasing height, was observed in 20 children with severe JIA, 17 of whom were on corticosteroid treatment (70). Positive results (lumbar BMD increase by 36.6%) were also observed in 13 JIA patients treated with GH for 3 years (71).

On the basis of these contradictory results, it is clear that long-term controlled studies are needed to determine the real impact of GH therapy on bone mass and bone turnover. It should also be considered that GH must be given almost every day by injection, is expensive, not free of potential side-effects, and there are legal limitations to its prescription in several countries.

Other Drugs

Calcitonin

Calcitonin inhibits bone resorption by osteoclasts and has been shown to reduce the risk of new vertebral fractures in adult patients. It can be administered by injection or intranasally. There is only one published study in 10 children with JIA, which showed a decrease in bone resorption markers and an increase in BMD ($7.2 \pm 9.5\%$/year) (72).

Teriparatide

Teriparatide (recombinant human parathyroid hormone, hPTH 1-34) is a relatively new drug, with unique anabolic properties on bone. While the majority of drugs used in osteoporosis are antiresorptive agents, teriparatide mainly stimulates bone formation. It is used in adult patients, also in glucocorticoid-induced osteoporosis (73,74). There are no published studies on its efficacy and safety in children. Great caution is recommended, since pharmacological stimulation of bone formation in the growing age might increase the risk for osteosarcoma.

SOME USEFUL WEBSITES ON OSTEOPOROSIS (PRIMARILY DESIGNED FOR ADULTS)

For Patients

1. Doctor's Guide to Osteoporosis—(www.pslgroup.com/OSTEO-POROSIS.HTM) Geared toward professionals this website features Medical News & Alerts, which provide the latest research and drug news on osteoporosis in one place.
2. Mayo Clinic, What Is Osteoporosis?—(www.mayohealth.org/mayo/pted/htm/osteopor.htm) Describes the disease, its causes, diagnosis, risk factors, prevention, and treatment information in a Q&A format.
3. International Osteoporosis Foundation—(www.osteofound.org/) The International Osteoporosis Foundation supports national osteoporosis societies to increase the awareness and understanding of the disease worldwide.
4. National Osteoporosis Foundation—(www.nof.org/) The National Osteoporosis Foundation's Web page is comprehensive and offers information for both professionals and consumers.
5. National Osteoporosis Society—(www.nos.org.uk/www.bonezone.org.uk) Designed for kids and teenagers a website where informations, quizzes, games and stories about healthy bones can be found.
6. National Osteoporosis Association—(www.osteoporosis.org.au/)

For Physicians

1. American Medical Association, Osteoporosis CME—(enet.ama-assn.org/public/cme/reg1.htm) This link goes directly to the American Medical Association's three-part CME course on managing osteoporosis.
2. American Society for Bone and Mineral Research—(www.asbmr.org) This Web site offers information on ASBMR's abstracts, grants, meeting information, job placement, publications, and events.
3. International Bone and Mineral Society—(www.ibmsonline.org) The International Bone and Mineral Society is a nonprofit organization that generates and disseminates knowledge of the basic biology and clinical science related to skeletal and mineral metabolism.
4. BoneKEy-Osteovision—(www.bonekey-ibms.org/) The Bone Knowledge Environment is provided by the International Bone and Mineral Society.
5. European Calcified Tissue Society (ECTS)—(www.ectsoc.org) The major organization in Europe for researchers and clinicians working in calcified tissues and related fields.

6. International Society for Clinical Densitometry—(www.iscd.org/) The International Society for Clinical Densitometry (ISCD) is a multi-disciplinary, nonprofit organization that provides a central resource for a number of scientific disciplines with an interest in bone mass measurement.

7. National Institutes of Health, Osteoporosis and Related Bone Disease—(www.osteo.org/) The Osteoporosis and Related Bone Disease Web site provides patients, professionals, and the public with information on metabolic bone diseases such as osteoporosis, Paget's disease, and others.

8. National Library of Medicine, Osteoporosis—(www.nlm.nih.gov/medlineplus/osteoporosis.html) The National Library of Medicine's MedlinePlus is a search function of medical information for consumers. This link takes users directly to topics found in MedlinePlus's database on osteoporosis, which includes links to information from various sources including the NIH, FDA, and national associations.

REFERENCES

1. Consensus Development Conference: Diagnosis, prophylaxis and treatment of osteoporosis. Am J Med 1993; 94:646–50.
2. World Health Organization; Assessment of fracture risk and its application to screening for postmenopausal osteoporosis. Technical Report Series 843. World Health Organization Geneva, Switzerland, 1994.
3. Marshall D, Johnell O, Wedel H. Meta-analysis of how well measures of bone mineral density predict occurrence of osteoporotic fractures. Br Med J 1996; 312:1254–9.
4. Cummings SR, Black DM, Nevitt MC, et al. Bone density at various sites for prediction of hip fractures. Lancet 1993; 341:72–5.
5. Kanis JA & the WHO Study Group Assessment of fracture risk and its application to screening for postmenopausal osteoporosis. Synopsis of a WHO Report. Osteoporos Int 1994; 4:368–81.
6. Goulding A, Jones IE, Taylor RW, et al. More broken bones: a 4-year double cohort study of young girls with and without distal forearm fractures. J Bone Miner Res 2000; 15:2011–8.
7. Skaggs DL, Loro ML, Pitukcheewanont P, et al. Increased body weight and decreased radial cross-sectional dimension in girls with forearm fractures. J Bone Miner Res 2001; 16:1337–42.
8. Ward LM, Glorieux FH. The spectrum of pediatric osteoporosis. In: Glorieux FH, Pettifor JM, Jüppner H eds. Pediatric Bone: Biology & Diseases. Amsterdam: Academic Press, 2003; 401–42.
9. Robson H, Siebler T, Stevens DA. Thyroid hormone acts directly on growth plate chondrocyte to promote hypertrophic differentiation and inhibit clonal expansion and cell proliferation. Endocrinology 2000; 141:3887–97.

10. Trotter M, Hixonw BB. Sequential changes in weight, density, and percentage ash weight of human skeleton from an early fetal period through old age. Anat Rec 1974; 179:1–18.

11. Bonjour JP, Theintz G, Buchs B, et al. Critical years and stages of puberty for spinal and femoral bone mass accumulation during adolescence. J Clin Endocrinol Metab 1991; 73:555–63.

12. Sabatier JP, Guaydier-Souquieres G, Laroche D, et al. Bone mineral acquisition during adolescence and early adulthood: a study in 574 healthy females 10–24 years of age. Osteoporos Int 1996; 6(2):141–8.

13. Lazcano-Ponce E, Tamayo J, Cruz-Valdez A, et al. Peak bone mineral area density and determinants among females aged 9 to 24 years in Mexico. Osteoporos Int 2003; 14(7):539–47.

14. Lu PW, Briody JN, Ogle GD, et al. Bone mineral density of total body, spine and femoral neck in children and young adults: a cross-sectional and longitudinal study. J Bone Miner Res 1994; 9:1451–8.

15. Gilsanz V, Kovanlikaya A, Costin G, et al. Differential effect of gender on the size of the bones in the axial and appendicular skeleton. J Clin Endocrinol Metab 1997; 82:1603–7.

16. Peacock M, Turner CH, Econs MJ, et al. Genetics of osteoporosis, Endocr Rev 2002; 23:303–26.

17. Morris FL, Payne WR, Wark JD. The impact of intense training on endogenous estrogen and progesterone concentrations and bone mineral acquisition in adolescent rowers. Osteoporos Int 1999; 10:361–8.

18. Cheng JC, Maffulli N, Leung SS, et al. Axial and peripheral bone mineral acquisition: A 3-year longitudinal study in Chinese adolescents. Eur J Pediatr 1999; 158:506–12.

19. Johnston CC, Miller JZ, Slemenda CW, et al. Calcium supplementation and increases in bone mineral density in children. N Engl J Med 1992; 327: 82–87.

20. Dent CE, Friedman M. Idiopathic juvenile osteoporosis. Quart J Med 1965; 34: 177–210.

21. Teotia M, Teotia SP, Singh RK. Idiopathic juvenile osteoporosis. Am J Dis Child 1979; 133:894–900.

22. Smith R. Idiopathic juvenile osteoporosis: experience of twenty-one patients. J Rheumatol 1995; 34:68–77.

23. Rauch F, Traves R, Norman ME, et al. The bone formation defect in idiopathic juvenile osteoporosis is surface-specific. Bone 2002; 31:85–9.

24. Cimaz R, Falcini F. Skeletal maturation and bone mineralization in the pediatric rheumatic diseases. In: Cassidy JT, Petty RP, eds. Textbook of Pediatric Rheumatology. 5th ed. Philadelphia, PA: Elsevier, 2005; 716–27.

25. Henderson CJ, Cawkwell GD, Specker BL, et al. Predictors of total body bone mineral density in non-corticosteroid-treated prepubertal children with juvenile rheumatoid arthritis. Arthritis Rheum 1997; 40:1967–75.

26. Henderson CJ, Specker BL, Sierra RI, et al. Total-body bone mineral content in non-corticosteroid-treated postpubertal females with juvenile rheumatoid arthritis. Frequency of osteopenia and contributing factors. Arthritis Rheum 2000; 43:531–40.

27. Zak M, Hassager C, Lovell DJY. Assessment of bone mineral density in adults with a history of juvenile chronic arthritis: a cross sectional long-term follow-up study. Arthritis Rheum 1999; 42:790–8.
28. Haugen M, Lien G, Flato B, et al. Young adults with juvenile arthritis in remission attain normal peak bone mass at the lumbar spine and forearm. Arthritis Rheum 2000; 43:1504–10.
29. French AR, Mason T, Nelson AM, et al. Osteopenia in adults with a history of juvenile rheumatoid arthritis. A population based study. J Rheumatol 2002; 29: 1065–70.
30. Chesney RW, Mazess RB, Rose, P, et al. Effect of prednisone on growth and bone mineral content in childhood glomerular disease. Am J Dis Child 1987; 132:768–72.
31. Naganathan V, Jones G, Nash P, et al. Vertebral fracture risk with long-term corticosteroid therapy: prevalence and relation to age, bone density, and corticosteroid use. Arch Intern Med 2000; 160:2917–22.
32. Bardare M, Bianchi ML, Furia M, et al. Bone mineral metabolism in chronic arthritis: the influence of steroids. Clin Exp Rheumatol 1991; 9(Suppl. 6):29–31.
33. Jones G, Ponsonby AL, Smith BJ, et al. Asthma, inhaled corticosteroid use, and bone mass in prepubertal children. J Asthma 2000; 37:603–11.
34. Sievanen H, Oja P, Vuori I. Precision of dual-energy X-ray absorptiometry in determining bone mineral density and content in various skeletal sites. J Nucl Med 1992; 33:1137–42.
35. Njeh CF, Samat SB, Nightingale A, et al. Radiation dose and in vivo precision in paediatric bone mineral density measurement using dual X-ray absorptiometry. Br J Radiol 1997; 70:719–27.
36. Koo WW, Walters J, Bush AJ, Technical consideration of dual-energy X-ray absorptiometry-based bone mineral measurements for pediatric subjects. J Bone Miner Res 1995; 10:1998–2004.
37. Warner JT, Cowan FJ, Dunstan FDJ, et al. Measured and predicted bone mineral content in healthy boys and girls aged 6–18 years: adjustment for body size and puberty. Acta Paediatr 1998; 87:244–9.
38. Rauch F, Tutlewski B, Fricke O, et al. Analysis of cancellous bone turnover by multiple slice analysis at distal radius: a study using peripheral quantitative computed tomography. J Clin Densitom 2001; 4:257–62.
39. Lewiecki EM, Watts NB, McClung MR, et al. Official positions of the International Society for Clinical Densitometry. J Clin Endocrinol Metab 2004; 89:3651–5.
40. McGartland C, Robson P, Murray L, et al. History of fracture and bone mineral density in adolescence: The N. Ireland young hearts project. Bone. 2005; 36(Suppl. 1):S39.
41. Szulc P, Seeman E, Delmas P. Biochemical measurements of bone turnover in children and adolescents. Osteoporos Int 2000; 11:281–294.
42. Tylavsky FA, Holliday K, Danish R, et al. Fruit and vegetables intake is an independent predictor of bone size in early-pubertal children. Am J Clin Nutr 2004; 79:311–7.
43. Brown SJ, Schoenly L. Test of an educational intervention for osteoporosis prevention with U.S. adolescents. Orthopaedic Nursing 2004; 23(4):245–51.

44. Ginty F, Prentice A. Can osteoporosis be prevented with dietary strategies during adolescence? Br J Nutr 2004; 92(1):5–6.

45. Henderson CJ, Lovell DJ. Nutritional aspects of juvenile rheumatoid arthritis. Rheum Dis Clin North Am 1991; 17:403–13.

46. Bonjour JP, Carrie AL, Ferrari S, et al. Calcium-enriched food and bone mass growth in prepubertal girls: a randomized, double-blind, placebo-controlled trial. J Clin Invest 1997; 99:1287–94.

47. Whiting SJ, Vatanparast H, Baxter-Jones A, et al. Factors that affect bone mineral accrual in the adolescent growth spurt. J Nutr 2004; 134:696S–700S.

48. McGartland C, Robson PJ, Murray L, et al. Carbonated soft drink consumption and bone mineral density in adolescence: the Northern Ireland young hearts project. J Bone Miner Res 2003; 18:1563–9.

49. Kalkwarf HJ, Khoury JC, Lanphear BP. Milk intake during childhood and adolescence, adult bone density, and osteoporotic fractures in US women. Am J Clin Nutr 2003; 77:257–65.

50. Crocombe S, Berry JL, Mughal MZ. Symptomatic vitamin D deficiency among non-Caucasian adolescents living in the United Kingdom. Arch Dis Child 2004; 89:197–9.

51. Whalen RT, Carter DR. Influence of physical activity on the regulation of bone density. J Biomech 1988; 21:825–37.

52. Slemenda WC, Miller JZ, Hui SL, et al. Role of physical activity in the development of skeletal mass in children. J Bone Miner Res 1991; 6:1227–33.

53. Warady BD, Lindsley CB, Robinson FG, et al. Effects of nutritional supplementations on bone mineral status of children with rheumatic diseases receiving corticosteroids. J Rheumatol 2004; 21:530–5.

54. Reed A, Haugen M, Patchman LM, et al. 25-hydroxyvitamin D therapy in children with active juvenile rheumatoid arthritis: short-term effects on serum osteocalcin levels and bone mineral density. J Pediatr 1991; 119:657–60.

55. Bianchi ML, Bardare M, Galbiati E. Bone development in juvenile rheumatoid arthritis. In: Schonau E, Matkovic V, eds. Paediatric Osteology, Prevention of Osteoporosis – A Paediatric Task ?: Singapore: Elsevier Science, 1998:173–81.

56. Brumsen C, Hamdy NA, Papopoulos SE. Long-term effects of bisphosphonates on the growing skeleton: studies of young patients with severe osteoporosis. Medicine (Baltimore). 1997; 76:266–83.

57. Van Persijn, Van Meerten EL, Kroon HM, et al. Epi- and metaphyseal changes in children causes by administration of bisphosphonates. Radiology 1992; 184: 249–54.

58. Shoemaker LR. Expanding role of bisphosphonate therapy in children. J Pediatr 1999; 134:264–7.

59. Srivastava T, Alon US. Bisphosphonates: from grandparents to grandchildren. Clin Pediatr 1999; 38:687–702.

60. Shaw NJ, Boivin CM, Crabtree NJ. Intravenous pamidronate in juvenile osteoporosis. Arch Dis Child 2000; 83:143–5.

61. Falcini F, Trapani S, Ermini M, et al. Intravenous administration of alendronate counteracts the in vivo effects of glucocorticoids on bone remodelling. Calcified Tissue Int 1996; 58:166–9.

62. Lepore L, Pennesi M, Barbi E, et al. Treatment and prevention of osteoporosis in juvenile chronic arthritis with disodium clodronate. Clin Exp Rheumatol 1991; 9(Suppl. 6):33–5.
63. Noguera A, Ros JB, Pavia C, et al. Bisphosphonates, a new treatment for glucocorticoid-induced osteoporosis in children. J Pediatr Endocrinol 2003; 16: 529–36.
64. Bianchi ML, Cimaz R, Bardare M, et al. Efficacy and safety of alendronate for the treatment of osteoporosis in diffuse connective tissue diseases in children. Arthritis Rheum 2000; 43:1960–6.
65. Cimaz R, Gattorno M, Sormani MP, et al. Changes in markers of bone turnover and inflammatory parameters during alendronate therapy in pediatric patients with rheumatic disease. J Rheumatol 2002; 29:1786–92.
66. Whyte MP, Wenkert D, Clements KL, et al. Bisphosphonate-induced osteopetrosis. N Engl J Med 2003; 349:457–63.
67. Simon D, Prewar A, Czernichow P. Treatment of juvenile rheumatoid arthritis with growth hormone. Horm Res 2000; 53:82–6.
68. Touati G, Ruiz JC, Porquet D, et al. Effects on bone metabolism of one year recombinant human growth hormone administration to children with juvenile chronic arthritis undergoing chronic steroid therapy. J Rheumatol 2000; 27: 1287–93.
69. Bechtold S, Ripperger P, Bonfig W, et al. Bone mass development and bone metabolism in juvenile idiopathic arthritis: treatment with growth hormone for 4 years. J Rheumatol 2004; 31:1407–12.
70. Rooney M, Davies UM, Reeve J, et al. Bone mineral content and bone mineral metabolism: changes after growth hormone treatment in juvenile chronic arthritis. J Rheumatol 2000; 27:1073–81.
71. Simon D, Lucidarme N, Prieur AM, et al. Effects on growth and body composition of growth hormone treatment in children with juvenile idiopathic arthritis requiring steroid therapy. J Rheumatol 2003; 30:2492–9.
72. Siamopoulou A, Challa A, Kapoglou P, et al. Effects of intranasal salmon calcitonin in juvenile idiopathic arthritis: an observational study. Calcified Tissue Int 2001; 69:25–30.
73. Neer RM, Arnaud CD, Zanchetta JR, et al. Recombinant human PTH (1-34) fragment [rh-PTH] reduces the risk of spine and non-spine fractures in postmenopausal osteoporosis. N Engl J Med 2001; 344:1434–41.
74. Quattrocchi E, Kourlas H. Teriparatide: a review. Clin Ther 2004; 26:841–54.

13

Health Issues of Adolescents

Donald E. Greydanus and Dilip R. Patel

*Michigan State University College of Human Medicine, Michigan State University/
Kalamazoo Center for Medical Studies, Kalamazoo, Michigan, U.S.A.*

INTRODUCTION

Adolescence is the critical process in which the child leaves childhood dependency and approaches a stage of human development in which dramatic changes develop leading to adulthood (1). It is a complex period with major physiologic, sociological, and psychological changes. The goal of adolescence is to allow the emergence of adults who are autonomous and ready to function at appropriate sexual, intellectual, and vocational levels and contribute to the society that hopefully nurtured them. Various terminology is used when discussing this age group, whether child (under the age of 18 years), adolescent (ages 10–19 years), youth (ages 15–24 years), or young people (ages 10–24 years) (2). There are over 1 billion adolescents on the planet, and 50% of the world's population is now under 25 years of age (3). Approximately 85% of adolescents live in developing countries.

HEALTH STATUS OF ADOLESCENTS

The World Health Organization's (WHO) Adolescent Health and Development Programme has identified four major causes of death, disability, and ill health among the world's adolescents: sexual and reproductive behavior, tobacco use, suicides, and road traffic accidents (3–5). The leading causes of mortality in 15- to 29-year-olds in the North America and Western Europe include motor vehicle accidents (and other unintentional injuries), suicide, homicide, cancer, and infection (including HIV/AIDS). Approximately one-third of youth have a chronic illness or disability, including 6% with a condition that causes daily limitations and 5% classified as having severe chronic illness or disability (Table 1) (6–9). About 70% have one condition, though about one in five have two diagnoses, and one in 10 have three or more conditions. Current estimates are that 13% to 18% of children in America have a special health care need (9). Over 90% of children with severe illness in America, England, and other developed countries now live past age 20 (10,11).

The impact that chronic illness has on the lives of our children and adolescents is considerable (12). All youth must go through the normal developmental processes of adolescence to become self-functioning adults. All adolescents, whether or not they have a chronic illness (as rheumatological disorders), are at a risk for difficulties in adolescence, such as complications of sexuality, substance abuse, mental health disorders, and various other medical disorders. Table 2 lists key adolescent health topics that are considered in this chapter.

SEXUAL BEHAVIOR

Statistics

The beginning of sexual (coital) behavior is in adolescence for most people in the world (13). The American 2005 Youth Risk Behavior Survey (YRBS) noted that 46.8% of all high school students (ages 13–18 years) are coitally sexually experienced, with a range of 67.6% for African-American youth, 51% for Hispanic youth, and 43% for Caucasians(14). This survey also comments that over 6.2% are sexually active before age 13 (4% in females and 9% in males) while over 14% have at least four sex partners—11% of the females and 17% of the males. Though parents and some clinicians assume that youth with chronic illness are not engaging in coital behavior, research has noted that chronic illness increases the risk for sexual behavior

Table 1 Prevalence of Chronic Illness in American Youth Aged 10 to 17 Years per 1000

Overall: 315/1000 adolescents, aged 10–17 years

Musculoskeletal diseases 20.9
Asthma 46.8
Headaches (frequent, severe) 45.8
Heart disease 17.4
Deafness and hearing loss 17.0
Blindness and vision impairment 16.0
Speech defects 18.9
Diabetes mellitus 1.5

Source: Adapted from Refs. 6–9.

Table 2 Selected Adolescent Health Topics

Sexuality
  Adolescent pregnancy
  Sexually transmitted diseases
Substance abuse disorders
Medical disorders
  Asthma
  Hypertension
  Diabetes mellitus
  Obesity
  Eating disorders (anorexia and bulimia nervosa)
  Others
Mental health
Mortality
  Motor vehicle accidents
  Homicide and suicide

in some youth who use sexual experimentation as a way of proving their normalcy (15).

Individuals who are sexually active early (i.e., during their adolescent years) tend to have multiple partners and often do not use condoms correctly or consistently; thus, they are at increased risk for unplanned (unwanted) pregnancy and sexually transmitted diseases (STDs). Having a chronic illness, such as a rheumatoid disorder, is not a situation that can be relied on to help avoid unplanned pregnancy or STDs. Most coital activity among adolescents in the world is unprotected by condoms (3). Sexually active adolescents tend to practice serial monogamy—that is, having one partner at a time. These youth with increased sexual behavior often have other high-risk behaviors as well, such as increased substance use and abuse, sometimes leading to involvement in survival sex as prostitutes living on the streets of the world.

Thus, the clinician caring for youth with or without rheumatic disorders, must inquire about each youth's sexual behavior. Such inquiry is imperative when prescribing teratogenic drugs such as mexthotrexate and with certain diseases, such as SLE, that have particular implications for reproductive health. It is always important to recommend sexual abstinence; however, the youth who is sexually active should be provided with appropriate contraception to allow them effective control over their fertility and prevention of unwanted pregnancy and abortion (15–18). Youth who wish to become mothers should learn how to space their children correctly so they can become better caretakers (19–25).

Adolescent Pregnancy

One in every six births in developing countries (one in 10 worldwide) is to a 15- to 19-year-old adolescent (18). Over half of females become mothers by

Table 3   Factors Contributing to Adolescent Pregnancy

Decreased age at menarche
Delay of marriage
Poverty
Lack of education
Inadequate contraceptive knowledge and availability
Cultural factors specific to that specific country/subpopulation
Sexual abuse

age 19 in developing countries. Over 14 million adolescent females give birth each year, with 5.7 million in Asia, 4.5 million in Sub-Saharan Africa, 2.1 million in the Middle East, as well as North Africa, and 1.3 million in developed countries (3,4,19,20). There are many factors involved in the rate of adolescent pregnancy in a country, as listed in Table 3. Table 4 notes percentages of adolescents aged 15 to 19 years giving birth in various countries (3).

About 9% of adolescent females in the United States become pregnant each year, with 5% delivering, 3% having an abortion, and 1% have a miscarriage or stillbirth (21–25).

Adolescent pregnancy under age 15 remains a relatively uncommon phenomenon throughout the world. Currently, approximately 43% of American adolescent females become pregnant at least once before age 20. Adolescent females account for 13% of all births in the United States (4,158,212 in 1992) and 26% of all abortions (about 400,000) (25). The 2004 birth rate of 41.1 per 1000 females aged 15 to 19 years in the United States is the highest among all developed nations and is in stark contrast to Japan (4 per 1000), the Netherlands (7 per 1000), France (10 per 1000), Canada (25 per 1000) or the United Kingdom (28 per 1000) (21,26,27). Though there has been some decline in adolescent birth rates in the United States from the 1990s through 2004, the U.S. rate remains the highest of any developed country (Table 5). Adolescent sexual behavior is similar in the United States and other developed countries; however, there is less access to comprehensive sexuality

Table 4   Adolescents Aged 15 to 19 Years
Giving Birth in Various Counties

1% in Japan
2% in China and Europe
4% in Asia
5% in North America
12% in Africa
18% in Pakistan
28% in India

Source: Adapted from Ref. 3.

Table 5 Birth Rates Among American Adolescents Aged
15–19 Years per 1000

Highest rates: 1950s–1960s
1970: 66
1986: 50.2
1990: 60
1997: 53
2000: 48.5
2001: 44.9
2004: 41.1 (ranging from 18.2 in New Hampshire to 62.6 in Texas)

Source: Adapted from Refs. 22 and 23.

education and contraception in the United States than in Western Europe and other regions of the world. Significant declines in adolescent pregnancy are primarily related to improved contraceptive patterns by adolescents (28).

SEXUALLY TRANSMITTED DISEASES

There are many types of STDs which can affect youth and over half of STDs occur to adolescents (1,3,29–31). The majority of STDs involve individuals aged 15 to 29 years. Each year, 1 in 20 adolescents in the world obtains a curable STD (3). STDs can be asymptomatic and youth often do not seek treatment even if symptomatic. Adolescents are less likely than adults to use protection (i.e., condoms). The most common STDs among youth are infections due to human papillomavirus (HPV), herpes simplex virus, *Chlamydia trachomatis*, *Neisseria gonorrhoeae*, and *Trichomonas vaginalis*. HPV is main cause of cervical cancer in females under 30 years of age and the recently developed HPV vaccine can prevent 70% of these cervical cancers.

Worldwide, the WHO estimates there are over 300 million curable STDs (Table 6), including an estimated 12 million cases of syphilis; 62 million cases of gonorrhea; 89 million cases of chlamydial infections; and 170 million cases of trichomoniasis (31). Every day, 725,000 STD cases develop: 360,000 trichomoniasis; 140,000 chlamydial infections; 84,000 HPV; 70,000 gonorrhea; 56,000 HSV; 10,000 syphilis; 5000 chancroid (3,31). Globally, 250,000 adolescents are infected with a STD each day (3).

Table 7 lists factors involved in the development of high rates of STDs in adolescents. Youth at the highest risk for STDs are runaways, involved in sex for survival (prostitution), housed in jails or detention centers, involved in male homosexual behavior, those who have been abused, are mentally retarded, or have a history of STDs (32). The cost in terms of *preventable* health care spending is staggering and the complications of STDs are severe, especially for females—chronic pelvic pain, ectopic (tubal) pregnancy and poor pregnancy outcomes, among others (32,33).

Table 6 Estimated Number of Curable STDs by Regions of the World

Region	Annual
North America	14
Western Europe	16
Australasia	1
Latin America and the Caribbean	36
Sub-Saharan Africa	65
Northern Africa and Middle East	10
Eastern Europe and Central Asia	18
East Asia and Pacific	23
South and Southeast Asia	150
Total	333

Source: Adapted from Ref. 32 (www.who.int/asd/figures/global_report.html).

It is important to provide STD services to adolescents around the world in a confidential manner that provides enough time to manage the youth properly. *Primary* prevention involves confidential youth counseling about STDs; proper immunizations (including hepatitis A and B as well as the HPV vaccine); encouragement of abstinence; and, if sexually active, use of latex condoms (32,34–36). *Seconary* STD prevention involves regular STD screening, proper STD treatment, and partner notification if an STD is identified (30,32,35,36).

SUBSTANCE ABUSE

Alcohol and illegal drug use among adolescents in the world are major health problems facing society in the 21st century (3,29,37). Young adolescents tend to start their drug experimentation with inhalants (aerosols, glue, petrol, or volatile solvents). However, the most chemicals widely used

Table 7 Factors in Adolescent STDs

High rate of coital rates
Multiple sex partners
Immature cervix (cervical ectropion)
Failure to use condoms
Use of needles for use of substance abuse
Other patterns of needle injury (self-mutilation, body piercing, tattoos)
Magical thinking (feeling that high-risk behavior will not hurt one)
Distrust of the "adult" world
Limited knowledge in dealing with the medical system

Source: Adapted from Ref. 32.

and abused by youth remain marijuana, tobacco, and alcohol. Adolescents have many other illicit drugs to choose from, whether heroin, cocaine, methamphetamine, and others (37).

There is a 3% to 4% prevalence rate for substance abuse or dependence in American 14- to 16-year-olds; this rises to 10% in 17- to 19-year-olds. In 2005, a survey of over 50,000 high school adolescents noted that 15.8% reported a past-month use of illicit drugs in contrast to 19.4% in 2001 (38). Table 8 reports on a 2003 drug use survey of adolescents in Europe (39). High-risk sexual practices, violence, and injuries are noted especially in adolescent males using such drugs. Intravenous use leads to additional complications, such as the spread of HIV/AIDS.

Approximately 50% of adolescent males and 40% of females drink alcohol (40). Alcohol use contributes to approximately half of deaths in adolescents and young people due to motor vehicle accidents or suicides (40,41). Alcohol abuse leads to increased risk-taking behavior, increased sexual behavior, unplanned pregnancy, sexually transmitted diseases, violence, adult alcoholism, and disorders as adults: heart disease, cirrhosis, peptic ulcer disorders, and various cancers (37). The younger the individual begins using and abusing alcohol, the greater the risk for development of a clinical alcohol disorder as an adult (3.37).

Between 15% and 30% of adolescents in the world use tobacco, often leading to a life-long addiction and major health risks (37,42). As with alcohol, there is the widespread global advertisement of tobacco and society's acceptance of tobacco (42–45). There are over 150 million adolescents who smoke tobacco in the world and over half of these young individuals will eventually die a premature death from lung cancer, emphysema, and heart disease (45). Health-care professionals working with youth need to seek to educate their patients about the dangers of all drug use, including tobacco. This is particularly pertinent when rheumatologists prescribe methotrexate for rheumatic conditions during adolescence in view of the known risks of concurrent alcohol and tobacco use with this drug.

MEDICAL DISORDERS

Asthma

As noted previously, 20% of youth have two chronic disorders and 10% have three or more. Thus, finding a youth with one condition (e.g., a rheumatic disorder) does not mean that other disorders are not present. Asthma prevalence in children increased 3.6% in 1980 and 5.8% in 2003 (46). Asthma is one of the most common medical conditions among adolescents, and its prevalence has increased over the past few decades, including 46% increase in Australia, 4.3% in the United States, 34% in New Zealand, and 4.6% in Japan (47). Though research has produced improved

Table 8　Epidemiology of Substance Abuse in Europe

Country	Lifetime use[a]			Lifetime use[a] of other illicit drugs			
	Cigarette smoking	Alcohol consumption	Cannabis	Amphetamines	LSD	Ecstasy	Inhalants
Bulgaria	35	27	21	2	2	3	3
Croatia	30	27	22	2	1	5	14
Czech Republic	39	46	44	4	6	8	9
Denmark	27	50	23	4	1	2	8
Estonia	35	32	23	7	2	5	8
France	..	22	38	2	1	3	11
Greece	20	35	6	0	1	2	15
Hungary	31	21	16	3	2	3	5
Ireland	27	39	39	1	2	5	18
Italy	25	24	27	3	3	3	6
Poland	26	27	18	5	2	3	9
Portugal	18	14	15	3	2	4	8
Romania	20	18	3	0	0	1	1
Slovak Republic	32	34	27	2	2	3	9
Slovenia	27	25	28	1	1	3	15
United Kingdom	22	43	38	3	2	5	12
The Netherlands	27	45	28	1	2	4	6

[a] Lifetime use ≥40 times.
Source: Adapted from Ref. 39.

medications for asthma treatment, asthma mortality has continued to increase throughout the world. For example, from the mid-1970s to the mid-1980s, there was an increase in asthma-related deaths for 5- to 34-year-olds of staggering proportions: 34% increase in Japan, 17% increase in Singapore, and 111% increase in the United States (47). The causes of this increase in morbidity and mortality are unclear, but linked to the complex interaction of such factors as local medical care practices, local environmental Issues (i.e., pollution, tobacco use, dust mites, allergens, infections), and genetics (9,46,47).

Hypertension

A well recognized high-risk factor for cardiovascular, neurovascular, and renal disease is systemic arterial hypertension (40,47). Research over the past several decades has revealed that coronary heart disease, a major cause of morbidity and mortality in adults, may begin in adolescence. Research is now looking at prevention of adult disorders by preventing or effectively managing disorders in adolescents that may become serious problems in the adult population. Thus, adolescents should be screened for coronary heart disease, looking for such factors as obesity, hypertension, cigarette use, hyperlipidemia, and lack of exercise. The importance of such screening in SLE is discussed in Chapter 8.

Diabetes Mellitus

Diabetes mellitus is the most common endocrine disorder in youth and research notes that its type I diabetes is increasing by 2.5% to 3% each year throughout the world (48). The projected incidence is 50 per 100,000 a year in Finland and over 30 in many countries for an overall increase of 40% from 1998 to 2010; this will result in an incidence of 22 per 100,000 in the United States and 36.7 in Western Australia (48). Type 2 diabetes mellitus is increasing even faster because of such factors as the major increase in obesity (49).

Other Medical Disorders

There are many other disorders noted in adolescents (40). Two more are considered here—headaches and epilepsy. One of the most common concerns of youth is that of headaches, affecting 75% in Western countries, including four or more headaches per month reported by 10% of females and 5% of males in the United States (50,51). Approximately 25% of adolescents in the United States and Europe consult a clinician at least once in their teenage years because of headaches, whether tension (chronic daily or muscle contraction) or migraine types. Tension headaches are three times more common than migaine headaches. The prevalence of migraines varies from 8% to 12% of the population in various countries and there is a 1:3.5 male to female ratio (52). Migraines that begin in childhood often resolve by adulthood, while those that begin in the teen years often continue throughout the adult years.

Epilepsy affects 1% of the population and nearly 25% are under age 18 years of age. The annual incidence of epilepsy is 24.7 per 100,000 for 10- to 14-year-olds and 18.6 for 15- to 19-year-olds (53). Data from 1935 to 1967 in Rochester, Minnesota noted an incidence of newly diagnosed seizure disorder as 36 to 48 per 100,000 in the 10- to 19-year-old population (53). The disorder in adolescents may be a carryover from childhood or a chronic illness beginning in the teen years (54). Problems that youth with epilepsy must deal with include teratogenic potential of some anticonvulsant medication, choice of contraceptives for sexually active youth, video game-induced seizures, implications of seizures and driving, and other issues (40).

Obesity

Surveys note a prevalence of over 20% in the United States, England, other European countries, China, and other areas (55–57). Obesity is one of the most important health problems of children, adolescents, and adults in the world, with major negative health implications on physical and psychological health (58). Obesity prevalence among Americans aged 18 to 29 is 14% and increases to 21% if they have spent time in a college or university; perhaps 25% of American college students are overweight (59–60). An obese young teen is 20 times more likely than a teen of normal weight to become an overweight adult; 80% of overweight adolescents become overweight adults (61).

The causes of obesity are implicated in the reduction in physical activity and increase in fatty foods noted in children and adolescents of the last part of the 20th century and the early part of the 21st century. The reduction in physical activity over the past 30 years has been seen as more adolescents forsake exercise for time spent sitting while playing or working at computers, attending movies, and other sedentary activities (60,61). Pregnancy factors are noted, such as limited nutrition during the first trimester and smoking by the pregnant mother (9). Thus, obesity has become a lifestyle disorder that leads to depression, poor self-image, and poor adjustment in the school or work environment for many overweight or obese youth (61–64). It also leads to various medical conditions, including type 2 diabetes mellitus, arthritis, cardiovascular disorders, and various cancers in adolescent or adult years (61,65,66). Any successful management must include improvement in nutrition intake as well as physical activity (66,67).

Management of overweight or obesity starts with a careful look at underlying causes. In less than 5% of cases, there will be an underlying endocrine cause, such as polycystic ovary syndrome, Prader-Willi syndrome, congenital adrenal hyperplasia. As noted, genetics and lifestyle are the main factors in most cases of overweight or obese youth. The precise role of behavioral modification, pharmacologic agents, and bariatric surgery remain unclear at this time and are not appropriate for most youth (61,68,69). Most appropriate in the care of these patients is a vigorous attempt by clinicians to prevent major weight gain by measures to improve poor nutrition and increase physical activity through organized and unorganized sports activity (66,70,71). Any type of physical activity is good if the youth enjoys the sport. Water-based sports may be the best choice for many overtly obese youth, but nearly any type of activity is important. The key to effective physical activities is that the youth enjoys them, and the clinician should not be surprised if choices change from time to time. The key principle is to use sports as a way of encouraging adolescents to make regular physical exertion a part of their lives as children, adolescents, and adults.

PHYSICAL ACTIVITY

In the United States, according to the 2005 YRBS (Youth Risk Behavior Survey), 35.8% of high school students had been physically active for one hour per day on more than five out of 7 days preceding the survey. Nationwide, 9.6% of high school students had not participated in any kind of moderate or vigorous physical activities during the seven days preceding the survey. Twenty-one percent of students engaged for three or more hours per day on an average school day in playing video or computer games and 37.2% of the students watched television for three or more hours per day on an average school day. At total of 54% of the students participated in physical education classes on one or more day in an average week when they were in school, and 33% of students participated in physical education classes for five days in an average week when they were in school. Among the 54.2% of the students who participated in physical education classes, 84% actually exercised or played sports for more than 20 minutes during an average class. Overall 56% of the students had played on one or more sports team (run by school or community groups) during the 12 months preceding the survey. Among the 78.8% of the students who exercised or played sports during the 30 days preceding the survey, 22.2% had had to seek medical attention for an injury related to their participation in exercise or sports.

Eating Disorders

Adolescents, especially females, may develop disordered eating behavior out of a desire to have a thin appearance (73–76). Western culture teaches youth that females must be very thin to be beautiful, a concept persistently advocated by movies and magazines glamorizing the ultrathin woman (73,74). Approximately 0.5% females in the United States, the United Kingdom, and other countries in Europe develop anorexia nervosa, often between 13 and 15 years of age (74). It is the third most common chronic disease of adolescent females, after obesity and asthma. Lifetime prevalence for bulimia nervosa varies in different surveys of Western countries, usually from 1% to 4% (74,76). Bulimia nervosa usually develops between 17 and 25 years of age. Eating disorders develop from a complex mixture of genetics, biology, and sociocultural phenomona. (74).

MENTAL HEALTH

Surveys note that 20% to 33% of disability in adolescents is due to mental disorders (77–80). Major depression is found in 9 of every 1000 preschool children, 20/1000 of school-age children, and nearly 50/1000 adolescents and nearly 50/1000 adults (78). There is a 1:1 male to female ratio in children with depression, but a 1:2 male to female ratio is noted in adolescents. Depression can be noted with various comorbid conditions, such as anxiety disorders, disruptive behavioral disorders, substance abuse disorders and others. Potential consequences of depression are listed in Table 9. Depression may occur with chronic illness and complicate compliance with treatment recommendations.

YOUTH VIOLENCE

General

Violence is a major cause of psychosocial and physical morbidity and mortality among adolescents in the world (1,81–83). Consequences of violence may be especially noted in male adolescents who are taught to be self-reliant, violent as other males, abuse females, abuse chemicals, and avoid care for their mental health or medical problems. Both males and females can be the victims of abuse, whether it is overt neglect, physical abuse, emotional abuse, or sexual abuse (29,84,85). American studies note

Table 9   Sequelae of Depression in Adolescents

Abuse
Academic dysfunction (failing grades, school dropout behavior)
Aggressive behavior
Disruption of intimate relationships and friendships
Sexual dysfunction
Sexual promiscuity with unplanned adolescent pregnancies and STDs
Substance abuse disorders
Suicide attempts and suicide completions
Others

that 10% of adult males and 20% to 25% of adult females have been sexually abuse sometime in their childhood or adolescence (84). In Canada, 33% of males report sexual abuse under age 18 (29). Abuse leads to many negative behaviors, including injuries, bullying behavior, dating violence, (up to 60% prevalence in adolescent and young adult females), STDs, unwanted pregnancies, and others (29,87).

Violence and Mortality

Nearly 1.5 million adolescents die each year because of potentially preventable causes, such as suicide, injuries (motor vehicle accidents, wars), homicide, drug abuse, and others (18). Violence is the factor behind 75% of deaths in those aged 15 to 24 years (3,82,83,89). In the United States, for example, three-fourths of deaths among those aged 10 to 24 years are from four causes: motor vehicle accidents (30%), other unintentional injuries (10%), homicides (10%), and suicides (13%) (90–97). The second and third leading causes of death in American males aged 15 to 19 years are suicide and homicide, while they are the third and fourth leading cause of death in 15- to 19-year-old females. Homicide is the third leading cause of death in American youth aged 10 to 14, and suicide is the fourth for this age cohort in America.

Motor Vehicle Accidents

Motor vehicle accidents (MVAs) are the leading cause of death in adolescents in developed countries; drugs, especially alcohol, are involved in 50% or more (41,91). MVAs are also major or leading causes of adolescent deaths in other countries as well. These deaths are related to many factors, including the magical thinking of youth, fast driving, mixing driving with drug use, failure to use seat belts, vehicles not in good repair, combination effects of several adolescent passengers in a car driven by a teen male driver, poorly maintained roads, and others. Enforcement of various factors can improve this situation, including prolonged driver education for youth, monitoring of seat belt use, limiting the number of teens in a car with a male teen driver, and others (41,91).

Suicide

Approximately 2 million people of all ages die each year from homicide or suicide, including nearly 900,000 suicides each year (29,92). At least 90,000 adolescents (10–18 years of age) commit suicide each year and as many as 200,000 15 to 24 year olds commit suicide each year (29,89,92). The ratio of suicide attempt to completions ranges from 40 to 500: 1 and factors involved in suicide include depression, chronic illness, abuse, homo-sexuality, and others (90–98). Twenty to twenty-five percent of American adolescents seriously consider suicide each year and 9% have tried suicide at least once (90,93).

Suicide is third leading cause of death in older teens and fifth in those 5 to 14 years of age in the United States. The estimated suicide rate in 2000 is 10/100,000 in the United States, leading to 2000 suicides in those 15 to 19 years of age and 2000 in those 20 to 24 years of age each year; this included a suicide rate of 14.6 for the male and 2.9 for females 15 to 19 years of age (93). More American adolescents and young adults die from suicide than from the combination of cancer, heart disease, HIV/AIDS, chronic lung disease, birth defects, cerebrovascular accidents, pneumonia, and influenza. Suicide rates of 15 to 24 year olds are over 30/100,000 in such countries as Finland, Lithuania, New Zealand, and the Russian Federation (93). The World Health Organization complied a comparison of deaths by suicide of 15 to 24 year olds from 1991 to 1993 in various countries (Table 10).

Homicide

In Latin America, homicide is the leading cause of death for young males (3,99). In the United States, homicide is the second leading cause of death for adolescent males 15 to 19 years living in inner cities (100). Homicide becomes more likely to occur in the city and suicide in suburban America. The relative easy access to guns is a contributing factor in both types of deaths for American youth. Each year, four to five thousand 15- to 24-year-olds are murdered in the United States, for a death rate of 14–15 per 100,000; this is in contrast to a rate of 5.9 in 1960 (79,82).

Table 10   Suicide Deaths per 100,000 15- to 24-Year-Olds from 1991 to 1993

Country	Rate in males	Rate in females
United Kingdom	12.2	2.3
France	14.0	4.3
Ireland	21.5	2.0
United States	21.9	3.8
Canada	24.7	6.0
Australia	27.3	5.6
Finland	33.0	3.2
New Zealand	39.9	6.2
Russian Federation	41.7	7.9
Lithuania	44.9	6.7

Source: Adapted from World Health Organization data (www.unicef.org/pon96/insuicid.htm).

SUMMARY

The one billion adolescents of the world are potentially subject to considerable morbidity and mortality. Many complex issues face youth of today as they grow up with or without a chronic illness. This chapter has reviewed some of them, such as sexuality (including pregnancy and sexually transmitted diseases), substance abuse, various medical disorder, mental health disorders, and violence. The latter may be seen in such complex issues as suicide, homicide, and motor vehicle accidents. Clinicians are challenged to help these valuable individuals survive their adolescence and become autonomous and healthy adults making contributions to the society that bore and sustained them.

REFERENCES

1. Greydanus DE, Tsikika A, Hutchins E, Patel DR. Adolescent health. In Wallace HM, Green G, Jaros KJ, eds. Health and Welfare for Families in the 21st Century. 3rd ed. Sudbury, MA: Jones and Bartlett Publishers, Unit 3-Article 6, 2008:289–314.
2. Convention on the Rights of the Child. Guide to WHO Documents Concerning Adolescent Health and Development. Geneva, Switzerland: WHO: Department of Child and Adolescent Health and Development, Family and Community Health, WHO, 2001:5.
3. Williams G. The Second Decade: Improving Adolescent Health and Development, 1-20. Geneva, Switzerland: World Health Organization, 2001.
4. Murray CJL. Lopez AD. Mortality by cause for eight regions of the world. Global burden of disease study. Lancet 1997; 349:1269–76.
5. The Second Decade. Guide to WHO Documents Concerning Adolescent Health and Development. Geneva, Switzerland: WHO: Department of Child and Adolescent Health and Development, Family and Community Health, WHO, 2001:6.
6. Darroch JE, Singh SS, Frost JJ, et al. Differences in teenage pregnancy rates among five developed countries: The roles of sexual activity and contraceptive use. Fam Plann Perspect 2001; 33(6):244.
7. Newacheck PW, McManus MA, Fox HG. Prevalence and impact of chronic illness among adolescents. Am J Dis Child 1991; 145:1367–73.
8. Newacheck PW, Halfon N. Prevalence and impact of disabling chronic conditions in childhood. A J Public Health 1998; 88:610–7.
9. Newacheck PW, Wong ST, Galbraith A, et al. Adolescent health care expenditures: A descriptive profile. J Adolesc Health 2003; 32S:3–11.
10. Newacheck PW, Rising JP, Kim SE. Children at risk for special health care needs. Pediatrics 2006; 118:334–42.
11. Consensus Statement on Health care transitions for young adults with special health care needs. American Academy of Pediatrics, American Academy of Family Physicians and American College of Physicians-American Society of Internal Medicine. Pediatrics 2002; 110(Suppl. 6):1304–6.

12. Gortmaker SI, Perrin JM, Weitzman M. et al. An unexpected success story: Transition to adulthood with chronic physical heath conditions. J Res Adolesc 1993; 3:317–36.

13. Greydanus DE, Pratt HD, Patel DR (Eds). Behavioral Pediatrics, 2nd Edition. Vol. 2. NY & Lincoln, Nebraska: iUniverse Publishers, 2006; p. 864.

14. Sex and Youth. Guide to WHO Documents Concerning Adolescent Health and Development. Geneva, Switzerland: WHO: Department of Child and Adolescent Health and Development, Family and Community Health, WHO, p. 8, 2001

15. Centers for Disease Control and Prevention: Youth Risk Behavior Surveillance – United States, 2005. MMWR 2006; 55:SS–5.

16. Greydanus DE, Rimsza ME and Newhouse PN. Sexuality and disability in adolescence. Adolesc Med 2002; 13:500–14.

17. Greydanus DE, Patel DR, Rimsza ME. Contraception in the adolescent: An update. Pediatrics 2001; 107:562–73.

18. Greydanus DE, Rimsza ME, Matytsina L. Contraception for college students. Pediatr Clin No Am 2005; 52:135–61.

19. WHO, UNICF: A Healthy Start in Life. Report on the Global Consultation on Child and Adolescent Health and Development. March 12–13, 2002. Stockholm, Sweden. WHO: Geneva, Switzerland, 2002.

20. Creatsas GC. Adolescent Pregnancy in Europe. Int J Fertil Menopausal Stud 1995; 40(Suppl. 2):80–4.

21. Kulin HE. Adolescent Pregnancy in Africa. World Health Forum. 1990; 11(3): 336–8.

22. Greydanus DE. "Teen Pregnancy and Contraception" In: Course Manual for Adolescent Health. Part I. Eds: DE Greydanus, DR Patel, H Pratt & S Bhave. Delhi, India: Cambridge Press (Kashmere Gate) & Indian Academy of Pediatrics, ch 20, 2002; 299–324.

23. Martin JA, Hamilton BE, Sutton PD, et al. Births: final data for 2004. Natl Vital Stat Rep 2006; 55(1):1–5.

24. Quickstats: Birth rates among females aged 15–19 years, by states—United States, 2004. MMWR 2007; 55(51):1383.

25. Kaunitz AM. Long-acting hormonal contraceptives—indispensable in preventing teen pregnancy. J Adolesc Health 2007; 40:1–3.

26. Greydanus DE. "Adolescent pregnancy and abortion" IN: Adolescent Medicine, Third Edition. Eds: AD Hofmann & DE Greydanus. Stamford, CT: Appleton & Lange. ch. 27, 1997; 589–604.

27. Ventura SJ, Mathews MS, Hamilton BE. Births to Teenagers in the United States, 1940–2000. National Vital Statistics Report, Vol. 49, No. 10, September 25, 2001.

28. Darroch JE, Singh S. Why is Teenage Pregnancy Declining/The roles of abstinence, sexual activity, and contraceptive use. [Occasional Report, no. 1] New York: Alan Guttmacher Institute, 1999.

29. Santelli JS, Lindberg LD, Finer LB, Singh S. Explaining recent declines in adolescent pregnancy in the United States: The contribution of abstinence and improved contraceptive use. AJPH 2007; 97(1):150–6.

30. Barker G. What About Boys: A Literature Review in the Health and Developent of Adolescent Boys. WHO Department of Child and Adolescent Health and Development. Geneva, Switzerland, 58 pagers, 2000 (WHO/FCH/CAH/00.7.

31. Workowski KA, Berman SM. Sexually transmitted diseases treatment guidelines, 2006. MMWR 2006; 55(RR-11):1–94.

32. World Health Organization (WHO): An Overview of Selected Curable Sexually Transmitted Diseases, Geneva: WHO, 1995.

33. Greydanus DE, Patel DR. "Sexually Transmitted Diseases in Adolescents" In: Current Pediatric Therapy, 18e. Eds: Burg FD, Ingelfinger JR, Polin RA, Gershon AA. Philadelphia, PA: Elservier, Section 6, 2006; 326–9.

34. Germain A, et al. (eds). Reproductive Tract Infections: Global Impact and Priorities for Women's Reproductive Health. New York: Plenum Press, 1992.

35. Committee on Infectious Diseases. Recommended immunization schedules for children and adolescents—United States, 2007. Pediatrics 2007; 119:207.

36. Johnson J. "Sexually transmitted diseases in adolescents." In: Essentials of Adolescent Medicine. Eds: DE Greydanus, DR Patel, HD Pratt. New York: McGraw-Hill Medical Publishers, chapter 24:511–542, 2006.

37. National Institutes of Allergy and Infectious Diseases: Workshop Summary: Scientific evidence on condom effectiveness for sexually transmitted diseases (STD) prevention. http://www.niaid.nih.gov/dmid/stds/condomreport.pdf, 2001

38. Greydanus DE, Patel DR. Substance Abuse in Adolescents: Current Concepts. Disease-a-Month 2005 (July); 51(7):392–431.

39. Johnston LD, O'Malley PM & Bachman JG. The Monitoring the Future Study on Adolescent drug use: Overview of key findings. 2005. National Institutes of Health Publication No. 04–5506. Bethesda, Maryland, USA: National Institute on Drug Abuse, 2006.

40. ESPAD– The European School Survey Project on Alcohol and Other Drugs (Report, 2003).

41. Greydanus DE, Patel Dr, Pratt HD. (eds): Essential Adolescent Medicine, NY: McGraw-Hill Medical Publishers, p. 800, 2006.

42. Patel DR, Greydanus DE & Rowlett JD. Romance with the automobile in the 20th Century: Implications for adolescents In a new millennium. Adolesc Med 2000; 11:127–39.

43. Mackay J, Eriksen, M. The Tobacco Atlas. Geneva, Switzerland: WHO, p. 128, 2002.

44. Strasburger VC & Donnerstein E. Children, adolescents, and the media in the 21st century. State of the Art Reviews: Adolescent Medicine 2000; 11(1): 51–68.

45. Warren C, Riley L, Asma S, et al. Tobacco Use by Youth: A Surveillance Report from the Global Youth Tobacco Survey Project. Bulletin of the World Health Organization. 2000; 78(7):868–76.

46. Wellman RJ, Sugarman DB, DiFranza JR, Winickoff JP. The extent to which tobacco marketing and tobacco use in films contribute to children's use of tobacco. Arch Pediatr Adolesc Med 2006; 160:1285–96.

47. Eder W, Ege MJ, von Mutius E. The asthma epidemic. N Engl J Med 2006; 355:2226–35.
48. Grant EN, Wagner R, Weiss KB. Observations on emerging patterns of asthma in our society. J Allergy Clin Immunology 1999; 104(2 pt.2):S1–9.
49. Onkamo P, Karvonen M, et al. Worldwide increase in incidence of Type I diabetes-the analysis of the data on published Incidence trends. Diabetologica 1999; 42:1395–403.
50. Rowell HA, Evans BJ, Quarry-Horn JL, et al. Type 2 diabetes mellitus in adolescents. Adolesc Med 2002; 13:1–12.
51. Lewis DW. Migraine headaches in adolescents. Adolesc Med 2002; 13:413–32.
52. Pakalnis A. Nonmigraine headaches in adolescents. Adolesc Med 2002; 13: 433–42.
53. Sakai I. Migraine headaches in Japan. JAMA, 1999.
54. Hauser WA, Rich SR, Annegers JF, et al. Seizures after a first unprovoked seizure: an extended follow-up. Neurol 1990; 40:1163–70.
55. Paolicchi MJ. Epilepsy in adolescents: Diagnosis and treatment. Adolesc Med 2002; 13:443–9.
56. Kiess W, Boettner A. Obesity in the adolescent. Adolesc Med 2002; 13:181–90.
57. Livingstone B: Epidemiology of childhood obesity in Europe. Eur J. Pediatr 2000; 159(Suppl. 1):14–34.
58. Ogden CL, Carroll MD, Curtin LR, et al. Prevalence of overweight and obesity in the United States, 1999–2004. JAMA 2006; 295(13):1549–55.
59. Obesity: Preventing and Managing the Global Epidemic. Guide to WHO Documents Concerning Adolescent Health and Development. Geneva, Switzerland: WHO: Department of Child and Adolescent Health and Development, Family and Community Health, WHO, p. 33, 2001.
60. Mokdad AH, Ford ES, Bowman BA, et al. Prevalence of obesity, diabetes and obesity-related health risk factors, 2001. JAMA 2003; 289:76–9.
61. Lowry R, Galuska DA, Fulton JE, et al. Physical activity, food choice and weight management goals and practices among U.S. college students. Am J Prev Med 2000; 18:18–27.
62. Rowlett JD. "Obesity in the adolescent" In: Essential Adolescent Medicine. DE Greydanus, DR Patel, HD Pratt (Eds): New York: McGraw-Hill Medical Publishers. ch. 31, 2006; 651–65.
63. Strauss RS & Knight J. Influence of the home environment on the development of obesity in children. Pediatrics 1999; 103:127.
64. Hill J, Peters J. Environmental contributions to the obesity epidemic. Science 1998; 280:1371–4.
65. Franklin J, Denyer G, Steinbeck S, et al. Obesity and risk of low self-esteem: A statewide survey of Australian children. Pediatrics 2006; 118:2481–7.
66. Hossain P, Kawar B, El Nahas M. Obesity and diabetes in the developing world—A growing challenge. N Engl J Med 2007; 356:213–5.
67. Greydanus DE, Bhave S. Editorial, Obesity in Adolescence. Indian Pediatrics 2004; 41:545–50.
68. Young DR, Phillips JA, Yu T, et al. Effects of a life skills intervention for increasing physical activity in adolescent girls. Arch Pediatr Adolesc Med 2006; 160:1255–61.

69. Yanovski SZ. Pharmacotherapy for obesity—promise and uncertainty. N Engl J Med 2005; 353:2187–9.
70. Xanthakox SA, Daniels SR, Inge TH. Bariatric surgery in adolescents: an update. Adolesc Med 2006; 17:589–612.
71. Sothern MS. Childhood and adolescent obesity: exercise as a modality in the treatment of childhood obesity. Pediatr Clin No Amer 2001; 48:1–17.
72. Bar-Or O, Baranowski T. Physical activity, adiposity and obesity among adolescents. Pediatric Exerc Sci 1994; 6:348–60.
73. Bar-Or O. The juvenile obesity epidemic: Is physical activity relevant? Sports Sci Exchange 2003; 16:1–6.
74. Brown JD, Witherspoon EM. The mass media and American adolescents' Health. J Adolesc Health 2002; 31(Suppl):153–70.
75. Golden NH. "Eating disorders: Anorexia nervosa and bulimia nervosa in the adolescent." In: Essential Adolescent Medicine. Eds: DE Greydanus, DR Patel, HD Pratt. NY: McGraw-Hill Medical Publishers, ch. 30. 2006; 635–50.
76. Friedman HL. Culture and adolescent development. *Journal of Adolescent Health* 1999; 25:1–6.
77. Reijonen JH, Pratt HD, Patel DR. et al. Eating disorders in the adolescent population. J Adolesc Res 2003; 18(3):209–22.
78. Manderscheid R & Somenschein MA, (eds). Mental Health, United States. Washington, DC: Center for Menal Health Services, U.S. Government Printing Office, 1996.
79. Elliott GR & Smiga S. Depression in the child and adolescent. Pediatric Clin No Amer 2003; 50(5):1093–106.
80. Greydanus DE, Pratt HD, Patel DR. et al. The rebellious adolescent. Pediatr Clin North Am 1997; 44:1460.
81. WHO World Mental Health Survey Consortium. Prevalence, severity, and unmet need for treatment of mental disorders in the World Health.
82. Juvenile Violence in the Americas: Innovative Studies in Research, Diagnosis and Prevention, Sept, 1998. Guide to WHO Documents Concerning Adolescent Health and Development. Geneva, Switzerland: WHO: Department of Child and Adolescent Health and Development, Family and Community Health, WHO, p. 27, 2001.
83. Pratt HD & Greydanus DE. Adolescent violence: Concepts for a new millennium. Adolesc Med 2000; 11:103–25.
84. U.S. Department of Health and Human Services: *Youth Violence: A Report of the Surgeon General.* Rockville, Maryland, U.S. Department of Health and Human Services, Centers for Disease Control and Prevention, National Center for Injury Prevention and Control; Substance Abuse and Mental Health Services Administration, Center for Mental Health Services; and National Institutes of Health, National Institute of Mental Health, 2001 (www.surgeongeneral.gov/library/youthviolence).
85. Finkelhor V, Hotaling G, Lewis I. Sexual abuse in a national survey of adult men and women: Prevalence, characteristics and risk factors. Child Abuse Negl 1990; 14:9.
86. Mitchell KJ, Finkelhor D & Wolak J. Risk factors for and impact of online sexual solicitation of youth. JAMA 2001; 285:3011–4.

87. Centers for Disease Control and Prevention. Homicide among 15 to 19 year old males-United States 1963–1991. Morb Mort Week Rep 1994; 43:725–7.

88. Pratt HD & Greydanus DE. Violence: Concepts of its impact on children and youth. Pediatr Clin No Am 2003; 50:1–24.

89. Center for Disease Control: Suicide Contagion and the Reporting of Suicide: Recommendations from a National Workshop. Morbidity and Mortality Weekly Report, 1994; 43(RR-6):9–18.

90. Brown P. Choosing to Die – A Growing Epidemic Among the Young. Bulletin of the World Health Organization 2001; 29(12):1175–7.

91. Advance Data-Vital Health Statistics. Atlanta, GA. Centers for Disease Control and Prevention, 1999. Organization World Mental Health Surveys. JAMA 2004; 291:2581–90.

92. Committee on Injury, Violence, and Poison Prevention. American Academy of Pediatrics. The teen driver. Pediatrics 2006; 118:2570–81.

93. Mann JJ, Apter A, Bertolote J, et al. Suicide prevention strategies: A systemic review. JAMA 2005; 294:2064–74.

94. Greydanus DE, Calles JL. Suicide in children and adolescents. Prim Care: Clin in Office Pract 2007; 34(2):222–45.

95. Suicide and attempted suicide. MMWR 2004; 52:471.

96. Kessler RC, Bergland P, Borges G, et al. Trends in suicide ideation, plans, gestures, and attempts in the United States, 1990–1992 to 2001–2003. JAMA 2005; 293:2487–95.

97. Maris RW. Suicide. Lancet 2002; 360:319–26.

98. Zamekin A, Alter MR, Yemini T. Suicide in teenagers: Assessment, management, and prevention. JAMA 2001; 268:2120–5.

99. Eisenberg ME, Resnick MD. Suicidality among gay, lesbian and bisexual youth: The role of protective factors. J Adolesc Health 2006; 39:662–8.

100. Falbo G, Buzzetti R, Cattaneo A. Homicide in Children and Adolescents: A Case–Control Study in Recife, Brazil. Bulletin of the World Health Organization. 2001; 79(1):2–7.

101. Moskowitz H, Laraque D, Doucette JT, Shelov E. Relationships of US youth homicide victims and their offenders, 1976–1999. Arch Pediatr Adolesc Med 2005; 159:356–61.

---------------------------- **14** ----------------------------

Walking the Talk: Parenting Adolescents with a Chronic Condition

Helena Fonseca

Pediatric Division, Hospital de Santa Maria, Faculdade de Medicina de Lisboa, Lisboa, Portugal

Marcelle de Sousa

University College Hospital, University College London Hospitals NHS Foundation Trust, London, U.K.

INTRODUCTION

The concept of family has evolved over time. Today there is a huge diversity of family structures/organizations and contexts (cultural, religious, socio-economic, etc.). Moreover, the way we were brought up may influence the way we deal with family issues. Family connectedness, family role models, family concern for the well-being of the child and autonomy at home are all identified factors that foster resilience in young people and should be encouraged and affirmed (1), especially during adolescence. Conversely, lack of parental support at this time has been associated with negative outcomes, for example, greater nonadherence to medication (2). This chapter will address the issues surrounding the parenting of adolescents with chronic rheumatic conditions from both a theoretical and a practical viewpoint.

FAMILY DYNAMICS AND ADOLESCENT DEVELOPMENT

Adolescents are the product of their genetic inheritance, family, and the society in which they live (3). Of course, they can change neither the genes they received from their parents nor the world in which they live. They cannot change the fact of living in specific contexts such as having to deal with a chronic condition, either.

The Role of Parents During Adolescent Development

Parents can help their adolescent cope with growing up, provide a good example, establish consistent firm limits, being always involved and warm (4). Parents are the child's and adolescent's first role model and teacher. From his/her parents, the child will learn that he/she is unique and deeply loved. These feelings can last a lifetime. Parenting involves the care, teaching, and guidance that enable adolescents to make appropriate decisions for themselves.

Adolescents are still immature in their formal thinking (the brain is only fully mature after age 20), and they may rebel or believe they are more capable than they really are. And that is were they can get into trouble. Parents should be able to discuss their choices with them and advise them on how to improve their own decisions (5). They (the parents) should give reasons for their decisions and not be afraid to say no. Moreover, they should prepare them to be independent, responsible adults, and not expect more from their adolescents than what they can realistically accomplish.

The impact of a chronic condition on the fulfillment of the developmental tasks of the adolescence may be huge (6). Throughout adolescence new competencies are acquired: Physical development including sexual (pubertal changes, body image); cognitive (development of abstract thinking and identity construction), and social (development of autonomy: change in the relationship with parents and peers, planning for the future). However, and above all, an adolescent with a chronic condition is an adolescent.

The main adolescent developmental tasks are the building of autonomy and identity. The adolescent with a chronic rheumatic condition may face additional challenges in fulfilling these tasks. The development of independence may be interrupted as the child retains childish behavior while becoming adherent to treatment regimes, leading to a compliant but still childish adolescent. On the other extreme, frustration and anger may lead to nonadherence and rebellion.

Regarding peer involvement, there might be fear of rejection and segregation from peers leading to increased absence from school and other activities and social segregation. As far as identity is concerned, an inferior self-image with lower self-esteem, sometimes depression, may lead to concerns about the future and their emerging sexuality. Of course, both the severity of the condition and personal and family history are major influences. Family becomes then a critical element. Health professionals may also play an important role. They need to understand the family in this new life-cycle stage, how family dynamics may influence the adolescent's development and how they may facilitate communication among the different elements of the family system. Assessment of the adolescent psychosocial maturation and autonomy is a priority when dealing with teenagers and is covered further in Chapters 2 and 4.

Patterns of Family Functioning

Once an adolescent with a chronic condition comes to the rheumatology clinic with his/her family, the health professional should be able to identify the impact of the dominant patterns of family functioning on the developmental aspects of the adolescent–parent relationship. Sometimes the adolescent is a symptom carrier for the family, and the health professional should wonder whose problem it is. The health professional should also:

1. Modulate empathy towards the adolescent and his/her parents
2. Raise questions in an nonjudgmental and open way
3. Support the parents and the adolescent in clarifying their respective demands
4. Enable and empower each person to express him or herself
5. Pay attention to nonverbal communication

A variety of theoretical models dealing with a systems perspective on the family have been developed by researchers, focusing independently on variables related to the cohesion, adaptability, and communication dimensions of the family dynamics.

Olson's circumplex model (7) was developed in an attempt to bridge the gap that typically exists between theory and practice. Clinically, it is used for identifying types of family systems and for planning treatment intervention. There are types of therapeutic techniques and interventions that are most and least effective with various types of systems. Moreover, the dominant patterns of family functioning may influence the developmental aspects of the adolescent-parents relationship. Olson's model is mainly based in the adaptability and cohesion dimensions. The *adaptability dimension* is defined as the ability of the family system to change (change role relationships, rules, and the power structure in response to situational and developmental stress). The four levels of adaptability range from *rigid* (very low): authoritarian leadership, roles seldom change, strict discipline, too little change to *structured* (low to moderate): leadership sometimes shared, roles stable, somewhat democratic discipline, change when demanded to *flexible* (moderate to high): shared leadership, role sharing, democratic discipline, change when necessary to *chaotic* (very high): lack of leadership, dramatic role shifts, erratic discipline, too much change. Central levels of adaptability (structured and flexible) are more conducive to family functioning.

The *cohesion dimension* is defined as the emotional bonding that family members have toward one another. There are four levels of cohesion, ranging from *disengaged* (very low): little closeness, lack of loyalty, high independence to *separated* (low to moderate): little loyalty, interdependent, more independence than dependence to *connected* (moderate to high): some loyalty, interdependent, more dependence than independence to *enmeshed* (very high): high loyalty, high dependency). Based on this model, high levels of cohesion (enmeshed) and low levels of cohesion (disengaged) might be problematic for relationships. Again, the central levels of cohesion (separated and connected) make for optimal family functioning.

Family communication is the third dimension in this model and is considered a facilitating dimension. Because of its specific dimension, communication is not graphically included in the model along with cohesion and adaptability. Positive communication skills include empathy, reflective listening, supportive comments. These skills enable families to share with each other their needs and preferences as they relate to the other two dimensions: cohesion and adaptability. Negative communication skills include criticism, double messages and binds. They minimize the ability of family members to share their feelings.

Chronic conditions have a significant impact on families because the ongoing care and management of the condition rests primarily with the family (8). The Family Adjustment and Adaptation Response Model developed by McCubbin and Patterson (9) is especially useful for examining both the impact of the condition on the family and what resources and coping behaviors in the family facilitate a successful adaptation. Throughout the life cycle the family, like all social systems, attempts to maintain balanced functioning by using its capabilities (resources and coping behaviors) to meet its demands (stressors and strains). According to these authors (10), a stressor is defined as a life event that occurs at a discrete point in time and produces or has the potential to produce change in the family system. A strain is defined as a condition of felt tension associated with the need or desire to change something. Strain may emerge from the unresolved tension associated with prior stressors. An adolescent's chronic rheumatic disease is a stressor. The seriousness and chronicity of the condition will influence the intensity of the demand and how much it upsets the family's homeostatic state. When the family is unable to accept the situation in a positive way or when it is impossible to resolve the stressor completely, there is a residue of tension that is carried along by the family over time as a part of their "list" of demands. The outcome of the family's efforts to achieve balanced functioning is conceptualized in terms of family adjustment or family adaptation, ranging on a continuum from good to poor. A crisis is a state of disequilibrium, emerging in the family system when the nature and/or number of demands exceed the existing capabilities of the family, and this imbalance persists. It may arise, for instance, at the moment of the teenager's diagnosis of a chronic, severe, rheumatic disease. During the adaptation phase, the family attempts to restore homeostasis by either acquiring new resources and coping behaviors or reducing the demands they must deal with. The multidisciplinary team may play a crucial role in facilitating the acquisition of new resources and the development of coping behaviors.

KEY ELEMENTS IN THE ASSESSMENT OF THE ADOLESCENT–PARENT DYNAMICS IN THE CONTEXT OF A CHRONIC CONDITION

A Psychosocial Family History

A fundamental aspect of the assessment of the adolescent–parent dynamics in the context of a chronic condition is a thorough family history extending beyond the traditional family history to ascertain inherited conditions. This can come under the Home component of the HEADSS acronym (Home, Education, Activities, Drugs, Sex, Suicide) (11) and includes such information as who lives with whom, who has contact with whom, where are the close or difficult relationships, the preferential and/or close bonds and who are the influential family members etc.

Acknowledging Different Perspectives

The different perspectives of the adolescent and their parent(s)/caregiver(s) need to be considered by health professionals involved in the triadic consultations of child-centered health services. Within the generic literature, the most comprehensive study of parents as proxies of adolescents has been conducted by Waters et al. who examined the relationship between 2096 Australian adolescents (aged 12–18 years) and their parents using the Childhood Health Questionnaire (12). This study demonstrated strong overall agreement for physical health. However, adolescents were less optimistic than their parents with respect to their mental health, well-being, general health, and impact of health on family activities. Moreover, these discrepancies increased when the adolescent had an illness.

Within the "chronic illness" literature, only a few studies of child-parent agreement pertain to childhood onset rheumatic diseases (13–20). These have found mixed (and often contradictory) findings including reports of no agreement (17) or poor agreement for pain (14); fair to good agreement for general health (14); fair to excellent agreement for functional disability (14,15,17) and fair agreement for health related quality of life (14,16,19). As such, they generally follow the pattern found in the wider literature, which suggests that parents and children tend to agree about easily observable behaviors compared with less overt phenomena (12). In a study which specifically addressed agreement between adolescents (with juvenile idiopathic arthritis, JIA) and their parents, approximately half did not show agreement in ratings for pain, general health perception, functional ability, and health-related quality-of-life (21). Agreement was associated with better disease-related outcome variables, but not significantly influenced by demographic factors.

Agreement between adolescents and parents was dependent on the level of disease outcome and the health domain under scrutiny and was less for those with moderate disease outcomes (as compared to mild or severe) and for less visible phenomena, e.g., pain, global well-being. These findings are consistent with the considerable changes in family dynamics which occur during adolescence, with young people becoming increasing emotionally autonomous from parents and wanting to spend more time away from home (22,23).

Assessment of Parental Needs

In a study using focus group methodology, parents of adolescents with JIA acknowledged that they found it difficult to "let go" of their son/ daughter but realized that it was important for them to become their own advocates (24). They suggested that health care providers could help them to facilitate increasing autonomy for their son/daughter by encouraging self-advocacy skills training for the adolescent. The parents suggested that the health professionals should actively involve the young person during the consultation and, ideally, ensure that he/she is able to see the same professional at each visit if the young person so chooses (i.e., continuity). Once parents realized that their son/daughter was capable, they could then gradually withdraw from the consultation and eventually wait outside the clinic room for part or all of the visit. The parents also saw this as an ideal opportunity for their own needs to be met (24). Meeting the parents' needs has been emphasized in the recent major policy documents on both sides of the Atlantic (25,26). These needs include support and preparation for transition and transfer to adult care; developing an understanding of adolescent development in the context of the chronic condition and their own important, dynamic role in the process as parents; provision of advice about the negotiation of boundaries, informational resources, and support services available both within the hospital and the local community. The resources in terms of staffing and clinic space required to meet these needs, however cannot be ignored with respect to such intervention, albeit integral to adolescent health care.

Assessing Parental Advocacy

The challenge of negotiating the appropriate extent of parental involvement is an integral component of adolescent health care whatever the setting. Parental overprotectiveness has been reported in the context of JIA (27) as in other chronic conditions (28–31). In a national survey of rheumatology health professionals, parental overprotectiveness was reported to put adolescents with JIA at risk of transitional difficulties (27). Geenen reported a significant discrepancy between the perceived age for commencing self-management skills training between parents of young people with special health care needs and their health care providers (30).

STRATEGIES FOR WORKING WITH PARENTS IN ADOLESCENT RHEUMATOLOGY CLINIC SETTINGS

Transitional care must include parents, acknowledging the dynamics of parents' evolving role as the young person moves from childhood through adolescence and, ultimately, into adulthood. In a national survey of professionals, a fifth of respondents reported difficulties with parents with respect to over protectiveness, adolescent-parent conflicts, denial of transitional issues, and consent during the transition process (27).

There are many simple strategies that health professionals can employ to limit the impact of and/or avoid such difficulties thereby facilitating a smooth transition through adolescence for young person and parent alike. Examples of these strategies are detailed in Table 1, and a few of these are discussed in detail below.

Environmental Aspects

The seating arrangements are of vital importance to ensure effective adolescent health care provision. The professional should always invite the young person to take the seat that allows direct eye contact, emphasizing the young person's central importance in the consultation. Similarly the parent should be invited to take the seat which is slightly out of direct eye contact, ensuring that the health professional will have to deliberately turn his or her head to respond to them. The ventriloquist parent will easily be identifiable with such arrangements! As the professional waits for the young person to respond, it will be the parent's voice coming from elsewhere in the room they will hear!

Specific Communication Strategies

When dealing with difficult situations such as those in which communication is damaged, when negotiation is difficult or there are false secrets, some pieces of systemic therapy may be useful. The professional should keep in mind that her/his neutrality should be preserved at all cost by challenging everyone or everything while siding with no one. This does not come easily, so take time to think before you speak.

Turn-Taking

One possible technique is "turn-taking," that is, involving each family member in turn, avoiding questions that invite yes/no responses, checking back with each participant to ask how they see something on which others have commented.

Table 1   Top "Six-Teen" Tips for Dealing with Parents of Adolescents with Chronic Rheumatic Conditions

---

1. Gain a good working knowledge of the social history and family dynamics. It is invaluable—never assume anything! (e.g., who is the person the young person talks to most in the family?)
2. Remember to direct your questions to the patient, NOT the parent
3. If conflict is evident, play for time e.g., unscrew pens, flick through notes, etc.
4. Be aware of the adolescent and/or the parent manipulating you
5. Consider the seating arrangement and make sure direct eye contact is possible between you and the young person
6. Remember that adolescents will not always talk openly in front of parents, especially regarding medication
7. Aim for continuity of professionals between visits to help gain the adolescent's confidence—and the parents' as they learn to let go
8. Never stop supporting the parents—even if they are out of the consultation room
9. Plan—start talking about the concept of seeing adolescent independently well in advance, all the time emphasizing the vital role of the supportive parent
10. Be clear about your intention to have time alone with the adolescent
11. Remember the relationship between parent and young person and health professional is dynamic and may vary from visit to visit throughout adolescence
12. Include ALL team members—another colleague can be seeing the parents while you are giving space to the young person. Confidentiality must be assured in all consultations
13. Encourage the parent to sustain the expectation that their child can/will work and live fulfilled and independent lives
14. Encourage the parents to ensure their child's attainment of functional independence, development of autonomy and self-advocacy skills could and should be equivalent to their peers
15. Address any educational/informational needs of the parents as well as the young person and make sure they know of resources available in the community. This means you have to know what there is to offer
16. Don't forget the dads, who may not be present in clinic

Circular Questioning

Circular questioning may also be helpful as used in family therapy. For example, if we want to see clearly what the definition of the problem is for each family member, we may ask: "What do you think X will say is the problem? ... Who agrees with him? ... Who disagrees? How would you put it?" Then, "In what way is this problem a problem? ... What makes the problem a problem? ... How is it a problem for you? ... Who is it most a problem for?"

   Problem-solving can also promote resilience. By asking each party "If you could change one thing ..." negotiation can be facilitated. Ideally the adolescent/family create the solutions but if not, the health care provider can propose one for discussion!!

Preparation for Clinic Visits

This aforementioned ventriloquist parental role described above often comes from a real need to ensure that the doctor knows everything that has gone on at home and the strong belief that something will be missed if the young person is allowed to speak for themselves. One strategy to address this is to encourage the parent to prepare for each visit. A simple exercise is detailed in Table 2 to aid such discussions and is based on templates used in the OnTrac program at the Children's Hospital in Vancouver (32) and the adolescent rheumatology transition program described by McDonagh et al. (33).

Concurrent Visits for Parents

The ideal albeit costly solution to address parental needs would be for parents to be seen by another person while the young person is having their appointment (24). Imperative to such visits is both informing the adolescent that their parent wishes to talk over their concerns to another member of the team whilst they are being seen. Furthermore, both the young person and the parent should be made aware of their rights to confidentiality. Nurse specialists often take on this role. Another solution is to facilitate a parents support group that takes place for the duration of the clinic, where support and education could be provided. This may be facilitated by a

Table 2 Preparing for Adolescent Rheumatology Clinic Appointments as a Parent

Before the appointment			
I talked about the appointment with my son/daughter the night before	Not at all	A little bit	A lot
I made a list of questions to ask with my son/daughter	Yes	No	
At the appointment			
I let my son/daughter talk about his/her ideas, questions, and concerns	Not at all	A little bit	All the time
I let my son/daughter be seen alone	For none of the visit	For part of the visit	For all of the visit
After the appointment			
I talked about the appointment with my child afterwards	Not at all	A little bit	All the time
My questions were all answered and/or my concerns were all listened to	Not at all	A little bit	All the time

Note: Some parents find it difficult to let their son/daughter take charge of his or her own health care. Think about what happened at your last clinic appointment and circle the best response, then discuss it with a team member.

volunteer from a charitable group or it could be another health care professional. This is an invaluable opportunity for parents/carers. Remember that they will always be wondering what is happening in the room with the doctor.

The Importance of Planning

One of the key attributes of components of transition, and indeed of adolescence itself, is envisioning a future for the young person (34). In the context of a chronic condition, planning is essential for success. Individualized transition plans have been advocated for young people by several authors (25,27,35), but it is worth considering similar plans for parents as their son/daughter moves through adolescence. An example of such a plan for parents of adolescents in the 14- to 16-year-old age group is shown in Table 3. Such plans were considered to be important to use by rheumatology professionals (27) and were successfully completed by the majority of parents in an evaluation of a transitional care programme involving 10 U.K. centers (33).

Parental Role in Self-Advocacy Skills Training for Adolescents

Negotiating the balance between under and over protectiveness, thereby facilitating the development of self-advocacy skills, can be challenging for all parents of adolescents but particularly those who have a chronic condition. A useful tool for facilitating discussions with parents and adolescents regarding advocacy is shown in Table 4 and is based on a theoretical leadership model of care (36).

Signposting Resources for Parents

An important aspect of care of parents of adolescents with chronic rheumatic diseases is the provision of information. An understanding of normal adolescent development and how it can potentially be affected by a chronic condition is core to such information provision. A useful book that addresses normal adolescent development for parents is *"Teenagers: The Agony, the Ecstasy, the Answers"* (36).

Finally do not see your role as the divider/separator of the young person and their family. You have an important and crucial role of seeing a young person develop control and independence, within the context of the family, under your care, before moving to adult services. Table 5 provides examples of web-based information for use with and/or by parents of young people with chronic rheumatic disease.

Table 3 Adolescent Rheumatology Mid Transition Plan for Parents

Name:
Start date:

Transition skills	Yes, I can do this on my own and don't feel I need any extra advice	I would like some extra advice/help with this	Action/ date
I understand the medical terms/ words and procedures relevant to my son/daughter's condition			
I feel confident for my son/ daughter to be seen on their own for some/all of each clinic visit			
I understand my rights and responsibilities as a parent to information, to privacy and in decision-making and consent			
I understand my son/daughter's rights and responsibilities to information, to privacy and in decision-making and consent			
I am able to help my son/daughter manage their fatigue (tiredness)			
I am able to help my son/daughter when they find it difficult to sleep well			
I am able to help my son/daughter manage any pain they may have			
I understand what each of my son/ daughter's medications are for and their side effects			
I encourage my son/daughter to be responsible for their own medication at home			
I know what each member of the rheumatology team can do for my son/daughter			

(Continued)

Table 3   Adolescent Rheumatology Mid Transition Plan for Parents (*Continued*)

Transition skills	Yes, I can do this on my own and don't feel I need any extra advice	I would like some extra advice/help with this	Action/ date
I understand the differences between pediatric and adult health care			
I understand the importance of exercise/activity for both my son/daughter's general health and their condition			
I understand what foodstuffs are good for young people like my son/daughter			
I know how to access reliable accurate information for parents about sexual health for young people			
I understand the risk of drugs, alcohol and smoking to the health of young people			
I encourage my son/daughter to be responsible for a particular household chore(s) at home			
I encourage my son/daughter to be self-caring at home, e.g., dressing, bathing/showering, etc.			
I know about resources that offer support for young people with my son/daughter's condition and their families			
I know how to access I know how to access advice and/or help with my son/daughter experiences unwelcome comments/bullying			
I know how to deal with any discomfort my son/daughter has about the way he/she looks to others			

(*Continued*)

Table 3 Adolescent Rheumatology Mid Transition Plan for Parents (*Continued*)

Transition skills	Yes, I can do this on my own and don't feel I need any extra advice	I would like some extra advice/help with this	Action/ date
I know my son/daughter has someone they feel able to talk to when they feel sad/fed-up			
I Know how to access advice and/ or help with my son/daughter's education			
I know what my son/daughter wants to do when they leave school			
I understand the importance of work experience for future career development of young people like my son/daughter			
I am aware of any potential impact of my son/daughter's condition to their education and/or work opportunities			
Please list anything else you would like help or advice with:			

Table 4 Shared Leadership Model

Increasing age/time	Provider	Parent/family	Young person
↓	Major responsibility	Provides care	Receives care
↓	Support to parent/family and young person	Manages	Participates
↓	Consultant	Supervisor	Manager
↓	Resource	Consultant	Supervisor

Note: Each person identifies where he/she is functioning on this table and then discuss what needs to happen to get to the ultimate goal of care management for that individual young person.
Source: From Ref. 35.

Table 5 Useful Web-Based Resources for Parents

Disease-specific information:

www.ccaa.org.uk

Chat 2 Parents booklet specifically for parents of adolescents with arthritis

General information for patients:

www.arthritis.org/communities/juvenile_arthritis/about_ajao.asp

The website of the American Juvenile Arthritis Organization – a council of the U.S.-based Arthritis Foundation – offers generic information for parents of adolescents

www.tsa.co.uk

The U.K.-based Trust for the Study of Adolescence, which produces a wide range of useful resources in various formats for parents of adolescents

www.parentlineplus.org.uk

A U.K.-registered charity that offers support to anyone parenting a child – the child's parents, stepparents, grandparents, and foster parents

www.youngminds.org.uk

A U.K.-registered charity with useful resources for parents of adolescents, with an emphasis on mental health

www.rcpsych.ac.uk/mentalhealthinformation/childrenandyoungpeople.aspx

The website of the U.K.-based royal College of Psychiatrists. Useful factsheets for parents re:child and adolescent mental health, including "Surviving adolescence"

www.aacap.org/index.ww

The website of the American Academy of Child and Adolescent Psychiatry. Useful information sheets on normal adolescent development.

www.dh.gov.uk

"Consent – What You Have a Right to Expect. A Guide for Parents"

A leaflet about consent for parents of children and young people published by the U.K. Department of Health.

Support groups:

www.ccaa.org.uk

U.K.-based Children with Chronic Arthritis Association

www.kidswitharthritis.org

U.K.-based charity for families with children with arthritis

www.cafamily.org.uk

U.K.-based charity (Contact a Family) for families of disabled children

---

SUMMARY

The role of the health care provider is therefore to empower families to improve their coping behaviors, encourage advocacy skills and to enhance their ability to bounce back, "family resilience." In doing this, health care providers should be nonjudgmental, listen to both adolescent and parent, promote resilience, enable and empower each person to express him or herself, pay attention to nonverbal communication between adolescent and parent and to facilitate communication between adolescent and his/her family.

REFERENCES

1. Patterson J, Blum RJ. Risk and resilience among children and youth with disabilities. Arch Pediatr Adolesc Med 1996; 150:692–98.
2. Lurie S, Shemesh E, Sheiner PA, et al. Nonadherence in pediatric liver transplant recipients—an assessment if risk factors and natural history. Pediatr Transplant 2000; 4:200–6.
3. Greydanus D. American Academy of Pediatrics. Parenting an Adolescent. In: Caring for your Adolescent: Ages 12 to 21. 1st ed. New York: Bantam Books, 1991:3–40.
4. Steinberg L, Mounts N, Lamborn S, Dornbusch S. Authoritative parenting and adolescent adjustment across varied ecological niches. J Res Adol 1991; 1:19–36.
5. Gellerstedt ME, leRoux P, Litt D. Beyond anticipatory guidance-parenting and the family life cycle. Pediatric Clinics of North America 1995; 42:65–78.
6. Coupey S, Neinstein L, Zeltzer L. Chronic Illness in the Adolescent. In: Neinstein LS. Adolescent Health-care-A Practical Guide. 4th ed. Philadelphia: Lippincott Williams & Wilkins, 2002:1511–36.
7. Olson D. Circumplex Model: Systemic Assessment and Treatment of Families. In: Circumplex Model of Family Systems VIII: Family Assessment and Intervention. The Haworth Press, Inc. 1989:7–49.
8. Patterson J, Blum RW. Risk and resilience among children and youth with disabilities. Arch Pediatr Adolesc Med 1996; 150:692–8.
9. McCubbin HI, Patterson J. The Family Stress Process: The Double ABCX Model of Family Adjustment and Adaptation. In: McCubbin HI, Sussman M, Patterson JM, eds. Social Stress and the Family: Advances and developments in family stress theory and research. New York: Haworth, 1983.
10. Patterson J. Families Experiencing Stress: I. The Family adjustment and adaptation response model; ii. applying the FAAR model to health-related issues for intervention and research. Fam Syst Med 1988; 6:202–37.
11. Goldenring JM, Cohen E. Getting into adolescent heads. Contemp Pediatr 1988; July:7590.
12. Waters E, Stewart-Brown S, Fitzpatrick R. Agreement between adolescent self-report and parent reports of health and well-being: results of an epidemiological study. Child Care Health dev 2003; 29:501–9.
13. Palmero TM, Zebracki K, Cox S, Newman AJ, Singer NG. Juvenile Idiopathic Arthritis: Parent-child discrepancy on reports of pain and disability. J Rheumatol 2004; 31:1840–6.
14. Brunner HI, Klein-Gitelman MS, Miller MJ, Trombley M, Baldwin N, Kress A, et al. Health of children with chronic arthritis: relationship of different measures and the quality of parent proxy reporting. Arthritis Care Res 2004; 51:763–73.
15. Cuneo KM, Schiaffino KM. Adolescent self-perceptions of adjustment to childhood arthritis: the influence of disease activity, family resources, and parent adjustment. J Adolesc Health. 2002; 31:363–71.
16. Varni JW, Seid M, Smith Knight T, Burwinkle T, Brown J, Szer IS. The PedsQL™ in pediatric rheumatology. Reliability, validity, and responsiveness of the Pediatric Quality of Life Inventory™ Generic Core Scales and Rheumatology Module. Arthritis Rheum 2002; 46:714–25.

17. Doherty E, Yanni G, Conroy RM, Bresnihan B. A comparison of child and parent ratings of disability and pain in juvenile chronic arthritis. J Rheumatol 1993; 20:1563–6.

18. Singh G, Athreya B, Fries J, Goldsmith DP, Ostrov BE. Measurement of health status in children with juvenile rheumatoid arthritis. Arthritis Rheum 1994; 37:1761–9.

19. Duffy CM, Arsenault L, Watanabe Duffy KN. Level of agreement between parents and children in rating dysfunction in juvenile rheumatoid arthritis and juvenile spondyloarthritides. J Rheumatol 1993; 20:2134–9.

20. Howe S, Levinson J, Shear E, et al. Development of a disability measurement tool for juvenile rheumatoid arthritis. The Juvenile Arthritis Functional assessment Report for children and their parents. Arthritis Rheum 1991; 34:873–80.

21. Shaw KL, Southwood TR, McDonagh JE. Growing up and moving on in Rheumatology: parents as proxies of adolescents with Juvenile Idiopathic Arthritis. Arthritis Care Res 2006; 55(2):189–98.

22. Coleman JC, Hendry L. The Nature of Adolescence. London, UK: Routledge; 1999.

23. Heaven PCL. Contemporary Adolescence: A Social Psychological Approach. Basingstoke, UK: The MacMillan Press, 1994.

24. Shaw KL, Southwood TR, McDonagh JE. Users' perspectives of transitional care for adolescents with juvenile idiopathic arthritis. Rheumatology 2004; 43: 770–8.

25. American Academy of Pediatrics, American Academy of Family Physicians, American College of Physicians-American Society of Internal Medicine. A consensus statement on health care transitions for young adults with special health care needs. Pediatrics 2002; 110:1304–6.

26. Department of Health. Getting the right start: National Service Framework for Children, Young People and Maternity Serivces: Standard for Hospital Services. April 2003.

27. Shaw KL, Southwood TR, McDonagh JE. Developing a Programme of Transitional Care for Adolescents with Juvenile Idiopathic Arthritis: Results of a Postal Survey. Rheumatology 2004; 43:211–9.

28. Durst CL, Horn MV, MacLaughlin EF, Bowmand CM, Starnes VA, Woo MS. Psychosocial responses of adolescent cystic fibrosis patients to lung transplantation. Pediatr Transplant 2001; 5:27–31.

29. Ehrich JHH, Rizzoni G, Broyer M, et al. Rehabilitation of young adults during renal replacement therapy in Europe 2. Schooling, employment and social situation. Nephrol Dial Transplant 1992; 7:573–8.

30. Geenen SJ, Powers LE, Sells W. Understanding the role of health care providers during transition of adolescents with disabilities and special health care needs. J Adolesc Health 2003; 32:225–33.

31. Gold L, Kirkpatrick B, Fricker F, Zitelli B. Psychosocial issues in pediatric organ transplantation: parent's perspective. Pediatrics 1986; 77:738–44.

32. Paone MC, Wigle M, Saewyc E. The ON TRAC model for transitional care of adolescents. Prog Transplant 2006; 16:291–302.

33. McDonagh JE, Southwood TR, Shaw KL. Growing up and moving on in rheumatology: development and preliminary evaluation of a transitional care programme for a multicentre cohort of adolescents with juvenile idiopathic arthritis. J Child Health-care 2006; 10(1):22–42.

34. Reiss JG, Gibson RW, Walker LR. Health-care transition: youth, family, and provider perspectives. Pediatrics 2005; 115:112–20.

35. Royal College of Nursing. Adolescent transition care: guidance for nursing staff. 2004, London (www.rcn.org.uk).

36. Kieckhefer GM, Trahms CM. Supporting development of children with chronic conditions: from compliance toward shared management. Pediatr Nursing 2000; 26:354–63.

37. McPherson A, MacFarlane A. Teenagers: the agony, the ecstasy, the answers. Time Warner: London, 2000.

15

Making Connections, Getting Connected: Peer Support and Chronic Rheumatic Disease

Janine Hackett and Bernadette Johnson

Department of Paediatric and Adolescent Rheumatology, Birmingham Children's Hospital, Birmingham, U.K.

INTRODUCTION

Friendships are important to us all and enhance our lives by providing emotional, practical, and social support. For young people, who spend long hours at school and also have large amounts of free time available, close friendships and peer relationships play an important role in their social and emotional development. Friendships help young people to develop an identity that is separate from their family and offer an opportunity to develop social skills, as well as providing companionship and fun. For those with chronic illness, however, establishing stable, peer support networks can be disrupted by such intrinsic factors such as poor self-esteem, reduced self-confidence, and impaired body image as well as by extrinsic factors including periods of hospitalization, frequent therapy appointments, overprotection by family members, and poor availability of transport. All of these may compound the development of friendships and limit opportunities to consolidate social skills and develop self confidence (1). Society may also be reluctant to accept those with disabilities into particular peer groups (2).

CHRONIC ILLNESS AND FRIENDSHIP

For a young person with a chronic rheumatic disease like juvenile idiopathic arthritis (JIA), maintaining friendships outside the family may pose additional challenges. This may be a direct consequence of the disease, such as pain, stiffness, and fatigue or secondary consequences such as limited knowledge and/or inaccurate beliefs about their condition and the benefits of social and sporting activities. Fear of hurting themselves or making worse their condition may lead to self-imposed limitations. These behaviors may be inadvertently reinforced by family, friends, school personnel as well as health care professionals. Fatigue may also limit opportunities to join friends in a number of social arenas including shopping and sports. However fatigue is not necessarily related to disease activity, and it may be necessary to consider other factors. Young people with chronic rheumatic disease may be less physically active compared to their healthy peers, resulting in deconditioning, decreased exercise tolerance, lower aerobic capacity, and muscle weakness (3,4). In addition Miller et al. (5) reported that children and young people with JIA report functional difficulties even in the absence of active signs of the disease. Careful assessment of the young persons function including social activities should therefore be documented by health professionals regardless of disease activity.

The relationship between friendship and social activity is not always straightforward however. A Canadian study (6) reported that young people with physical disabilities between the ages of 11 and 16 were less socially active and involved in fewer intimate relationships despite reporting good self-esteem, strong family relationships, and many close friends compared to national statistics. Other factors may therefore be relevant. Adolescents with JIA have reported increased social support from parents and teachers, which could perhaps be interpreted as having a potentially negative impact on the development of social activities. Overprotectiveness by parents, teachers, and health professionals often results in a delay in the development of self-advocacy, separation from family, as well as the challenging of authority, all of which are necessary to achieve independence from parents.

Disease experience has been shown to correlate with levels of self-competence, including physical attractiveness and global self worth, even after controlling for disease severity (7) suggesting psychosocial factors such as friendships can play an important role in disease outcome. Peer support may therefore be particularly important for this group and act as a buffer against the stresses of the disease.

Various authors have studied the significance of peer relationships in the context of chronic illness during adolescence. Friends of adolescents with chronic illnesses are often younger and nondisabled (8). Wolman et al. (9) reported that 32% of the variance in the emotional well-being of adolescents with chronic condition was explained by concern about peer relationships along with body image and family connectedness. When data of young people with visible versus invisible conditions were compared, there was no difference (9).

WHY SHOULD PROFESSIONALS BE INTERESTED?

A U.K. study involving national focus groups of young people with JIA highlighted the need to consider social aspects of the young person's life alongside their physical and psychological needs (1). Young people reported an overwhelming need to meet similar others with JIA and the need for health professionals to pay increased attention to issues such as bullying, social isolation, and the loss of valued social activities. In a health care setting discussion of such topics can help develop rapport and build trusting relationships. In addition the development of interventions to address these issues may prove invaluable. Developing a supportive client-centered relationship that is seen as responsive and motivating may improve adherence, as has been demonstrated in young people with diabetes, comparing a client-centered approach with doctors who were "expert" decision makers who adopted a traditional medical model (10). Health care workers may therefore need training to ensure that their consultations are adolescent friendly and not dominated by disease monitoring tasks (see Chapters 4 and 17).

The development of psychosocial interventions is also important as social groups are a useful mechanism for sharing feelings they would not normally disclose to others (11). Social groups may therefore be an important tool for screening for mental health issues. Mood has also been shown to play an important role in the reporting of disease symptoms, including pain and fatigue, and that mood enhancing activities could have a positive effect on such symptoms (12). It could therefore be inferred that social isolation and the lack of peer support could have an effect on mood and the subsequent reporting of symptoms in clinic. Health professionals therefore need to be cognisant of the benefits of psychosocial interventions when managing physical symptoms as well as the more traditional medical treatments for symptom relief.

Adherence

Support from close friends can be an important resource when adhering to treatment regimes. Since non-adherence contributes to increased morbidity, health professionals need to pay close attention to this area. Asking a young person about their friends is not only a good way to build rapport and demonstrate an interest in them as a young person and not simply a patient, but also it is a useful method of identifying those who are socially isolated as well as determining potential health risk behaviors. Members of particular peer groups tend to be similar in health risk behaviors, therefore asking about friends may be revealing about the young person themselves (13). Young people with chronic illness sometimes feel "different" and therefore in order to "fit in" may be discordant with medical treatment or ignore lifestyle advice regarding diet, exercise, alcohol, drugs, etc.

Adherence to therapy and disease management may prove challenging to some young people during this stage of development (14). The challenge for health care professionals is to engage young people as active participants in their disease management and in informed decision making regarding their treatment. Encouraging young people to bring a friend along to clinic may prove useful in increasing the friend's knowledge of the condition, as well as increasing awareness of the constraints and challenges it poses for the young person. Subsequently this may result in increased practical support with health related behaviors. Integral to success and quality in this area of health care is the design of holistic, developmentally appropriate and innovative interventions which best meet the psychosocial needs of young people and facilitate their evolving independence. Adherence is discussed further in Chapter 5.

Disclosure

Friendships may facilitate an adolescent's adjustment to a chronic disease or their ability to cope with a difficult medical treatment (2,15,16). However, this is very difficult if peers are unaware of their friend's condition. For some young people with chronic illness the fear of disclosing their illness and the impact they perceive this will have on how others respond to them means that they will sometimes try to keep their diagnosis secret. However disclosure can be a great relief and can foster both practical and emotional support. It is also an important skill to develop for later life, as they may want to disclose their condition to partners and potential employers. A review of the literature (17) reported that conditions under which is best to disclose illness are not yet fully understood. In some cases it has been found that disclosure to classmates as a whole resulted in little or no impact on the popularity of the child (18) and in other cases has adversely affected relationships (19). Disclosure to close friends however for children with HIV resulted in improved functioning compared to that of children who had not disclosed their HIV status (20). On balance it would appear that disclosure of a young person's chronic illness to carefully chosen friends can be helpful and can provide a sense of relief that their condition is no longer secret and support can be elicited (2). Health professionals may need to offer advice and support to facilitate the process of disclosure since some young people may not possess the skills and confidence to ensure a successful outcome, which may hinder future disclosure.

PEER SUPPORT IN HOSPITAL SETTINGS

Hospitals can play an important role in facilitating peer support. One very successful programme is the Chronic Illness Peer Support (ChIPS) programme in Melbourne, Australia, which has been effective in creating peer support networks for young people with chronic illness (21). ChIPS is a generic program recognizing that young people with any chronic illness face many similar psychosocial issues irrespective of illness type. Initially the program begins with an eight- week group for eight- young people with a variety of diagnoses. The group is run by a health professional and a trained peer leader and during these sessions they are able to discuss what it's like to live with a chronic illness. As a follow-up from this program, an ongoing social and recreational timetable is planned by participants. Activities include movie nights and newsletter production. A leadership training program is also offered to graduates of the program who then become co-facilitators and leaders of other activities. A qualitative evaluation study of the ChIPS program reported a positive impact on well being of young people with a reduction in social isolation, an improved acceptance of illness and improved adherence to treatment (21). Other research by Clark et al. (22) reported their monthly peer support group involving adolescents with cancer, hematological diseases and healthy high school students resulted in improved coping skills and improved quality of life for the patients. In the healthy adolescents a positive attitudinal change and intended behavior toward peers with chronic illness was also reported.

Organizing less structured programs such as vacation social groups, bowling trips, Christmas parties, or inviting local cosmetic companies in for a "pamper day" may serve to increase self-confidence levels and facilitate the development of peer support networks. In addition, therapy groups such as hydrotherapy or gym groups involving similar others may also serve to facilitate social networks. Careful selection of patients by health professionals may further enhance this process, by considering age, interests, problems, and personalities.

Outpatient Settings

Designated adolescent clinics may also be useful in developing peer relationships. A welcoming outpatient waiting area with seats arranged strategically and adolescent-friendly reading materials may also lead to social intercourse with other patients. A youth worker or other volunteer could be instrumental in introducing young people to one another. When friendships are evidently developing, these can be facilitated by scheduling appointments at the same time in order to maintain contacts (Fig. 1).

In-Patient Settings

During in-patient admissions, it is important to ensure young people are placed in an appropriate environment where they are able to meet similar others to ensure continued social interaction with their peer group. Having a designated adolescent common room with developmentally appropriate leisure activities may assist in establishing friendships within the hospital

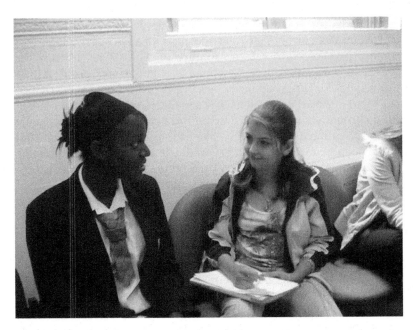

Figure 1 Potential of clinic waiting areas in peer support.

environment. In order to maintain outside friendships, visiting times should be flexible enough to allow visits from school friends who may only be able to visit late afternoon, particularly when it is a prolonged admission. Young people should perhaps be encouraged to bring mobile phones with them to maintain ongoing contact with friends while an inpatient. Hospital policies banning the use of mobile phones however may need to be relaxed in clinical areas where it is not detrimental to the health of other patients in order to facilitate this. Providing access to the internet and e-mail within the hospital ward should also be considered as a way of sustaining friendships.

RESIDENTIAL CAMPS

Summer camps are another way of addressing peer support, and they have been shown to be a valuable way of addressing psychosocial issues including locus of control (23), self-esteem (24), physical fitness (24,25), independence from parents, health care self-management and an opportunity to meet similar others (23). Many rheumatology centers throughout the world, including Melbourne, Vancouver, San Diego, and Newcastle (U.K.) run their own summer camps. Each differs in content; however, all are seen as a valued adjunct to conventional therapy and are a valuable method of assessing psychological well-being.

Birmingham, U.K. Model

Designed for young people with a chronic rheumatological condition between the ages of 12 and 16 the Birmingham Residential Program has been running for the past 10 years and takes place during the summer holiday in order to avoid absence from school (26). Self-catering accommodation in a rural location is selected for its proximity to public transport networks and shopping facilities, as well as the availability of adventure activities such as canoeing, climbing, abseiling and team building challenges. Participants are invited to a pre-meeting at the hospital a number of weeks before the trip in order to meet each other and plan the program. The young people are given a range of activities to choose from in the locality of the hostel, and are asked to vote on their preferred activities. All meals are planned by participants and the house rules are also agreed. Characteristics of the residential program are detailed in Table 1.

In a recent evaluation of this trip (26), friendship development was one of the major benefits perceived by young people. At follow-up four months later, the majority had stayed in touch with at least one other person with more girls staying in touch than boys. This may suggest that females either have a greater need for social support or that they may be more socially skilled. For male participants, social stereotype may have prevented them from maintaining contact. Difficulties in the relationships of young adult males with JIA have been reported (27). Health professionals should therefore bear in mind this evidence of gender differences and specifically consider provision of opportunities for young males with rheumatic diseases to meet other young people. In this study mobile phones played an important role in maintaining social contact and may have a role to play in health care for communicating with teenagers, as well as peer support networking. Overall the program was perceived as a valuable experience and offered the young people the opportunity to develop informal peer support networks. Examples of the feedback from a recent camp in Birmingham are detailed in Table 2. Residential camps as described may play an important role in the psychosocial care of teenagers with rheumatic disease and provide a forum for facilitating peer support.

SCHOOLS

Since young people spend a considerable amount of time at school it is very important to have knowledge of and communication with individual schools. Schools can play a significant role in fostering positive peer relations and have a variety of initiatives at their disposal to assist those with difficulties in this area. The school's prevailing ethos is fundamental and sets the tone for the dominant atmosphere around school. A culture which is

Table 1 Characteristics of the Birmingham, U.K., Residential Summer Camp Model

Characteristic	Features	Rationale
Staffing	4 members of rheumatology MDT	Low profile staffing to facilitate peer interaction
Program	Self-directed program, agreed at pre-meeting	Increase decision making and independence skills
	House rules determined by participants	Promote sense of ownership
Meals	Planned by young people	Catering for "fussy eaters" who might otherwise not attend
Chores	Shopping	Exposure to daily chores
	Cooking and cleaning	Increase mobility
		Promote team work
		Facilitate independence in acitivities of daily livings
Activities	Canoeing, team challenges, bowling, etc.	Teamwork
		Promote self-esteem and confidence
		Social interaction
		Fun
Transportation	Train	Confidence in use of public transport
Medication	Self-medicating	Facilitate responsibility for disease self-management and decisions regarding risks/ benefits of adherence
Therapy regimes	No formal therapy provided by staff	As above
Leisure	Unstructured leisure time	Facilitate interaction and structure own leisure time
	Daily challenge	Facilitate teamwork

Abbreviation: MDT, multidisciplinary team.
Source: Adapted from Ref. 26.

inclusive and makes young people feel listened to and valued with clear policies around collaborative learning and anti bullying will help to make all young people feel safe and supported.

The Role of Teachers

Peer support can mean many different thing to different people and there are many different ways that this can be facilitated both formally and informally. First, teachers play a valuable role in acting as a good role model

Table 2   Residential Trips

What young people say

I have felt isolated at times as I know nobody else with the same condition. When I met other people with arthritis, whilst on a recent trip to the Peak District, I found the whole experience uplifting. I had the opportunity to meet other people my age and talk freely about arthritis. It brought home to me that many other young people suffer the same pain and frustration. I made friends and found we have a lot in common. Following the trip, I plan to stay at one girl's house in the near future. I would definitely recommend other people with arthritis or similar conditions to take the opportunity of going on a trip of this nature. I would say everybody was able to benefit from the experience.

(Caroline, aged 14)

At first I was extremely nervous about going on the trip and the pre-meeting made me a bit more nervous. When we were on the train I made friends instantly. Kaz, Karan and I talked the whole journey. We talked about what medications we took and how we were affected. For the first time I heard people my age talking about something familiar, arthritis. The trip helped me a lot, talking how they overcame their pain, just being in their company was a comfort. I had never met any young people with arthritis and it was a great help to spend 4 days with people who had similar problems. It opened my eyes and showed me that I am quite lucky compared to some. Now I am happy with my arthritis and I have finally learned to cope with it. I am very grateful to the hospital and the team who gave me a great 4 days.

(Georgina, aged 14)

What one parent says

Writing as a parent, I thought the idea of a group of teenagers all suffering from arthritis going off to the Peak District to take part in outdoor activities sounded brilliant and so it proved to be with my daughter Georgina.

After a wretched year for her when she had been very low at times and almost reclusive, she arrived home from the "Get a Grip Trip" a different person! She had found the whole experience hugely beneficial and it had made her realise that she was not alone in how she felt. She had the opportunity to meet new friends, some of whom had the illness much more severely than herself, to discuss with them how she felt and what had happened to her. I think it was a huge relief and having had loads of fun and with a huge smile on her face. The trip has helped her to regain her confidence, which had been gradually ebbing away over the past few years. Moreover, she got on particularly well with Kaz, whose family were kind enough to have her to stay with them for a few days at the end of August. We are hoping that Kaz can come and stay with us soon; in any event we hope to see her in Birmingham at the beginning of January. We were very lucky to be offered this chance and I would encourage any teenager to go on the trip if the opportunity comes their way.

(Georgina's mother)

for young people. Those who are open, supportive, and seek the views of young people and encourage them to express their views sends a clear message to students that they are valued and it is acceptable to disclose any problems. Secondly, flexibility and creativity which fosters inclusivity of all young people (including those with special needs) in all activities (including physical exercise classes) sends a clear message to students to be inclusive and supportive. Finally teachers can also play a role in encouraging students to work cooperatively by considering environmental factors, for example, creative seating arrangements in a class setting as well as the use of partners in classes such as art, drama, and music.

Activity Clubs

Activity clubs can provide a "safe" space during the long lunch hour for those who find this period difficult. Groups are often organized around particular activities such as art or computers and offer opportunities to socialize or excel in a particular activity. Encouraging young people to attend before and after school clubs may also serve to facilitate peer relations. Alongside learning, leisure facilities and clubs may be available to the wider community outside regular school hours providing opportunities for young people to further develop social networks.

Peer Support Schemes

More formal schemes may be in operation in some schools, each with their own unique title however these broadly fall into the following categories.

Student Councils

This is a formal arena recognized by staff and pupils where young people are elected to represent the views of their peers on a wide range of topics. This creates an environment where young people feel valued and listened to and provides an opportunity to get items of concern on the school agenda. Standing for election for such a position also offers a valuable opportunity for young people to improve their self confidence and self esteem.

Peer Mentors

This type of scheme can be valuable in reducing social isolation for vulnerable young people. Training is often provided for mentors who can act as a positive role model and be-friend students and help them to fit in. This type of scheme can work extremely well when older students act as "buddies" to younger students who may be vulnerable during the transition from primary to secondary school, which may be a very stressful time.

Peer Mediators

This type of scheme focuses on young people resolving conflicts before they escalate further. Training is provided to mediators in order to help young people express their views, see both sides and come to an acceptable compromise, thus facilitating the maintenance of friendships.

Peer Counselors

Training is provided to students who volunteer to become counselors. At specified times a common room or classroom is staffed by counselors on a rota which enables students to drop in and discuss their difficulties in a confidential setting. This is often useful as young people may find it easier to discuss problems with their peers. Those with a chronic illness may be particularly suited to act as a counselor as they may be particularly empathetic and/or demonstrate superior communication skills.

Anti-Bullying Policies

All schools should have a robust anti-bullying policy with clear systems in place that are communicated to staff and students regarding to how bullying is dealt with. Often the main focus is to eliminate the climate of bullying and tackle bystander behavior. This involves not only intervention for the victim or bully but for all young people, who learn that bullying is not acceptable behavior.

The peer support of friends and school-initiated policies may also be a positive way of dealing with bullying. When mechanisms are available to students, they are more likely to discuss and tackle their problems at an early stage before they escalate. Talking to someone of a similar age who understands allows the young person to enlist support and help in dealing with the bully. Without peer support, the victim may eventually tell teachers, however this is usually happens much later in order to avoid being accused of 'tattle-telling' and usually the matter has become more serious and young people feel desperate. In view of the reported associated negative psychosocial and psychosomatic health problems (28), young people who are being bullied should be encouraged to seek help.

Role of Other School Personnel

Schools have a variety of staff who can play a significant role in pastoral care. Form teachers and heads-of-year can often do much to promote peer support. Many schools will also have a range of support staff including learning mentors who can provide support to vulnerable, disaffected, or underachieving young people. Although schools may be able to meet all the needs of young people, peer isolation may create difficulties in emotional well being, and they may therefore need to draw on the skills of outside agencies, such as educational psychologists who may be able to help schools set up specific interventions that meet the needs of the individual.

Role of Health Professionals

Hospitals also have role to play in facilitating peer relations, and, if at all possible, interventions should be avoided around the time of transfer from primary to secondary school. During this time friendships are quickly developed which makes coming into already established peer networks very difficult and can make the young person feel isolated and vulnerable.

ROLE OF PARENTS

Parents also have a role to play in reinforcing friendships including those developed at school. Encouraging young people to have friends over for tea or to "hang out", allowing them to use the telephone or helping them out with transport arrangements can help young people further cement their friendships particularly during school holidays.

MODERN TECHNOLOGIES AND PEER SUPPORT

The last decade has seen a significant increase in the use of technologies such as mobile phones and the internet by young people. Such technologies are now recognized as an integral part of the support network of adolescents with chronic disease (29) and will now be discussed further.

Mobile Phones

Mobile phones have become an integral part of adolescent culture for expressing identity and style. They are vital in most young people's social lives for arranging meetings with friends, chatting up a potential girlfriend/boyfriend, and also for getting information via the internet. Mobile phones also provide a sense of security for young people and their parents (30). In 2005, a U.K. study found that 97% of females and 92% of males aged 11–21 have access to a mobile phone (31) Texting was by far the most common form of communication with 9 out of the 10 young people texting daily and 54% texting more than five times a day. Males were more likely to talk to their friends on their phone than females. Texting is preferred for nearly all social activities and is regarded as being more private.

Since mobile phones play such an important part in young people's lives, the potential of text messaging in the hospital environment should be considered with respect to the development of peer relationships and support. Health professionals can once again be instrumental in helping to establish relationships between young people in gaining their permission to exchange phone numbers as well as encouraging them to bring their phones to group activities where opportunities may arise for the young people themselves to exchange numbers.

The "Sweet Talk" project (32) has demonstrated the usefulness of text messaging in improving adherence in a population of adolescents with diabetes. Similarly Pal (33) demonstrated its usefulness with an adult population of patients with arthritis, offering exciting opportunities for future developments in adolescent rheumatology.

The Internet

In this technological era young people thrive on using technology as a way to communicate with others. The use of email and instant messaging now allows young people to communicate with others quickly and easily at the touch of a button, despite living miles apart. This can be a useful tool for harnessing the skills of young people with arthritis who can act a positive role model and can offer support and advice to others, particularly when there are no similar others who live in the area or where young people have difficulty accessing transport to meet up with friends and peers. However it should be remembered that not all young people have access to the internet at home, but liaising with the school to gain permission for the young person to be able to access the internet during the school day, is one way to overcome this problem. In any discussion of internet use, professionals need to raise awareness of online personal safety particularly in chat rooms. Awareness of recognized sites specifically for young people with chronic illness and/or disability is useful in this regard, for example, www. ablelink.org (Toronto,Canada) and www.arthritiscare.org.uk/GetInvolved/ Discussionforum/Youngpeoplezone (United Kingdom).

Although letter writing may be viewed by many to be rather old-fashioned some young people will still consider it as a means of communicating with their peer group. Health professionals can once again play an important role in helping to establish links between such young people, finding those of similar age and interests to put in contact with one another if they so desire.

SUPPORT GROUPS

Support groups for young people with chronic rheumatic disease arthritis may be available in your area so it is worth exploring resources that may be able to offer social support. The United Kingdom alone has a number of organizations including Arthritis Care (www.arthritiscare.org.uk/ LivingwithArthritis/Youngpeople) which offers "positive future", workshops which are designed to enable teenagers to meet others with long term medical conditions, for support and fun. The Children's Chronic Arthritis Association (www.ccaa.org.uk) caters for young people up to the age of 16 and also offers residential trips for young people and their families, which allows them to meet others from all over the country and to participate in a wide range of challenging leisure activities. Many countries have similar support groups.

Table 3   Trigger Questions to Determine Levels of Peer Support
in Clinic Setting

Who are your best friends? What are they called? How old are they?
Tell me about your other friends?
What do you like to do with your friends out of school?
Have you ever stayed over at a friend's house?
Do you know any one else with your condition?
Who knows about your arthritis/SLE, etc.?
What do your friends think of you having this illness?

CONCLUSION

Peer support can enhance the lives of young people, facilitate resilience and act as a buffer against potential consequences of chronic illness. Whilst it should be recognized that not all young people will respond to all modalities of peer support health professionals need to be innovative in creating a variety of opportunities to meet similar others. Health professionals need to develop their communication skills to enable them to determine levels of peer support as this may have an impact on outcome (Table 3). This should be viewed as an integral and important aspect of assessment and steps should be taken to remedy social isolation and exclusion, rather than accept it as a fact of life. Such interventions are further enhanced by collaboration with other agencies such as youth services, school personnel and voluntary agencies. Since friends are so intrinsic to healthy adolescent development, psychosocial interventions addressing peer support should be acknowledged as a major component of holistic, multidisciplinary, adolescent rheumatology health care.

REFERENCES

1. Shaw KL, Southwood TR, McDonagh JE. Users' perspectives of transitional care for adolescents with juvenile idiopathic arthritis. Rheumatology 2004; 43: 770–8.
2. La Greca AM. Social consequences of pediatric conditions: fertile area for future investigation and intervention? J Pediatr Psychol 1990; 15:285–307.
3. Henderson C, Lovell D, Specker B, et al. Physical Activity in Children with Juvenille Rheumtoid Arthritis, quantification and evaluation. Arthritis Care Res 1995; 8(2):114–25.
4. Gianni M, Protas E. Aerobic capacity in juvenile rheumatoid arthritis patients and health children. Arthritis Care Res 1991; 4:131–5.
5. Miller M, Kress A, Berry C. Decreased physical function in JRA. Arthritis Care Res 1999; 12(5):309–13.
6. Stevens SE, Steele CA, Jutai JW, et al. Adolescents with physical disabilities: some psychosocial aspects of health. J Adolesc Health 1996; 19:157–64.

7. Ennet S, Devellis B, Earp J, et al. Disease experience and psychosocial adjustment in children with juvenile rheumatoid arthritis; children versus mothers reports. J Pediatr Psychol 1991; 16(5):305–10.
8. Blum R, Resnick M, Nelson R, et al. Family and peer issues among adolescents with spina bifida and cerebral palsy. Pediatrics 1991; 88:280–5.
9. Wolman C, Resnick MD, Harris LJ, et al. Emotional well-being among adolescents with and without chronic conditions. J Adolesc Health 1994; 15: 199–204.
10. Kyngas H, Hentiness M, Barlow J. Adolescents perceptions of physicians, nurses, parents and friends: help or hindrance in compliance with diabetes self care? J Adv Nurs 1998; 27:760–9.
11. Barlow JH, Shaw KL, Harrison K. Consulting the 'experts': children's and parents' perceptions of psycho-educational interventions in the context of juvenile chronic arthritis. Health Educ Res 1999; 14:597–610.
12. Schanberg L, Sandstrom M, Starr K, et al. The relationship between mood and stressful events to symptoms in juvenile rheumatic disease. Arthritis Care Res 2000; 13(7):33–41.
13. Seiving RE, Perry CL, Williams CL. Do friendships change behaviors, or do behaviors change friendships? Examining paths of influence in young adolescents' alcohol use. J Adolesc Health 2000; 26:27–35.
14. McDonagh JE, Southwood TR, Ryder CAJ. Bridging the Gap in Rheumatology: Ann Rheum Dis 2000; 59:575–84.
15. Burroughs TE, Harris MA, Pontious SL, et al. Research on social support in adolescents with IDDM: a critical review. Diabetes Educ 1997; 438–48.
16. Varni JW, Babani L, Wallander JL, et al. Social support and self-esteem effects on psychological adjustment in children and adolescents with insulin-dependent diabetes mellitus. Child Fam Behav Ther 1989; 11:1–17.
17. La Greca AM, Bearman KJ, Moore H. Peer relations of youth with pediatric conditions and health risks: promoting social support and healthy lifestyles. Dev Behav Pediatr 2002; 23:271–80.
18. Guite JW, Walker LS, Smith CA, Garber J. Children's perceptions of peers with somatic symptoms: the impact of gender, stress and illness. J Pediatr Psychol 2000; 25:125–35.
19. Bell SK, Morgan SB. Children's attitudes and behavioural intentions toward a peer presented as obese: dies a medical explanation for the obesity make a difference? J Pediatr Psychol 2000; 25:137–45.
20. Sherman BF, Bonanno GA, Wiener LS, Battles HB. When children tell their friends they have AIDS: possible consequences for psychological well-being and disease progression. Psychosom Med 2000; 62:238–47.
21. Olsson CA, Toumbourou JW, Bowes G. Chronic Illness Peer Support (ChIPS). Aust Fam Physician 1997; 26:500–1.
22. Clark HB, Ichinose CK, Meseck-Bushey S, et al. Peer support group for adolescents with chronic illness. Child Health Care 1992; 21:233–8.
23. Stefl ME, Shear ES, Levinson JE. Summer camps for juveniles with rheumatic disease: do they make a difference? Arthritis Care Res 1989; 9:35–41.
24. Page CJ, Pearson J. Creating therapeutic camp and recreation programs for children with chronic illness and disabilities. Pediatrician 1990; 17:297–307.

25. Milliet J, Carman D, Browne R. Summer Camp: Effects on function of children with autoimmune diseases. Arthritis Care Res 1996; 9(4):309–14.

26. Hackett J, Johnson B, Shaw K, et al. Friends United: An evaluation of an innovative residential self-management programme in adolescent rheumatology. Br J Occupat Ther 2005; 68(12):567–73.

27. Ostensen M, Almberg K, Koksvik HS. Sex, reproduction and gynecological disease in young adults with a history of juvenile chronic arthritis. J Rheumatol 2000; 27:1783–7.

28. Fekkes M, Pijpers FI, Frediks AM, Vogels T, Verloove-Vanhorick SP. Do bullied children get ill or do ill children get bullied? A proscpective cohort study on the relationship between bullying and health related symptoms. Pediatrics 2006; 117:1568–74.

29. Kyngas H. Support network of adolescents with chronic disease: adolescents' perspective. Nurs Health Sci 2004; 6:287–93.

30. Australian Psychology Society. Psychosocial aspects of mobile phone use amongst adolescents. Nov (2004) (www.psychology.org.au/news/mobilephoneresearchreport.pdf, last accessed 2 October 2006).

31. Haste H. Joined-Up texting: The role of mobile phones in young people's lives Nestle Social Research Programme (2005), report no. 3, 1–19 (http://www.spreckley.co.uk/nestle/NSRP-4-TEXTING.pdf, last accessed 2 October 2006).

32. Franklin V, Walker A, Pagliari C, et al. "Sweet Talk": text messaging support for intensive insulin therapy for young people with diabetes. Diabetes Technol Ther 2003; 5:991–6.

33. Pal B. The doctor will text you now: is there a role for the mobile telephone in health care? Br Med J 2003; 326:607.

16

Growing Up: Transition from Adolescence to Adulthood

Patience H. White

Departments of Medicine and Pediatrics, The George Washington University School of Medicine and Health Sciences, and Arthritis Foundation, Washington, D.C., U.S.A.

INTRODUCTION

Today over 90% of all young people with special health care needs (SHCN), a group that includes youth with chronic illnesses, such as rheumatic diseases and asthma, survive into adulthood. This is exemplified by the improved long-term survival of young people with rheumatic diseases. The focus of outcome is now on the quality of their lives and not just their survival. There are three critical junctures for young people with SHCN: diagnosis, puberty, and school completion. Perhaps the most challenging of these is the transition to adulthood, a period of complex biological, social, and emotional change. This transition involves learning to move from (*i*) school to work, (*ii*) home to community, and (*iii*) pediatric- to adult-oriented health care. This chapter focuses on the steps involved for the young person with rheumatic disease as he or she moves into adulthood and the how a health care professional can help the successful transition of an individual with rheumatic disease from adolescence to adulthood.

From the perspective of a young person include, the goals of transition include: (*i*) being valued as a human being and treated with dignity; (*ii*) having opportunities for social experiences, dating, community involvement, recreation, and worship; (*iii*) obtaining education and/or job training; (*iv*) becoming interdependent, and (*v*) finding meaningful work for reasonable pay. To attain these goals, young people with rheumatic diseases will have to, first and foremost, attend to their health, including careful management of their condition and attention to preventive care issues. Health care professionals often pay more attention to the chronic illness than to assisting the young person with the skills they need to manage their illness. Studies in the United Kingdom have shown that young people want health care providers to acknowledge their lives beyond their disease and to assist them in preparing for transition (1,2). This chapter will explore the general principles of transition and then discuss the major areas of self-determination, school to work and post-secondary education, and pediatric to adult health care.

GENERAL PRINCIPLES OF TRANSITION

Transition is defined as "the purposeful, planned movement of adolescents and young adults with chronic illness/disability from child-centered to adult-oriented systems" (3). Successful transition planning is the result of partnerships among the individual, his or her family, school personnel, the health care system, local community and adult service organization representatives, and interested others. The goal is to maximize lifelong functioning, social participation, and human potential. Several general principles of successful transition are summarized below:

1. Transition is a process, not an event. Planning should begin as early as possible on a flexible schedule that recognizes the young person's increasing autonomy and capacity for making choices. Transition to adult services should occur prospectively rather than during a crisis and when the young person's rheumatic disease is under good control.
2. The transition process should begin at diagnosis and include long term sequential planning toward goals of independence and self management.
3. Coordination between health care, educational, vocational, and social service systems is essential. It is particularly important to recognize the complex interplay between health and social outcomes as young people age into employment and, in the United States, into an employment-based health insurance system.
4. As the role of the young person changes in transitioning to adult systems, the families' and the health care professionals' roles also should change. Pediatricians, other health care professionals, and the family should appreciate the young person's change in status as they move from adolescence to adulthood.
5. Self-determination skills should be fostered throughout the transition process. Practice standards for transition services call for a young person–centered and asset-oriented approach that involves young people as decision makers for the entire transition process (3). The key elements of transitional care have been highlighted by policy statements in the United States, Canada, and the United Kingdom (4–10) and are summarized in Table 1.

Table 1 Key Elements of Transition

- An orientation that is future focused, proactive and flexible
- An early start
- An approach that fosters personal and medical interdependence and creative problem solving
- A written transition policy agreed upon by all members of the multidisciplinary team and target adult services, posted for families and young people to see
- A key worker identified to attend to the transition needs of the young person
- Liaison personnel in both the pediatric and adult health-care teams
- A flexible policy on the timing of events, with the anticipation of change
- A preparation period for youth and parent
- An educational program for young people and their families which addresses medical, psychosocial, and educational/vocational aspects of care
- A written individualized health-care transition plan by age 14, created with the young person and his/her family and updated as needed
- Identified network of relevant community agencies, adult primary and subspecialty care providers
- A portable, continuously updated, medical summary
- Training program for pediatric and adult providers on transition and adolescent issues
- Provision of appropriate primary preventive care
- Affordable continuous health insurance coverage

SELF-DETERMINATION

Self-Determination Through Childhood and Adolescence

Self-determination is a combination of attitudes and abilities that lead people to set goals for themselves, and to take the initiative to reach these goals (11). The capabilities needed to become self-determined are learned through real-world experience (including mistakes) and an open, supportive acknowledgement of their chronic illness/disability (12). Too often families, teachers, and other well-intentioned people protect young people with SHCN from making mistakes and avoid discussing the ramifications of their illness/disability. This approach can set the child up for failure or can result in "learned helplessness." Teachers and those providing assistance to families can and should begin preparing children with rheumatic disease for independence as early as possible. For example, young children between three and five years of age can begin to incorporate chores into their daily routine. Families that give children opportunities to demonstrate competence through developmentally appropriate household chores send a clear message of support, capability, and that they are being treated like everyone else, without a chronic illness/disability. In a classic longitudinal study of at-risk children, Werner found that involvement in household chores promoted resilience and positive social outcomes in adulthood (13). Subsequent studies have documented the important role of family dynamics and parental expectations on social outcomes (14). By the developmental age of 6 to 11 years, children should begin assuming responsibility for their self-care. For example, school-aged children with juvenile idiopathic arthritis (JIA) should be ready to plan and ask their physician some questions about their arthritis and their health. Self-determination skills should be used to help identify and meet self-care goals by early adolescence. During mid-adolescence, self-determination skills can be focused on identifying and meeting educational and vocational goals (15,16). In late adolescence, these skills can then be used to identify and meet goals related to independent living.

Tools for Shared Management in Clinical Practice

To help families and health care providers understand the new roles they will assume as the young person matures, several tools such as the shared management model tool (see Table 4, Chapter 4) described in detail by Kieckhefer and Trahms (17), or check lists, examples of which can be found on the websites listed in Table 2. Each family member, the health care team, and the young person can assess their level of involvement in the transition process using the shared management tool, and the results can be used to discuss how to move to the next stage. Discussing everyone's expectations as the young person moves into self-management of their illness can be a clarifying experience and give everyone a good idea as to their ultimate role in the process. For example, discussing the family's ultimate goal of

Table 2   Examples of Web-Based Resources for Transition

United States and Canada
   http://www.htrw.org
   http://www.door2adulthood.com
   http://hctransitions.ichp.edu
   http://depts.washington.edu/healthtr/index.html
   http://chfs.ky.gov/ccshcn/ccshcntransition.htm
   http://www.communityinclusion.org/transition/

United Kingdom
   http://www.transitioninfonetwork.org.uk
   http://www.dh.gov.uk/transition
   http://www.dreamteam-uk.org
   http://www.transitionpathway.co.uk
   http://www.youngminds.org.uk/publications/booklets/adulthood.php
   http://www.tsa.uk.com

Australia
   http://www.rch.org.au/transition

becoming consultants in their son or daughter's medical care, which means answering only when asked during clinic sessions, can be a helpful experience for families.

SCHOOL TO POST–SECONDARY EDUCATION AND WORK

School

Graduation from school is associated with the greatest social disruption. The end of formal education, the end of the structured schedule provided by school attendance, and the rising expectation for work and independent living place increasing stress on the young person at this time. Increasing levels of education predict better a chance of labor force participation and higher level of income (18). Thus, making post-secondary education a key goal for the young person with rheumatic disease is important to his or her future success in the marketplace. Yet people with physical disabilities and other health impairments have lower graduation rates than those without impairments. Scal et al. found that graduation rates in the United States declined based on severity of condition: among the general population of adults aged 18 to 30 years old, 82.6% graduated from high school, and, for those even with mild disabilities, the graduation rate fell to 79.5% (19). Awareness of laws that that outline important educational practices in secondary school can foster successful adult outcomes for students with special health care needs. In the United States, these include the Individuals with Disabilities Education Act (IDEA), the School to Work Opportunities Act, and the Workforce Investment Act.

Higher and Further Education

Similar findings are seen in the percentage of young persons with SHCN that attain higher education (19). While nearly 85% of all young people in the United States will pursue some form of higher education, those with orthopedic and other health impairments go on to any post-secondary school at the rate of 46.3% and 56%, respectively (19). Key to making the post-secondary education experience successful is referring the young person to a disability support service (or the equivalent) in college. Most colleges and universities in the United States and the United Kingdom have either a Disability Support Services (DSS) office or some other office or individual designated to assist students with disabilities. To receive assistance or request accommodations for disability-related needs, a student must take the lead by disclosing his or her disability, providing documentation of the disability, and identifying needed accommodations. Documentation of the disability must support the requested accommodations. Examples of accommodations for young people with rheumatic disease that can be requested of DSS include allowing extra time to get to class when the young person is on a big campus or having an elevator available for dormitory rooms on higher floors. The DSS office should be able to assist a student with disclosing the disability to instructors; requesting accommodations; identifying support services and assistive technology; and addressing other disability-related needs presented by the student. There is a great deal of variability among schools as to the steps undertaken on behalf of the student with the disability as well as to the types of accommodations provided.

Role of Vocational Rehabilitation Agencies

Linking schools with systems of care that serve adults with chronic illnesses/ disabilities, including vocational rehabilitation (VR) agencies, strengthens the transition process. Knowing the laws that support adults with chronic illnesses, such as The School-to-Work Opportunities Act of 1994 in the United States that provide workplace mentoring and skill certificates for youth with SHCN, can improve the outcome for the young person in the workplace and, ultimately their independence. The Workforce Improvement Act of 1998 links education, employment, and training services to a network of resources in local areas called One-Stop Career Centers (20). Similarly, transition planning mandated under IDEA 2004 stipulates that vocation/ rehabilitation counselors must participate in transition planning if needed before the student exits the school system. Parents and students can request participation as early as age 14 through One-Stop Career Centers (21) or the schools. In the United Kingdom, a similar transition plan is required at age 14 under the Statement of Special Educational Needs implemented by the local educational authority (22). This helps to provide a seamless transition from school to adult service provision. Vocational agencies can provide or arrange for a host of training, educational, medical, and other services individualized to the needs of the person. VR services are intended to help individuals acquire and maintain gainful employment. A VR counselor works with young adults to assess their disability and help him or her develop an individualized plan for employment. This plan will identify an employment goal and the means for achieving it, often including some form of post-secondary education or training. Although VR counselors can provide direct services to the young adult, they more often refer the individual to appropriate community-based agencies for self-advocacy training, development of employment-readiness skills, adaptive driving evaluation and instruction, and job coaching.

Success in the job market and the world of work are critical to successful long-term employment for youths with rheumatic disease. Previous work experience is a prerequisite for many jobs. Unfortunately, most young people with SHCN enter the workforce later than their nondisabled peers. Work activity of a nationally representative sample of nondisabled U.S. high school students who were interviewed between 1997 and 2003 revealed that 41% of high school freshman and 85% of high school seniors had regular jobs either during the school year or during summer months (23). Keeping young people with rheumatic disease on the same developmental milestone trajectory for employment as those without disabilities is essential to their long term independence and well being. The implications of limited early job experience on work-force readiness, long-term employment, economic status, and social functioning in adulthood are profound. In 2004, employment rates for the 14 million U.S. adults with a disability (7.9% of adults aged 18–64 years) were substantially lower than for the nondisabled population (19% vs. 77%). The correlate to this is a poverty rate for adults who have a disability that is substantially higher than that of the nondisabled population (28% vs. 9.2%) (24).

Limited provision of careers counseling in U.K. pediatric rheumatology services has been reported (25) despite evidence that young people themselves want such support (1,26,27). A lack of awareness of such aspects by health care professionals may also be at play (28). A national survey of occupational therapists (OTs) has reported that although OTs felt it was important and appropriate to address the vocational issues of adolescents with a chronic illness, they reported limited perceived knowledge, confidence, and significant unmet training needs (29).

HOME TO INDEPENDENCE

Legalities of Adulthood

In most countries there is an age when young people become legal adults. In the United States the natural guardianship of parents ends when children reach age 18. When the young person reaches 18 years of age, parents no longer have the legal right to make decisions and sign consent forms for their child or to see their child's medical record, unless the young person is in agreement. The health care professional must address this directly with the young person. In cases where the intellectual capacity of the young person is such that a legal guardian needs to be appointed, the parents submit an application for guardianship through the court system. In the United States, two pre-requisites should exist before a court appoints a guardian: (*i*) young people must be incompetent in at least one important area of their lives, such as health care decisions or financial matters; and (*ii*) there must be a present need for the guardianship.

Financial Implications

In addition, it is important to address several key financial issues prior to age 18 to avoid loss of income and/or services, to protect family assets, and to assure that young people with SHCN have suitable independent living options as they move from home to the community. Financial barriers are the most common reason young people with SHCN fail to transition to independent living in the community (30).

Social Security Support

If working is not an option to attain financial independence, the health care professional should guide the young person with rheumatic disease to look into social security supports. In the United States, it is called Supplemental Security Income (SSI), and it is a monthly payment for individuals with disabilities. To qualify for SSI, individuals must meet both disability and financial eligibility requirements. SSI eligibility is re-determined using adult criteria when adolescents turn 18 years old. Young people with rheumatic disease may lose their SSI at this time because individual rather than household income is used to determine income eligibility or because they do not meet the adult disability criteria. Generally speaking, adults in the United States who receive SSI cannot have assets greater than $1,500 and still remain eligible.

PEDIATRIC TO ADULT HEALTH CARE

Holistic View of Health

As a result of advances in medical technology and dramatic improvements in the delivery of acute health care, the vast majority of children with rheumatic diseases can now expect to survive to adulthood. As life expectancy for persons with rheumatic disease approaches that of the general population, socio-economic factors are increasingly being recognized as important determinants of health (31), and quality-of-life and social integration as meaningful health outcomes (32,33). The International Classification of Functioning, Disability, and Health (ICF), introduced by the World Health Organization in 2001, provides a framework for understanding the impact of the social and physical environment on health (34). Unlike mortality statistics, this framework looks at how people live with their disability. The ICF assesses health not solely in terms of body functioning and structure (i.e., impairment) but also in terms of activities, social participation, and the physical environment. Understanding the health of a person "in his/her own world" can help to identify a variety of strategies for improving health. For example, setting up ramps to make community swimming pools accessible is an effective way to "treat" the attitudinal and physical barriers that contribute to obesity in young people with rheumatic disease.

Health Transition

Ideally, health care transition should be "family-centered, continuous, comprehensive, coordinated, compassionate, and culturally competent and developmentally appropriate as it is technologically sophisticated" (4). Access to quality health care continues to be a major issue for all young people as well as those with rheumatic disease. In the United States, a national survey of adolescents with chronic illness and severe disability conducted between 1997 and 2002 established that nearly 35% of young adults had unmet health care needs due to costs, that 19% had unmet needs due to accessibility, that one in six had no usual source of care, and that nearly one in four young adults between ages 18 and 24 years were uninsured (32). In many countries but particular to the United States, funding for health care is often lacking during the critical years when transition from pediatric-oriented care to adult-oriented care should occur (35). Similarly, the quality of transitional care is also an issue (1,36,37). A major obstacle with transition to adult-oriented care is that young people have "nowhere to go" (38). In a study of the determinants of adolescent satisfaction with a transitional care program, provider characteristics were significantly more important that the physical environment and process issues (36). Low patient satisfaction with adult providers has been reported in terms of their availability, thoroughness, respect, and knowledge base (39). Adolescents also complain about the lack of privacy and of not being asked for their opinions about their own health care in pediatric practices (40).

Different Cultures of Care

What is particularly confusing to families and young people with chronic illnesses are the two contrasting cultures and systems of health care: the pediatric and adult health care systems (3). As in many aspects of the young person's life, there are times the young person wants to be treated like a child and other times when he/she wants to be treated like an adult. Thus the young person is faced with two different approaches to health care and needs guidance to navigate the two conflicting systems (41–43). Table 3 outlines some of the major differences between the two systems. The different possibilities and timing for moving to the adult-oriented systems must be discussed with the young person and family so the young person can be an integral part to the process. Adult-oriented systems focus on the individual with the rheumatic disease and are rarely structured to provide multidisciplinary care (3). The demands of treating young adults with chronic illnesses may outweigh the benefits in the eyes of some adult health care providers, especially if young adults with rheumatic disease are not prepared by the pediatric system to be their own health advocates, are nonadherent, and/or confused and demanding. In addition, systems of care (availability of case managers, social workers and mental health services) and financial reimbursement practices have not caught up with the numbers of young adults with chronic illnesses. In contrast, pediatric providers focus on the family, and many are

Table 3 Comparison of Pediatric to Adult Health Care Systems

	Pediatric	Adult
Age-related	Growth and development, future focused	Maintenance/decline: optimize the present
Focus	Family	Individual
Approach	Paternalistic, proactive	Collaborative, reactive
Shared decision making	With parent	With patient
Services	Entitlement	Qualify/eligibility
Nonadherence	>Assistance	>Tolerance
Procedural pain	Lower threshold of active input	Higher threshold for active input
Tolerance of immaturity	Higher	Lower
Coordination with federal systems	Greater interface with education	Greater interface with employment
Care provision	Interdisciplinary	Multidisciplinary
Number of patients	Fewer	Greater

inadequately mobilized to "let go" of their adolescent patients with SHCN (38). The U.S. National Survey of Children with Special Health Care Needs, conducted in 2000–2001 among 4332 households of adolescents aged 14 to 17 years, found that only one out of two pediatric health care providers had discussed transition issues with families, and only one out of six had discussed and developed a plan for addressing those needs (44). Similar results have been reported in Australia (45) and the United Kingdom (46).

Professional Training for Transition

To exacerbate the lack of transition readiness in providers, both pediatricians and adult providers feel unprepared for their roles in this transition process. A study of general pediatric practices in the Northeastern part of the United States showed that general pediatric practices were not ready for their patients to transfer. For example, most had not decided on transition policies for their practice or, if they had, did not post them. They had few office processes that supported transition and wanted help to become more competent (46). McDonagh et al. showed that rheumatology health care providers (pediatric and adult) would welcome more training in adolescent and transition issues (47). Table 4 presents a check list based on the U.S. Consensus Statement for pediatric practices to see how their practice measures up on transition processes developed for the Bureau of

Table 4 Checklist for Transition: Core Knowledge and Skills for Pediatric Practices

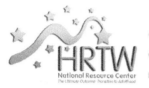

CHECKLIST FOR TRANSITION:

CORE KNOWLEDGE & SKILLS:

FOR PEDIATRIC PRACTICES

This checklist addresses one of the critical first steps to ensuring successful transitioning to adult-oriented health care: the need for core knowledge and skills required to provide developmentally appropriate health-care transition services to young people with special health-care needs.

The HRTW National Resource Center believes these skills apply to all youth with and without a diagnosis.

Core knowledge and skills checklist for practices policy   **Yes**   **No**

1. Dedicated staff position coordinates transition activities

2. Office forms are developed to support transition processes

3. CPT coding is used to maximize reimbursement for transition services

4. Legal health-care decision making is discussed prior to youth turning 18

5. Prior to age 18, youth sign assent forms for treatments, whenever possible

6. Transition policy states age youth should no longer see a pediatrician is posted

Medical home

1. Practice provides care coordination for youth with complex conditions

2. Practice creates an individualized health transition plan before age 14

3. Practice refers youth to specific family or internal medicine physicians

4. Practice provides support and confers with adult providers post-transfer

5. Practice actively recruits adult primary care/specialty providers for referral

(Continued)

Table 4 Checklist for Transition: Core Knowledge and Skills for Pediatric
Practices (*Continued*)

Family/youth involvement	Yes	No
1. Practice discusses transition after diagnosis, and planning with families/youth begins before age 14		
2. Practice provides educational packet or handouts on transition		
3. Youths participate in shared care management and self-care (calling for apppointments/Rx refills)		
4. Practice assists families/youth to develop an emergency plan (health crisis and weather or other environmental disasters)		
5. Practice assists youth/family in creating a portable medical summary		
6. Practice assists with planning for school and/or work accommodations		
7. Practice assists with medical documentation for program eligibility (SSI, VR, college)		
8. Practice refers family/youth to resources that support skill-building: mentoring, camps, recreation, activities of daily living, volunteer/ paid work experiences		

Health-care insurance

1. Practice is knowledgeable about state-mandated and other insurance benefits for youth after age 18		
2. Practice provides medical documentation when needed to maintain benefits		

Screening

1. Exams include routine screening for risk-taking and prevention of secondary disabilities		
2. Practice teaches youth lifelong preventive care, how to identify health baseline and report problems early; youth know wellness routines, diet/exercise, etc.		

Notes: The HRTW National Resource Center is headquartered at the Maine State Title V
CSHN Program and is funded through a cooperative agreement (U39MC06899-01-00) from the
Integrated Services Branch, Division of Services for Children with Special Health Needs
(DSCSHN) in the Federal Maternal and Child Health Bureau (MCHB), Health Resources and
Services Administration (HRSA), Department of Health and Human Services (DHHS).
Activities are coordinated through the Center for Self-Determination, Health and Policy at the
Maine Support Network. The Center enjoys working partnerships with the Shriners Hospitals
for Children and the KY Commission for CSHCN.

The opinions expressed herein do not necessarily reflect the policy or position nor imply
official endorsement of the funding agency or working partnership.

Maternal and Child Health Healthy and Ready to Work National Center. Health-care providers in the adult-care system have had little or no training in adolescent developmental issues or in diseases that, until recently, did not present to adult physicians. An American survey of 3066 physicians and other health care professionals showed major deficits in their knowledge of and skills in adolescent health care, including care for young with SHCN (48). Similar results have been reported in a more recent survey of the staff a large U.K. children's hospital providing tertiary care, where over a third of the patients at any one time are adolescents (49). Training is further discussed in Chapter 17.

TRANSITION MODELS—PROCESS AND PLANNING

Models of Transition

Models for improving transition care have been described for condition-specific diagnoses (50) within professional disciplines (3,51), for primary care settings (52) and non-disease-specific, non-medical programs (53). Only a few studies have been conducted to examine the effectiveness of various health care transition models on health status and health-related outcomes (54). Recently McDonagh demonstrated improved health-related quality-of-life, disease knowledge, satisfaction, and vocational readiness for adolescents with JIA (55) who participated in a subspecialty evidence-based transition program (51) in the United Kingdom. Wolf Branigin et al. showed increased quality-of-life and improved health and well-being for youth with all types of disabilities who participated in a career-readiness transition program (53). More studies are needed to demonstrate who needs what kind of transition program. Much of what is currently known about transition care is largely based upon descriptive summaries of models (56,57), qualitative studies with young people and families (58), and the expert opinion of health care professionals, such as the study by Rettig et al. for young people with rheumatic disease (59).

Key Components of Transitional Care Programs

Two important factors appear to influence the process and outcome of health care transition: cognitive ability and whether a disability is progressive. Young people and families tend to view transition as a developmental process composed of three stages: (*i*) "envisioning a future," which begins at diagnosis; (*ii*) "age of responsibility," during which children are taught and expected to carry out tasks of daily living and medical self-care; and (*iii*) "age of transition," which is associated with the same expectations and timeframes for independence as in the general population (38). The quality of parent-provider interactions correlates with the extent to which transition services are addressed by pediatric providers (44).

In the United States, a professional consensus statement between the pediatric and adult physician professional organizations was put forth in 2002 that delineated several first steps to ensuring successful transitioning to adult oriented health care for young people with special health care needs (4). These recommendations are incorporated into Table 1 and include:

1. Identifying a health care professional who acts as a transition coordinator in partnership with the young person/family
2. Educating health care professionals to provide developmentally appropriate transition services
3. Preparing and maintaining an up-to-date medical summary that is portable and accessible
4. Creating a written health care transition by age 14 together with the young person/family
5. Applying same guidelines for primary and preventive care;
6. Ensuring affordable, continuous health insurance coverage that includes compensation for transition planning and care coordination

Transition Planning

In line with the agreement on first steps, the transition process in health care should begin early and be developed in earnest with a transition plan by the age of 14. A study of young people with SHCN showed that after age 13–14 the gap between youth with disabilities and those without disabilities widened, and a transition program intervention was most successful if started by ages 11 to 14 years (51,53,55). The transition process should be a collaborative one between health care professionals, the young person, and the parents. The components of health care plan needed by the person with rheumatic disease should be identified, such as which professionals (e.g., occupational therapist, physical therapist) are needed to provide the necessary care and who the care manager will be.

Skills Training for Young People

In addition, health-related skills (e.g., learning to give their own injections) need to be identified so that the individual can manage his or her rheumatic disease once they have left home. Collaboration with other providers and across systems of care (including school and community-based service agencies) is the ideal during this complex time of physical and psychosocial change. The transition plan should involve not only the transfer of medical information from pediatric to adult providers but also the transition of responsibility for health-related issues from the parent to the individual with rheumatic disease. Adolescents are notorious for being nonadherent to the recommendations of health care providers and other authority figures. Young people with rheumatic disease can go "on strike" at this time and "rebel" by neglecting their self-care. To be ready to move to the adult system, the adolescent needs to be responsible for taking medications, to develop the ability to understand and discuss his or her disability, and to use required adaptive equipment or appliances. During this process, health care professionals should consider when to start seeing the individual alone and when to develop a confidential relationship with him or her. For many adolescents this is appropriately at age 12 to 13 years. Meeting independently with the provider sends a clear message to young people that their autonomy is respected and that active participation in their health care is expected. Studies have shown that adherence to medical recommendations improves when adolescents contribute to health care decisions, monitor their own care, and make their own appointments (60). Seeing health professionals independently of parents has also been reported to be associated with adherence to the first appointment in adult care (61). Providers can improve adherence by simplifying their recommendations and by being consistent, both in terms of availability and, if there are multiple providers, by coordinating appointments and recommendations. For further discussion re adherence, see Chapter 5.

Health- and Disease-Related Knowledge

As adolescents transition to adult-oriented care, it is also essential that they understand both their past medical history and current health care needs. It has been demonstrated that many young people with JIA score poorly on arthritis related knowledge (62), even long-term clinic attendees (63). Effective transitional care has shown to improve such knowledge (55). Thus, assisting the young person to be able to communicate their health care disease and needs is essential. Creating a health summary is one way that adolescents can prepare themselves for the transition to adult-oriented care (e.g., "My Health Passport" at www.sickkids.on.ca/myhealthpassport/). Numerous templates and tools such as youth health autonomy check lists are available to help youths and providers develop written health care transition plans and portable medical summaries and templates for medical visits. Examples of these can be found on the websites listed in Table 2.

As mentioned in Chapter 4, health care providers need to use age-appropriate preventive care approaches and be mindful of the risk-taking activities and the growing sexuality of the young person with rheumatic disease. In addition, young people with chronic illnesses may be at increased risk for developing mental health problems. Underdiagnosis of treatable psychiatric conditions such as anxiety and depression can be a common occurrence. It is important to question adolescents and their families about any physical symptoms of anxiety and depression, such as altered sleep and appetite. Excessive school absence is also a red flag.

Health Insurance

The final point on the U.S. joint pediatric and adult consensus statement was to ensure health insurance for all young people with SHCN. The health care provider should encourage the young person with rheumatic disease and his/her family to review, understand, and plan for the young person's future health insurance options. This is a particular problem for the United States and in a recent study the majority of young adults with disabilities reported gaps in insurance coverage, and many were uninsured for a substantial portion of the three-year study (64). Health insurance options in the United States center on public and private insurance options.

Data from the U.S. Census Bureau indicate that people with disabilities are more likely to have public health insurance and less likely to have private coverage than people who do not have disabilities. Among adults with disabilities aged 22 to 44 years, 22% have public insurance, almost 20% are uninsured, and 58% are privately insured. In contrast, in the same age group of nondisabled adults, 3% have public insurance, 17% are uninsured, and 80% are privately insured (65). There are a few ways in which young people with special health care needs can qualify for Medicaid when they transition to adulthood. As noted previously, young people who maintain SSI benefits on redetermination automatically qualify for Medicaid in most states. Second, some individuals who do not meet adult SSI eligibility criteria can continue to receive Medicaid as long as they are enrolled in an approved vocational rehabilitation program. Finally, some individuals who did not qualify for SSI as children due to family income may become income-eligible to receive SSI and Medicaid as an adult, single head-of-household. Young people with SHCN who are privately insured under family plans automatically lose coverage at age 19 years unless families pursue one of two available options to continue benefits. The most common option for maintaining coverage under a family insurance plan is to qualify for student status, which typically requires young people who attend college to maintain full-time schedules. Student coverage under most family plans is not available beyond ages 22 to 24 years. A second and usually not needed option for young people with rheumatic disease is that they be declared "dependent for life." This qualifies them for continued coverage as long as they have no gainful employment and meet annual recertification procedures for disability and dependent status. Young people who obtain private health insurance independently (young adult pays premium) have a variety of options, depending upon their particular circumstance: college student plans, group employments plans, Consolidated Omnibus Budget Reconciliation Act coverage if temporarily unemployed, Ticket-to-Work, and self-payment (66). The Health Insurance Portability and Accountability Act of 1996 helps to assure full coverage under private insurance plans by permitting young people with disabilities to purchase individual coverage when group coverage is terminated, regardless of pre-existing conditions (65).

CONCLUSION

Young people with rheumatic disease should expect to become happy and effective participants in the adult world. Their health care provider should provide them with opportunities to learn about their strengths, abilities, skills, needs, and interests as well as allow them to take certain risks and to learn from failure. They need to assume responsibility for themselves and to understand the difference between the protected world of school, pediatric health care, and home and the world of work, adult health care, and adult life. Most of all, they must believe they are capable of success. These goals can be accomplished by comprehensive young-person-centered transition planning, understanding the resources available to them, and their health care providers. Together, the transition process will become easier and a successful experience for all.

REFERENCES

1. Shaw KL, South wood TR, McDonagh JE. "User's perspectives of Transitional care for adolescents with Juvenile Idiopathic arthritis. Rheumatology 2004; 43: 770–8.
2. Shaw KL, Southwood TR, McDonagh JE. Transitional Care for Adolescents with Juvenile Idiopathic Arthritis: results of a Delphi Study. Rheumatology 2004; 43:1000–6.
3. Rosen DS, Blum RW, Britto M, Sawyer SM, Siegel DM, Society for Adolescent Medicine. Transition to adult health-care for adolescents and young adults with chronic conditions: position paper of the Society for Adolescent Medicine. J Adolesc Health 2003; 33(4):309–11.
4. American Academy of Pediatrics, American Academy of Family Physicians, & American College of Physicians-American Society of Internal Medicine. A consensus statement on health-care transitions for young adults with special health-care needs. Pediatrics 2002; 110(6 Pt 2):1304–6.
5. Canadian Paediatric Society. Care of adolescents with chronic conditions. Paediatr Child Health 2006; 11(1):43–8 (http://www.cps.ca/english/publications/AdolesHealth.htm).
6. Department of Health. Getting the right start: National Service Framework for Children. Standard for Hospital Services. 2003 (www.dh.gov.uk)
7. Department of Health. National Service Framework for Children, Young People and Maternity Services (Core Standard 4). 2004 http://www.dh.gov.uk
8. Department of Health. Transition: getting it right for young people. Improving the transition of young people with long-term conditions from children's to adult health services. Department of Health Publications, 2006, London www.dh.gov.uk/transition

9.   Royal College of Nursing. Adolescent transition care: guidance for nursing staff. 2004 London (www.rcn.org.uk)

10. Royal College of Paediatrics and Child Health. Bridging the Gap: Health-care for Adolescents. 2003 (http;//www.rcpch.ac.uk)

11. Ryan RM, Deci EL. Self-determination theory and the facilitation of intrinsic motivation, social development, and well-being. Am Psychol 2000; 55(1):68–78.

12. Bremer CD, Kachgal M, Schoeller K. Self-Determination: Supporting Successful Transition. Research to Practice Brief: Improving Secondary Education and Transition Services through Research (Electronic version). National Center on Secondary Education and Transition, 2003; Vol. 2. (Retrieved June 16, 2005, from http://ncset.org/publications/viewdesc.asp? id = 962).

13. Werner E, Smith R. Overcoming the odds: High risk children. Ithaca, NY: Cornell University Press, 1992.

14. Holmbeck GN, Johnson SZ, Wills KE, et al. Observed and perceived parental overprotection in relation to psychosocial adjustment in preadolescents with a physical disability: the mediational role of behavioral autonomy. J Consul Clin Psychol 2002; 70(1):96–110.

15. Malian I, Nevin A. A review of self-determination literature – Implications for practitioners. Remedial and Special Education 2002; 23(2):68–74.

16. Wehmeyer ML, Palmer SB, Agran M, Mithaug DE, Martin JE. Promoting causal agency: The self-determined learning model of instruction. Exceptional Children 2000; 66(4):439–53.

17. Kieckhefer GM, Trahms CM. Supporting development of children with chronic conditions: from compliance toward shared management. Pediatric Nursing 2000; 26:354–63.

18. Yamaki K, Fujiura GT. Employment and income status of adults with developmental disabilities living in the community. Intellectual disability. 2002; 40(2):132–41.

19. Scal PS, Larson MI, Blum RW. Young Adults with Childhood onset disability making their way into Adulthood. Pediatric Research 2002; 53:1287.

20. Barnow BS, King CT. Workforce Investment Act in Eight States, (Electronic version) United States Department of Labor Employment and Training Administration Occasional Reports 2005-1 (AK-12224-01-60). Retrieved June 16, 2005: www.doleta.gov/reports/searcheta/occ/papers/FINAL_DOL_ Workforce_Academy_Report.pdf

21. United States Department of Labor Employment and Training Administration. Map of State One-Stop Websites (2005). Retrieved June 16, 2005 from www. doleta.gov/usworkforce/onestop/onestopmap.cfm

22. Department for Education and Skills (DfES) Special Educational Needs Code of Practice. 2001. DfES, London, U.K.

23. United States Department of Labor, 2005. Work activity of high school students: Data from the National Longitudinal Survey of Youth 1997. (Electronic version) United States DL reports: 05-732. Retrieved on June 16, 2005 from http://www.bls.gov/news.release/pdf/nlsyth.pdf

24. Houtenville, Andrew J. Disability Statistics in the United States. Ithaca, NY: Cornell University Rehabilitation Research and Training Center on Disability

Demographics and Statistics (StatsRRTC), www.disabilitystatistics.org. 2005. Posted April 4, 2005. Accessed June 02, 2005.

25. McDonagh JE, Foster H, Hall MA, Chamberlain MA. Audit of rheumatology services for adolescents and young adults in the United Kingdom. Rheumatology 2000; 39:596–602.

26. Shaw KL, Hackett J, Southwood TR, McDonagh JE. Vocational issues in juvenile idiopathic arthritis. The adolescent perspective. Br J Occupational Therapy 2006; 69(3):98–105.

27. Beresford B, Sloper T. The information needs of chronically ill or physically disabled children and adolescents. Social Policy Research Unit, York, 2000.

28. Bateman BJ, Finlay F. Long term medical conditions: career prospects. Arch Dis Child 2002; 87:291–2.

29. Shaw KL, Hackett J, Southwood TR, McDonagh JE. The Prevocational and Early employment needs of adolescents with juvenile idiopathic arthritis: the occupational therapy perspective. British Journal of Occupational Therapy 2006; 69:497–504.

30. McPherson M, Weissman G, Strickland BB, van Dyck PC, Blumberg SJ, Newacheck PW. Implementing community-based systems of services for children and youths with special health-care needs: how well are we doing? Pediatrics. 2004; 113(5 Suppl.):1538–44.

31. Newacheck PW, Kim SE. A national profile of health-care utilization and expenditures for children with special health-care needs. Archives of Pediatrics & Adolescent Medicine. 2005; 159(1):10–7.

32. Anderson LL, Larson SA, Lakin KC, Kwak N. (2003). Health insurance coverage 30. and health-care expenses of persons with disabilities in the NHIS-D. DD Data Brief 5 (1). Minneapolis: University of Minnesota, Research and Training Center on Community Living 2003.

33. Liptak GS, Accardo PJ. Health and social outcomes of children with cerebral palsy. J Pediatr 2004; 145(2 Suppl.):s36–41.

34. World Health Organization. International classification of functioning, disability and health. Geneva: World Health Organization; 2001.

35. White PH. Access to health-care: health insurance considerations for young adults with special health-care needs/disabilities. Pediatrics 2002; 110(6 Pt 2): 1328–35.

36. Shaw KL, Southwood TR, McDonagh JE. Young People's satisfaction of transitional care in adolescent rheumatology in the United Kingdom. Child: Care, Health & Development 2007; 33:368–79.

37. Robertson LP, McDonagh JE, Southwood TR, Shaw KL. Growing up and moving on. A multicentre United Kingdom audit of the transfer of adolescents with Juvenile Idiopathic Arthritis JIA from paediatric to adult centred care. Ann Rheum Dis 2006; 65:74–80.

38. Reiss JG, Gibson RW, Walker LR. Health-care transition: youth, family, and provider perspectives. Pediatrics 2005; 115(1):112–20.

39. Larson S, Lakin C, Huang J. DD Data Brief: Service Use by and Needs of Adults with Functional Limitations or ID/DD in the NHIS-D: Difference by Age, Gender, and Disability. DD Data Brief 5 (2) p. 10. Minneapolis:

University of Minnesota; Research and Training Center on Community Living, 2003.

40. Reiss J, Gibson R. Health-care transition: destinations unknown. Pediatrics 2002; 110(6 Pt 2):1307–4.

41. Rosen D. Between Two Worlds: Bridging the cultures of Child health and adult medicine. J Adol Health 1995; 17:10–6.

42. Viner RM. Transition from Pediatric to Adult Care. Bridging the gaps or passing the buck? Arch Dis Childhood 1999; 81:271–5.

43. White PH, Gallay L. Youth with Special Health-care needs and Disabilities in Transition to Adulthood in On Your Own without a Net (Eds. D. Wayne Osgood, E Michael Foster, Constance Flanagan and Gretchen Ruth), Univ Chicago Press 2005, pp. 349–74.

44. Scal P, Ireland M. Addressing transition to adult health-care for adolescents with special health-care needs. Pediatrics 2005; 115:1607–12.

45. Lam PY, Fitzgerald BB, Sawyer SM. Young adults in children's hospitals: why are they there? Med J Aust 2005; 182(8):381–4.

46. White PH, Hackett P, Turchi R, Gatto M. The Needs of Pediatric Practices for Policy and Procedures to Facilitate Youth with Special Health-care Needs Transition to Adulthood. Presented Pediatric Academic Societies Meeting (abstract) May 2006.

47. McDonagh JE, Southwood TR, Shaw KL. Unmet adolescent health training needs for rheumatology health professionals. Rheumatology 2004 43:737–43.

48. Blum RW, Bearinger LH. Knowledge and attitudes of health professionals toward adolescent health-care. J Adol Health-care 1990; 11:289–94.

49. McDonagh JE, Minnaar G, Kelly KM, O'Connor D, Shaw KL. Unmet education and training needs in adolescent health of health professionals in a United Kingdom Children's Hospital. Acta Paediatrica 2006; 95(6):715–9.

50. Reeve DK, Lincoln NB. Coping with the challenge of transition in older adolescents with epilepsy. Seizure 2002; 11:33–9.

51. McDonagh JE, Southwood TR, Shaw Kl. Growing up and moving on in rheumatology: development and preliminary evaluation of a transitional care programme for a multicenter cohort of adolescents with Juvenile idiopathic arthritis. J Child Health-Care 2006; 10:22–42.

52. Scal P. Transition for youth with chronic conditions: primary care physicians' approaches. Pediatrics. 2002; 110(6 Pt 2):1315–21.

53. Wolf-Branigin M, Schuyler V, White PH. Improving Quality of Life and Career Attitudes of Youth with Disabilities: Experiences from the Adolescent Employment Readiness Center. Research on Social Work 2007; 17(3):324–33.

54. Betz CL. Transition of adolescents with special health-care needs: review and analysis of the literature. Issues in Comprehensive Pediatric Nursing 2004; 27(3):179–241.

55. McDonagh JE, Southwood TR, Shaw KL. The impact of a coordinated transitional care programme on adolescents with juvenile idiopathic arthritis. Rheumatology 2007; 46(1):161–8.

56. While A, Forbes A, Ullman R, Lewis S, Mathes L, Griffiths P. Good practices that address continuity during transition from child to adult care: syntheses of the evidence. Child: Care, Health and Development 2004; 30(5):439–52.

57. Chamberlain MA, Rooney CM, Young Adults with arthritis: meeting their transitional needs. Br J Rheumatol 1996; 35:84–90.
58. Beresford B. On the road to nowhere? Young disabled people and transition. Child: Care, Health and Development 2004; 30(6):581–7.
59. Rettig P, Athreya BH. Adolescents with Chronic Disease: transition to adult health-care. Arthritis Care and Research 1991. 4:174–80.
60. Liptak G. S. Enhancing patient compliance in pediatrics. Pediatrics in Review. 1996; 17(4):128–34.
61. Reid GJ, Irvine MJ, McCrindle BW, et al. Prevalence and correlates of successful transfer from pediatric to adult health-care among a cohort of young adults with complex congenital heart defects. Pediatrics 2004; 113(3):197–205.
62. Shaw KL, Southwood TR, McDonagh JE. What's in a name Disease knowledge in Idiopathic arthritis. Arch Dis Child 2004; 98(Suppl.):A44.
63. Berry SL, Hayford JR, Ross CK, Pachman LM, Lavaigne JV. Conceptions of illness by children with juvenile rheumatoid arthritis: a cognitive developmental approach. J Pediatr Psychol 1993; 18(1):83–97.
64. Callahan ST, Cooper WO. Continuity of Health Coverage Among Young adults with disabilities. Pediatrics 119:1175180.
65. Schulzinger R. Youth with Disabilities in Transition: Health Insurance Options and Obstacles. An occasional policy brief of the Institute for Child Health Policy, 2000, Gainesville, FL, p. 4.
66. Hackett P, Gallivan G. Public and private insurance plans: Understanding the options for YSHCN (Electronic version). Healthy and Ready to Work National Center Tip Sheet (2003). Retrieved June 16, 2005, from http://www.hrt.org/healthcare/hlth_ins.html

17

Education and Training Needs for Health Professionals in Adolescent Rheumatology

Lindsay Robertson

Department of Rheumatology, Derriford Hospital, Plymouth, U.K.

INTRODUCTION

The needs of adolescents require specific consideration by health care professionals. As outlined in the preceding chapters of this book, there are many aspects of health that are of particular importance in adolescence. In addition, young people today face issues and dangers that are more complex than in previous generations, often with less support. It is also a time in life that future behaviors are developed that can form the basis for lifelong conduct. Therefore with respect to health-related behavior, it is an ideal time to effectively promote and encourage positive practices and attitudes towards health for the future.

To be able to interact effectively with a young person when in a perceived position of authority requires particular skills and also awareness of the issues that are important to and affect the age group. During health care professional training, attention to these themes is certainly apparent for pediatrics and adult care specialties such as the care of the elderly. However, attention to the required skills and knowledge for effective and successful adolescent care has been lacking until relatively recently.

This chapter aims to outline the training needs of rheumatology health professionals for effective adolescent care and will summarize the evidence supporting this need, including regarding what is required to promote good practice in adolescent health care.

DIFFERENT PERSPECTIVES—YOUNG PEOPLE AND HEALTH PROFESSIONALS

Adolescent friendly services need to accessible, equitable, acceptable, appropriate, comprehensive, effective, and efficient (1). Provider behavior is an important determinant of adolescent satisfaction with their health care. In a survey of 124 adolescents attending a university-based general adolescent medicine clinic, pre-visit attitudes about provider style predicted satisfaction with the consultation, and visit satisfaction was associated with intention to keep follow-up appointments (2). When 188 young people in the United Kingdom were asked what they wanted from their general practice, 80% rated confidentiality as important; 50% having a doctor interested in teenagers; 40% same day appointments; 33% choice of doctor gender; 39% drop-in clinics; 30% friendly receptionists (3). However, young people perceive barriers to accessing health care (4). In 253 14- and 15-year-olds interviewed with semi-structured questionnaires, knowledge of available health services was found to be poor (5). In spite of this, they expressed clear views of what was required from health services were expressed, and, again, confidentiality was identified as very important (5). Furthermore, Beresford and Sloper reported that the experiences of chronically ill adolescents in communicating with doctors raised attitudinal, behavioral, and practical factors regarding the delivery of care that the young people felt negatively affected their interactions with the doctor. Adolescents were reluctant to raise personal or sensitive issues or to ask questions that revealed poor adherence (6).

Contrary to the perception that adolescence is not associated with health problems, visits to health care professionals appear to be frequent and often problematic. Balding found that 50% of 12–15 year olds reported visiting a general practitioner (GP) within the past 3 months, 85% in the past year with 27% of females reporting feeling quite or very uneasy about the consultation (7). Donovan et al. also found that among 4000 young people aged 15 to 16 years, 53% reported problems with GP consultations (8). There has been interest in the reasons for consultations with a GP and Churchill's group found that the commonest reasons were respiratory, dermatological and musculoskeletal complaints (9). Perhaps of concern, the proportion attending for mental health problems was very small—4%, which is not in keeping with the known prevalence rates of mental health disorders in adolescents, 9% to 13% of 11- to 15- year-olds (10), suggesting a reluctance of young people to consult about these issues.

Health professionals have also reported concerns regarding their own knowledge and skills in providing adolescent health services. Out of 57 GPs interviewed individually and participating in focus groups, 91% had no or little formal training and 75% had concerns about their own competence and knowledge in delivering adolescent health care. A range of barriers was identified including confidentiality, communication and cost (11). Similarly, in a survey of a pediatric advanced trainees to elicit satisfaction with developmental-behavioral training, more than half considered themselves to be ill informed about adolescent problems (12).

There have been similar findings within the nursing profession. A national U.K. survey of 212 hospital nurses found that that average nurse spends up to 20% of his/her time with teenage patients, but only 1 in 5 had specific training to manage the emotional needs and problems that may occur in this age group (13). Gregg et al. found that GP practice nurses were uncomfortable discussing psychological issues with teenagers such as depression as well as bullying, safe sex, and drug use (14). Examining a wider range of health professionals including doctors, nurses, social workers, psychologists, and nutritionists perceived competencies for key areas of adolescent health have also been found to be low (15). In a Swiss national survey of six medical disciplines involved in adolescent care, strong interest in adolescent medicine was expressed particularly for functional symptoms, acne, obesity, and communication. However, confidentiality/legal issues, injury prevention, and the impact of chronic conditions were rated as low priority areas, reflecting further educational and training needs in epidemiological and legal/ethical issues (16).

Approximately 10% to 20% of adolescents have a chronic condition, and many will need to be able to access adult health care services for their condition when they are older. Making the change from pediatric to adult health services can be difficult. Shaw et al. conducted focus groups of young people and their carers regarding this issue and found that this time was often fraught with difficulties, anxieties, and concerns (17). The young people reported feeling "dumped" or "tossed" by their pediatric teams without any preparation for coping with adult care. Their carers or parents also had great concerns about the quality of care for their children as they became older (17). Therefore this aspect of health care delivery—transitional care is crucial and appropriate training of health care professionals in key areas for affected adolescents is essential. In a survey of 263 health professionals involved in transitional care, McDonagh et al. found that there were many unmet needs in key areas of transition, and informational resources and transitional issues were the most frequently reported areas of need. Lack of training, lack of informational resources aimed at adolescents, and limited clinic time were also identified in a second smaller survey of 22 clinical personnel (18). (For further discussion of transition, see Chapter 16.)

In a more detailed study of a children's hospital staff ($n=159$) and trainee pediatricians ($n=54$), no specific training in adolescent health was reported by 60% of the former and 58% of the latter. The most common topic to have been covered in prior teaching was the definition of adolescence and of biopsychosocial development during adolescence, but practical issues around common adolescent problems such as acne, menstrual, and mental health and musculoskeletal problems, chronic pain, chronic fatigue, epidemiology, chronic illness, resilience, and risk behaviors were rarely addressed. These topics were rated as having either high or very high importance by the majority of respondents for 85% of topics (19). Reflecting this, perceived knowledge, confidence, and skill in these areas were reported as low. High knowledge was reported in one area, which was confidentiality. There was a significant relationship between prior teaching and perceived knowledge, confidence, and skill (19). There were no major differences between the unmet training needs of doctors compared to other health professionals [19] supporting the potential of multiprofessional training.

Most published information comes from survey work, which does have its limitations, including low completion rates, nonrespondent biases, respondents' anxieties about admitting ignorance and unawareness of educational/training needs. Only perceived knowledge/confidence and skills can be assessed, which may not reflect the results of assessment of actual competency.

LACK OF TRAINING—A PERCEIVED BARRIER TO ADOLESCENT HEALTH-CARE PROVISION

From the studies described above despite their limitations, it can be concluded that adolescent health care delivery has been highlighted as important and further attention is required in the training of current and future generations of health professionals to facilitate confidence and competence. However, there are also perceived barriers not only to gaining the necessary knowledge and skills but also in implementing them. Britto et al. found that pediatric rheumatologists had difficulties in promoting adolescent health in their clinics. Levels of screening young people for alcohol use and sexual activity was linked to lack of time, organizational problems, discomfort in dealing with the subject area, ambivalence as to whether the role was within the remit of a pediatrician, and doubts as to the relevance of the subject to their patient group (20). In units dedicated to the care of adolescents, Sawyer reported comorbidities such as underlying behavioral or mental health problems that can often affect the presentation to the hospital or, indeed, be the cause of an admission (e.g., overdose). In such units these issues can be more easily identified and managed and can give a focus for training and continuing professional development in the field that, in more general medical environments, is otherwise difficult to deliver (21).

With respect to involvement in transition, 45% of health professionals in a U.K. national survey cited lack of training to be a barrier to providing transitional services (18). In a survey of 743 parents of young people with special health care needs and 141 health professionals (primary pediatricians), Geenen et al. found that time, training, financial constraints, and other issues, such as discomfiture, lack of applicability, difficulty accessing resources were the barriers perceived by the health professionals. Furthermore, there were significant differences between providers and parents concerning both the level of provider involvement and the extent to which it was the provider's responsibility to assist in various transition activities. The health providers reported significantly more involvement than did parents perceived them to have for most transition activities (22).

EVIDENCE FOR EDUCATIONAL INTERVENTIONS FOR ADOLESCENT HEALTH CARE

Evidence is accumulating for the benefits of educational interventions in adolescent health care particularly in higher rates of desired clinical practices such as confidentiality, screening for health risk behaviors. Marks et al. found that out of 101 general pediatricians surveyed those with some training in adolescent medicine during residency were significantly more likely to provide care and anticipatory guidance related to sexuality and substance abuse (23). Pediatric residents at a university children's hospital were also more likely to screen for these issues and record them if they had some postgraduate-level experience and had been on a prior adolescent rotation (24). Key et al. in a survey of Canadian pediatricians reported a greater number of adolescents seen and a greater tendency for engagement in continuing education in adolescent health if adolescent medicine training was received during residency years (25).

A randomized controlled trial has been published of a multifaceted educational program delivered weekly for 2.5 hours for six weeks on the principles of adolescent health care for GPs in Melbourne, Australia. This showed sustainable, large improvements in knowledge, skill, and self-perceived competency in the group randomized to the education program compared to the controls, with the exception of rapport and satisfaction rating by the standardized patients. Competence was measured objectively with videotaped consultations (26). At 5-year follow up, scores were all higher than at baseline, improvements were sustained and 54% of doctors had been involved in further training (27).

The European Training in Effective Adolescent Care and Health (EuTEACH; www.euteach.com) working group has developed a curriculum that covers the main teaching areas in the field, such as basic skills (i.e. setting, rights and confidentiality, gender, and cultural issues) as well as specific themes (i.e., sexual and reproductive health, eating disorders, chronic conditions). It is a modular, flexible program, each module containing detailed objectives, learning approaches, examples, and an evaluation method. Evaluation after two summer schools was good overall, with most items surpassing three on a four-point Likert scale. However, some deficiencies were identified, and an increase in interactive sessions (role playing) and a better mix of clinical and public health issues were suggested as useful additional features of the course for future participants (28).

PRACTICAL ASPECTS OF TRAINING PROVISION

While comprehensive theoretical knowledge of a field is important for appropriate practice, experiential learning is crucial for consolidating theoretical knowledge and for the development of interviewing, counselling and examination skills. It also allows development of experience in answering questions from patients and/or their carers and facilitates reflective learning. A consultation needs to be of adequate length so that it is effective and worthwhile for the patient and also allows the health professional to use all the resources/knowledge and experience to benefit the patient and gain further experience. The Royal College of Pediatrics and Child Health has recognized that longer consultation times are required for adolescent than for either children's or adult clinics (29). A comparison of pediatric and adult rheumatology clinics found that on average the pediatric clinic consultations were twice as long (30). This difference was maintained when young people older than 12 years were compared to the adult clinics (Robertson, and McDonagh, unpublished). However, Jacobsen et al. found that when comparing 119 consultations with young people aged 11 to 19 years, with 781 consultations with other age groups, the consultations with young people were actually shorter by 23% (31). This may have been for many reasons, including difficulty establishing rapport with young people, inadequate time allotted to explore issues fully, and organizational difficulties within the clinic workspace.

Young people themselves have been found to have difficulty with the experiential learning of health care professionals. The extent of their trust in the service provided for them may be reduced by the presence of strangers (e.g., students, trainees) in a consultation. However, young people do realize that professionals need to gain experience and training. Young people have suggested sessions separate from consultations where they are "case study" so that their clinic appointments are kept as their time rather than for the benefits of students (18).

WHO ARE THE TEACHERS?

In North America and Australia there are recognized training programs in adolescent health. In the U.K. provision of training in adolescent health is limited. In 2006, there were still no formal training programs outside mental health in the UK and only one consultant in adolescent medicine in the country. Within hospital practice in the U.K. surveys of clinics have found no adolescent service provision to be available in two thirds of pediatric gastroenterology clinics (32), 47% of pediatric diabetes services

(33) and 82% of rheumatology units seeing children (34). Therefore it is unlikely that the majority of trainee rheumatology professionals have had much exposure to adolescent health. The Royal College of Physicians in the United Kingdom has stated that training in adolescent health should be mandatory for both undergraduates and the trainees of all Royal Colleges whose members may be involved in the care of young people" (29). Adolescent health and transitional care have now been integrated into the training curricula in both pediatric and adult rheumatology in the United Kingdom.

From the undergraduate perspective the newer medical schools in the United Kingdom are defining adolescent health as a subject within their curriculum (35). However in a 2003 survey of general medical textbooks available to medical undergraduates in Birmingham, U.K., only 5 out of 12 pediatric books had a chapter on adolescent issues, which represented 2% of the total pages, and none of the adult medicine textbooks were identified (36).

Examples of web-based curricula readily available are detailed in Table 1. The EuTEACH program aims to train individuals to be able to deliver training themselves in adolescent health care and the web-site acts as a resource for this (28). A multidisciplinary modular program based on the EuTEACH curriculum has recently commenced at Birmingham University, U.K.

The National Training Initiative in Adolescent Health (NTIAH) is a Canadian-based comprehensive multidisciplinary training program for professionals working with youth. It aims to incorporate a youth health curriculum as an essential component of fully accredited training programs for graduates and practicing professionals in a variety of health-related fields. It was developed after a review conducted by the Canadian Pediatric

Table 1 Examples of Adolescent Health Curricula for Health Professionals

Europe
    www.euteach.com
    European initiative to provide web-based teaching resources for adolescent health
    www.repch.ac.uk/Education/Adolescent.Health-Project U.K. initiative to develop
    e-learning packages for adolescent health
Canada
    National Training Initiative in Adolescent Health
    http://www.cps.ca/english/prodev/NTIAH/index.htm
Australia
    Centre for Adolescent Health, Melbourne
    www.caah.chw.edu.au
United States
    University of Southern California
    http://www.usc.edu/adolhealth/

Society of the adolescent medicine content of pediatric resident training programs in Canadian medical schools revealed serious inadequacies (37)

Recruiting professionals who are keen to develop skills in the adolescent health historically has been difficult. Blum conducted the first U.S. national survey of primary care physicians' perceptions of their competency in dealing with adolescents' health concerns. This found that only 27% of doctors were interested in further training despite reporting deficiencies in many key areas of knowledge (38). In a survey of medical practitioners in a large, multi-specialty, group practice, Klitsner et al. found that only a third of those surveyed which included pediatricians, internists, obstetricians, and gynecologists, family doctors actually reported that they liked caring for adolescents (39). More recently, though, reports have suggested increased awareness and interest in improving skills (15,16,18).

THE FUTURE

The continuing and increasing awareness of adolescent health needs to be encouraged and fostered in all disciplines. Publication in the general medical literature needs to be encouraged. In the 12 editions of "Archives of Disease in Childhood" only 4% and 8% of original and review articles, respectively, were adolescent health–related (36)

There is great scope for multidisciplinary involvement in creating appropriate adolescent health services that young people will want and be able to access easily. Involvement of young people in service development and training may be a key aspect to success. Involvement as case studies or as simulated patients using adolescent actors has been reported as successful (40,41). Collaboration of medical schools and postgraduate programs with secondary schools with drama departments may be fruitful in the teaching of adolescent medicine with special emphasis on communication skills with teenagers. The reliability and validity of an observation guide that incorporates adolescent psychosocial data collection with the physician's communication skills have recently been assessed using trained adolescent raters (42). Videos of simulated consultations have been developed for training purposes. The DIPEx charity has produced a unique, award winning website aimed at young people, their carers, family and friends, doctors, nurses, and other health professionals. Approximately 100 main illnesses and conditions are covered, including teenage health and childhood-onset chronic conditions (www.youthhealthtalk.org). Interviews with volunteers or actors are available to watch online and are potentially useful teaching aids for issues such as communication and confidentiality (43).

There is also potential for interdisciplinary education and training programs. Many issues faced by adolescents are generic and have the potential to occur in many disciplines. Surveys of different professionals show there are few differences between perceived importance, knowledge and confidence in most of the key areas of adolescent health (11–16,18). In addition, training disciplines together is potentially more cost-effective than each profession running its own program and will foster future collaboration either in the clinical or research arenas.

SUMMARY

The profile of adolescent health care is gradually gaining in prominence across many of the developed countries of the world. Concomitantly there is an increasing focus on the educational and training needs of health professionals working in environments where they may be involved in the care of young people. There is already some convincing evidence of this need and also of the benefits of responding to it. Further work to strengthen this evidence base is required and professionals working with adolescents all need to continue to promote this aspect of health care to commissioners and fund holders of health care budgets. By providing effective adolescent health care, a healthier, and consequently more productive, adult population will emerge, which will ultimately benefit our society.

REFERENCES

1. McIntyre P, Adolescent friendly services–an agenda for change. WHO 2003 http://www.who.int/child-adolescent-health/publications/ADH/WHO_FCH_CAH_02.14.htm (accessed 27 July 2006).
2. Freed LH, Ellen JM, Irwin CE Jr, Millstein SE. Determinants of adolescents' satisfaction with health-care providers and intentions to keep follow-up appointments. J Adolesc Health 1998; 22(6):475–9.
3. McPherson A. Primary health-care and adolescence. In A. MacFarlane, ed. Adolescent Medicine. London: Royal College of Physicians, 1996: 33–41.
4. Ginsburg KR, Slap GB. Unique needs of the teen in the health-care setting. Curr Opin Pediatr 1996; 8(4):337–7.
5. Oppong-Odiseng AC, Heycock EG. Adolescent health services–through their eyes. Arch Dis Child 1997; 77(2):115–9.
6. Beresford BA, Sloper P Chronically ill adolescents' experiences of communicating with doctors: a qualitative study. J Adolesc Health 2003; 33 (3):172–9.
7. Balding J. Young People in 2003. University of Exeter: Schools Health Education Unit, 2004.
8. Donovan C, Mellanby AR, Jacobson LD, Taylor B, Tripp JH. Teenagers' views on the general practice consultation and provision of contraception. The Adolescent Working Group. Br J Gen Pract 1997; 4:715–8.
9. Churchill R, Allen J, Denman S, Williams D, Fielding K, von Fragstein M. Do the attitudes and beliefs of young teenagers towards general practice influence actual consultation behaviour? Br J Gen Pract 2000; 50:953–7.
10. Meltzer H, et al. Mental health of children and adolescents in Great Britain. Office for National Statistics 2000. Stationary Office. London, 2000.

11. Veit FC, Sanci LA, Young DY, Bower G. Adolescent health-care: perspectives of Victorian general practitioners. Med J Aust 1995; 163(1):16–18.

12. Chee KY, Simpson JM, Hutchins P. Survey of developmental-behavioural training experiences of Australian advanced paediatric trainees. J Paediatr Child Health 1994; 30:478–82.

13. Norwich Union. The views of adolescent and nurses on the provision of health care in hospitals. Norwich Union, 2001.

14. Gregg R, Freeth C, Blackie D. Teenage health and the practice nurse: choice and opportunity for both? Br J Gen Pract 1998; 48(426):909–10.

15. Blum RW, Bearinger LH. Knowledge and attitudes of health professionals toward adolescent health-care. J Adolesc Health-care 1990; 11(4):289–94.

16. Kraus B, Stronski S, Michaud PA. Training needs in adolescent medicine of practising doctors: a Swiss national survey of six disciplines. Med Educ 2003; 37 (8):709–14.

17. Shaw KL, Southwood TR, McDonagh JE. The British Paediatric Rheumatology Group. User perspectives of transitional care for adolescents with juvenile idiopathic arthritis. Rheumatology (Oxford) 2004; 43(6):770–8.

18. McDonagh JE, Southwood TR, Shaw KL Unmet education and training needs of rheumatology health professionals in adolescent health and transitional care. Rheumatology (Oxford) 2004; 43(6):737–43.

19. McDonagh JE, Minnaar G, Kelly KM, et al. Unmet education and training needs in adolescent health of health professionals in a UK Children's Hospital. Acta Paediatrica 2006; 95(6):715–9.

20. Britto MT, Rosenthal SL, Taylor J, Passo MH. Improving rheumatologists' screening for alcohol use and sexual activity. Arch Pediatr Adolesc Med 2000; 154(5):478–83.

21. Sawyer S, Shea L, Patton G. Do we need specialist units for adolescents in hospitals? Such units are valuable in Australia. Br Med J 2001; 323 (7309):401–2.

22. Geenen SJ, Powers LE, Sells W. Understanding the role of health-care providers during the transition of adolescents with disabilities and special health-care needs. J Adolesc Health 2003; 32(3):225–33.

23. Marks A, Fisher M, Lasker S. Adolescent medicine in pediatric practice. J Adolesc Health-care 1990; 11(2):149–53.

24. Middleman AB, Binns HJ, Durant RH. Factors affecting pediatric residents' intentions to screen for high risk behaviours. J Adolesc Health 1995; 17 (2):106–12.

25. Key JD, Marsh LD, Darden, PM. Adolescent medicine in pediatric practice: a survey of practice and training. Am J Med Sci 1995; 309(2):83–7.

26. Sanci LA, Coffey CM, Veit FC, Carr-Gregg M, Patten GC, Day N, Bowes G Evaluation of the effectiveness of an educational intervention for general practitioners in adolescent health-care: randomised controlled trial. Br Med J 2000; 320(7229):224–30.

27. Sanci L, Coffey C, Patton G, Bowes G. Sustainability of change with quality general practitioner education in adolescent health: a 5-year follow-up. Med Educ 2005; 39:557–60.

28. Michaud PA, Stronksi S, Fonseca H, Macfarlane A, EuTEACH working group. The development and pilot-testing of a training curriculum in adolescent medicine and health. J Adolesc Health 2004; 35(1):51–7.
29. Royal College of Paediatrics and Child Health. Bridging the Gap: Health-care for Adolescents. June 2003. (www.rcpch.ac.uk accessed July 2006).
30. Robertson LP, Hickling P, Davis PJC, Bailey K, Ryder CAJ, McDonagh JE. Comparison of paediatric and adult rheumatology clinics. The doctor perspective. Rheumatology 2003; 42:97A.
31. Jacobson LD, Wilkinson C, Owen PA. Is the potential of teenage consultations being missed?: a study of consultation times in primary care. Fam Pract 1994; 11(3):296–9.
32. Davies IH, Jenkins HR. Transition clinics for adolescents with chronic gastrointestinal disease in the UK and Ireland. J Pediatric Gastroenterol Nutr 2003; 36:505–8.
33. Jefferson IG, Swift PG, Skinner TC, Hood GK. Diabetes services in the UK: third national survey confirms continuing deficiencies. Arch Dis Child 2003; 88 (1):53–6.
34. McDonagh JE, Foster HE, Hall MA, Chamberlain MA. Audit of rheumatology services for adolescents and young adults in the UK. British Paediatric Rheumatology Group. Rheumatology (Oxford) 2000; 39(6):596–602.
35. Pennisula Medical School, Universities of Exeter and Plymouth www.pms.ac. uk (accessed July 2006).
36. McDonagh JE, Walker V, Foullerton M, Robertson L, Gupta K, Diwakar V. Young People–Lost in Transition (letter). Arch Dis Child 2006; 91(2):201.
37. The National Training Initiative in Adolescent Health http://www.mcs.bc.ca/ ntiah.htm (accessed December 2007).
38. Blum R. Physicians' assessment of deficiencies and desire for training in adolescent care. J Med Educ 1987; 62(5):401–7.
39. Klitsner IN, Borok GM, Neinstein L, MacKenzie R. Adolescent health-care in a large multispecialty prepaid group practice. Who provides it and how well are they doing? West J Med 1992; 156(6):628–32.
40. Blake K, Greaven S. Recruiting and following adolescent standardized patients. Acad Med 1999; 74(5):584.
41. Hardoff D, Schonmann S. Training physicians in communication skills with adolescents using teenage actors as simulated patients. Med Educ 2001; 35 (3):206–10.
42. Blake K, Vincent N, Wakefield S, Murphy J, Mann K, Kutcher M. A structured communication adolescent guide (SCAG): assessment of reliability and validity. Med Educ 2005; 39(5):482–91.
43. DIPEx.org. Personal experiences of health and illness. www.dipex.com, www. youthhealthtalk.org, University of Oxford (accessed December 2007).

18

How Can We Develop Adolescent Rheumatology Care That Continually Improves Outcomes for Young People?

Boel Andersson Gäre

Futurum Academy of Health and Care, Jönköping County Council, Jönköping, and Department of Pediatrics, Linköping University, Linköping, Sweden

Marjorie M. Godfrey

The Dartmouth Institute for Health Policy and Clinical Practice, Dartmouth Medical School, Lebanon, New Hampshire, U.S.A.

We are not hosts in our organizations so much as we are guests in our patients' lives.

Don Berwick, 1999 (1)

Every system is perfectly designed to get the results it gets.

Paul Batalden, 1996 (2)

Integration is the key to quality: integrating systems and spirit, methods and motivation, and professional excellence with consumer service. Without integration, we do not use our resources to the best effect. We get technique without heart, and systems without soul, which do not heal or enable people a safe growth. Public health care can develop technical and human quality to give safe and soulful service.

John Övretveit, 1999 (3)

INTRODUCTION

Not only do adolescents who live with a rheumatic disease need to grow up and move on, the health care systems that provide care for them need to do the same. And we as professionals need to take an active part in that continuous work of improvement. This chapter gives a brief introduction to the background and philosophy of quality improvement in health care and how it can be applied to the "clinical microsystem" of pediatric adolescent rheumatology, that is, the place where adolescents with a rheumatic disease, their families, and health care professionals meet (4). The possibilities for improving outcomes for patients with rheumatic disease have increased tremendously during the last decades owing to new medications, improved methods for habilitation/rehabilitation, and improved methods for joint surgery. In addition, a more holistic way of providing care to children and adolescents with chronic disease has evolved based on interdisciplinary teams with the aim of meeting not only the medical but also the psychological and social needs of patients and families.

All these new possibilities and demands have made care much more complex. With the use of more effective and potent drugs, it has also become potentially more dangerous for patients. Safety related to the right drug in the right amount and potential side effects becomes a central focus for the interdisciplinary health care team. Much of the health care system is still organized as if we handle only acute disease and not chronic illness, which has significant implications for tracking patient outcomes, treatment plans, and coordinating care over time. We are organized around events, or in silos based on professional specialties, rather than on integrated long-term healing relationships with the patient in the center (5). Patients and their families are often still thought of as "guests" in our systems rather than health care professionals being guests in the lives of patients and families (1).

The Current Situation in Health Care—The "Quality Chasm"

Much has been written lately about the inadequate quality and safety in health care. A very strong whistleblower on safety issues was the report, "To Err Is Human: Building a Safer Health System," published by Institute of Medicine (IOM) in 2000. According to an estimate in that report, 7% of all hospitalized patients experience a serious medication error, and 44,000 to 98,000 Americans die in hospitals each year from care injuries (6). Similar figures from all parts of the western world have been published—the United Kingdom, Denmark, Australia, and other countries. The types of errors that occur can be divided into diagnostic, treatment, preventive (failure to provide prophylactic services) and other processes, for example, failures in communication. In pediatrics, we have also learned that our field is particularly at risk for medication errors, owing to the complexity dosing and administering of drugs to children and the scarcity of studies on children and drugs. Studies show that errors occur in 5 of 1000 medication orders in pediatrics, and the most prevalent is overdosing (6) The follow-up IOM report (2001) states, on the basis of numerous examples of underuse, overuse, and misuse of medical services, that there is not only a gap, but a *chasm* between the evidence-based knowledge and the actual performance and outcomes in health care. This happens despite the fact that everyone in health care tries their best to get it right. The reality of the current situation is that the problems are caused by the increased complexity in health care and the fragmentation of care processes—and only by changing the system can sustainable change be made with significantly improved measured outcomes (7).

What Is High-Quality Care?

The 2001 IOM report proposed that high-quality care should be:

- Patient centered—providing respectful, responsive, individualized care
- Safe—avoiding injury from care that is intended to help
- Timely—reducing waits and harmful delays in care
- Equal—providing equal care regardless of personal characteristics, gender, ethnicity, geography, or socio-economic status
- Effective—avoiding under use, overuse, or misuse of services
- Efficient—avoiding waste of all kinds

These suggested six aims have gained wide acceptance and have been incorporated into the national directives for health care in both Sweden and Norway.

Don Berwick, a pediatrician by training, and President, CEO of the Institute for Healthcare Improvement in Boston (www.ihi.org) has proposed the dimensions of high-quality care in a " 'No'-list" which is easily translated into daily clinical work. In health care there should be: No needless deaths, No needless pain, No helplessness, No unwanted waiting, No waste...for anyone (8).

What Is Quality Improvement?

Batalden and Davidoff recently proposed to define quality improvement as "the combined and unceasing efforts of everyone—health care professionals, patients and their families, leaders, researchers, payers, planners, educators—to make changes that will lead to better patient outcomes (health), better system performance (care), and better professional development (learning)" (Fig. 1) (9). This means that "quality improvement is not tools and methods. The tools and methods help us to work on the work of improving our work"(10). Quality improvement is not a project that starts and ends at certain times, and it is not for a special group of "quality people"—but a part of the daily work for *everyone*.

WHAT DO WE NEED TO KNOW FOR QUALITY IMPROVEMENT?

On the basis of the alarming reports and the evolution of a vision for high-quality health care systems, the movement for quality improvement in health care has grown stronger. The goal is to do the right thing for every

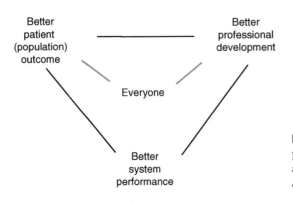

Figure 1 The aims of improvement need to be linked and to involve everyone. *Source*: Adapted from Ref. 9.

patient, every time. Theories, concepts, models, methods, and tools have been developed and adapted to suit health care needs. Many good examples to learn from have emerged, along with advice on how to use these methods and tools in everyday clinical practice (4,11–13). Much of the knowledge is generic and can be adjusted and adapted to many different care situations. If we, as caregivers in adolescent rheumatology, want to fulfill our goal of offering the best possible care and support for the young people and families we serve, every day to every patient, we need to embrace the idea that we have two jobs when we come to work every day: to do our job and to improve it (Table 1) (9). Quality is inherent in every moment in everyone's actions in health care and can not be delegated to a special office or to "quality people." However, in order to fulfill both our jobs we need not only

Table 1 Questions for Reflecting About Your Current Rheumatology Practice

Discuss the proposed aims of high-quality care and how they apply to your workplace:
  How does your workplace live up to "no needless care" delivery standard?
  Are procedures as pain free as they could be? How can you know?
  Are there waits for appointments with a pediatrician? For intra-articular steroid injections? How can you know?
  Does the teenager always know where to turn or is there a sense of helplessness? How can you know?
  Is the care safe and reliable? For example; are eye examinations timely according to guidelines? Are blood counts timely for patients on cytotoxic drugs according to recommendations? How can you know?
  Is access equal when needed? Are services and outcomes equal for patients from different social backgrounds? How can you know?
If, after you have reviewed these questions, you discover you do not know enough about the performance and outcomes of patients or our system of care delivery, what might you do to improve the current state? How might you "find" the answers to these questions?

to keep up with the evidence-based subject matter but we also need a new set of knowledge and skills, "the knowledge of improvement," which is usually not included in the basic training of health care professionals (Fig. 2) (14). The professional knowledge, here defined as knowledge of subject, discipline and values including ethical considerations needs to be combined with the second block of knowledge to create maximum value for our patients. This second block was described by Deming (15) as the knowledge of improvement and includes knowledge of system, variation, psychology, and theory of change. These knowledge domains will be further explored below and later put into improvement in the context where care is provided, or the "clinical microsystem" addressed in this book—the adolescent rheumatology clinic.

Professional Knowledge

Subject, Discipline, and Values

Improvements in health care depend on the subject knowledge (e.g., anatomy, pharmacology, pathology) and discipline (e.g., pediatric rheumatology, pediatric nursing, occupational therapy). In addition, the values of patients, families, and health care professionals need to be considered along with ethical considerations in society that drive improvement. Traditionally these domains have been or seemed sufficient to improve health care. Today, in the very complex health care system they still form the necessary basis for improvement but need to be combined with other knowledge domains

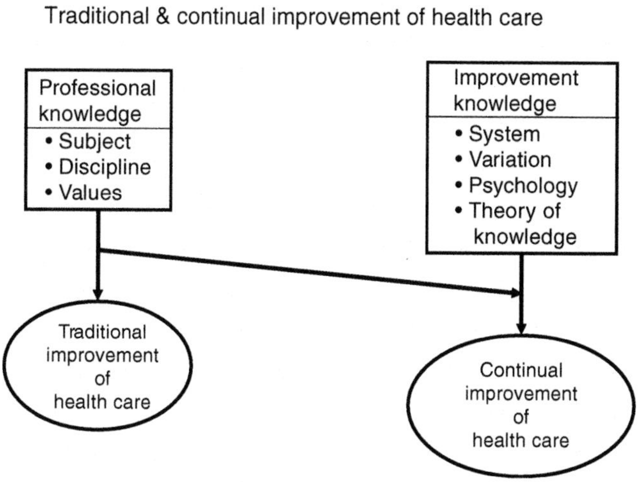

Traditional & continual improvement of health care

Figure 2 Knowledge that health care professionals need for improvement. *Source:* Adapted from Ref. 14.

in order to improve the performance of systems and resultant outcomes of care.

In this book the necessary subject- and discipline-specific areas of adolescent rheumatology are updated and expanded. Subjects covered, such as: adolescents as new users of health services, pharmacokinetics during adolescence; adolescent friendly health care, communication, strategies to facilitate adherence, opportunities for health promotion, peer support, information technology, transition, and training are all necessary components of high-quality care for adolescents with a chronic disease. However, to get all that knowledge in place every day for every patient challenges our current understanding of our particular context—the adolescent rheumatology clinic—and our ability to continuously and systematically improve our processes of care. This is where the knowledge of improvement enters our framework.

Improvement Knowledge

Knowledge of a System

The health care system has an *aim* to improve the health of the patients it serves. This care is "made" through several *processes*, such as diagnostic services, assessments, plans of care, and delivery of care at the ward or in the clinic. All these processes include many steps that need to be analyzed and understood in greater detail before we plan to change and redesign processes for improved performance and outcomes. The *clinical microsystems* are the essential building blocks of the larger health care systems. The microsystem is the local context where patients and families, health care teams, support staff, information, and processes meet to provide care for a particular group of patients. In a pediatric hospital there are many microsystems, such as allergy, rheumatology, and diabetes clinics, neonatal intensive care units, and units for infectious disease. These different microsystems will interact horizontally with each other in planned and unplanned ways. A rheumatology patient, for example, will mainly receive care in the pediatric rheumatology clinic but may sometimes need to be cared for in the inpatient unit, which is another microsystem. Examples of other linking microsystems for the same patient might be the ophthalmologist clinic, the department of radiology, the pharmacy, or physical therapy department. Using "system thinking" invites the challenge: to make the process for the patient and family smooth and seamless. The flow of information and data should be uninterrupted, and the process should not be dependent on which day of the week it is or which insurance-plan the patient has. A microsystem can be viewed as being embedded in a larger system called the mesosystem, which in turn is imbedded in an even larger system called the macrosystem. This is illustrated in the "systems of health care" (Fig. 3) (4).

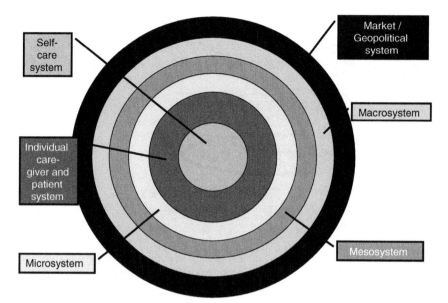

Figure 3 Systems of health care. Which system is the unit of practice, intervention, measurement, or policy? *Source*: Adapted from Ref. 4.

Another way to consider the systems of care (micro-, meso- and macrosystems) is through current organizational structures such the "multilayered health system diagram" (Fig. 4) (4). In order to improve care we need to have deep knowledge of the current system and know how to make improvements.

Knowledge of Measurement and Variation

The next dimension of improvement knowledge is variation. Processes often show variation, a lack of standardization of care, and steps in care. Understanding and studying variation over time is key to recognizing and identifying opportunities for improvement. In a stable process we still find some variation that occurs because of chance, *common cause variation*. But, there can also be *special causes* that we can discover when we follow data over time and action can be taken (16). If we react to common cause variation as if it were a special cause we might "tamper" with the system, resulting in poorer outcomes than intended. For example, blood sugar values in the normal ranges in a diabetes patient will always show some common variation. However, if we start to give extra insulin because of a higher value within the common variation, we might risk making the patient hypoglycemic, which

System levels   Example

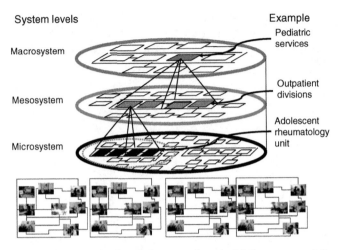

Figure 4 Organizational layers of embedded systems. Microsystems are the building blocks that come together to form macro-organizations. *Source*: Adapted from Ref. 4.

leads us to administer extra calories, resulting in too high a blood sugar level, that is, we "tamper" with the system unnecessarily.

In pediatric rheumatology, we can analyze variation at many levels. We can gain more insight into the patients and populations we serve, the performance of our system, and the outcomes of our patients by asking some questions.

- Do we get patients from some referral areas and not from others?
- Do patients come late, after onset of symptoms, from some areas and early from other areas?
- Does the frequency with which intra-articular steroids are given for the same kinds of patient vary between centers?
- Do the rates of given vaccinations, which are recommended by guidelines, vary between groups of our patients or between centers?
- Do outcomes differ between centers?

Only if we start to measure data over time and observe patterns in performance and outcomes can we begin to identify opportunities to improve care and through continued data measurement know if improvement activities lead to improved outcomes.

A disease registry can be an important source of information about the characteristics of the population of patients served, the performance of the provided care and multidimensional outcome measures as illustrated by examples from the Swedish Rheumatology Registry (Table 2) and disease

Table 2 The Swedish Rheumatology Registry

A "registry case": In Sweden, a web-based clinical quality registry for adult patients with rheumatoid arthritis that is used for several purposes has been created. It is built as a "feed-forward" system which means that the patient can enter data into the Health Assessment Questionnaire, get results from laboratory tests, and a joint evaluation *before* the visit to the rheumatologist. Thus, a patient over-view can be created and used as a template for the conversation between patient and provider to help guide decisions that need to be made. Since data are shown over time, it can help the patient and provider see trends in improvement or worsening of the disease. In addition, the data from the patients at the microsystem level can be aggregated, analyzed, and used for local learning and improvements. At the national level, unanimous patient data can be aggregated for comparison of performance measures and outcomes for benchmarking, learning, and improvement (Fig.5).

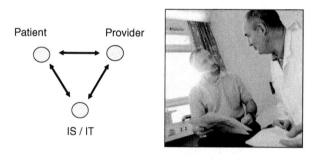

The clinical microsystem

Disease activity (DAS) over ten years at initial consultation
and at 6 and 12 months in recent onset rheumatoid arthritis

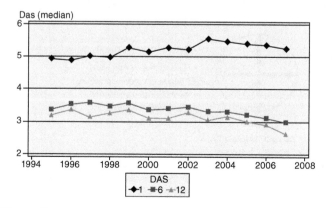

Figure 5 The Swedish rheumatology register. *Source*: Courtesy of Staffan Lindblad, MD, PhD, Karolinska Institute, Stockholm, Sweden.

activity data over a 12-year period from patients with adult rheumatoid arthritis detailed in Figure 5.

A pedagogic tool for illustrating measurements in multiple dimensions is the "Clinical Value Compass" (12). In adolescent rheumatology examples of measures in the different directions are illustrated in Figure 6.

A registry can give clues if and why health disparities occur about groups of patients and between geographic locations. An interesting study from Cinncinati Children's Hospital Medical Center (Cinncinati, Ohio, U.S.) using a prospective disease registry showed that children with Medicaid status who had been diagnosed with juvenile idiopathic arthritis had significantly lower health-related quality of life and higher disability than children with the same severity of disease and private insurance. The difference was present in spite of similar overall resource utilization. However, children with Medicare status were more likely to visit the emergency department and had fewer magnetic resonance images (17).

Knowledge of Psychology of Work and Change

The performance of a system can be attributed to multiple causes, including understanding health-professional behavior. Seeking knowledge about what nurtures curiosity and learning, joy, and pride in health care professionals can support leaders who are interested in engaging staff in change and improvement. Change theory and leading change knowledge is an important leadership responsibility.

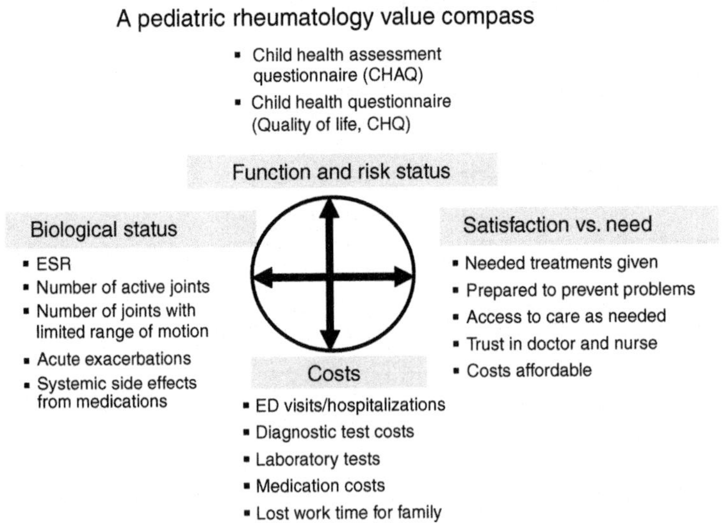

A pediatric rheumatology value compass

- Child health assessment questionnaire (CHAQ)
- Child health questionnaire (Quality of life, CHQ)

Function and risk status

Biological status

- ESR
- Number of active joints
- Number of joints with limited range of motion
- Acute exacerbations
- Systemic side effects from medications

Satisfaction vs. need

- Needed treatments given
- Prepared to prevent problems
- Access to care as needed
- Trust in doctor and nurse
- Costs affordable

Costs

- ED visits/hospitalizations
- Diagnostic test costs
- Laboratory tests
- Medication costs
- Lost work time for family

Figure 6 The clinical value compass: An example for adolescent rheumatology. *Source*: Adapted from Ref. 12.

Theory of Knowledge for Change

When we link theory and action we have the potential for learning and building knowledge, which forms the basis for continual improvement. This model is how clinicians work with patients, with a diagnosis as a theory and the tests with some treatment as the action—and then measurement and evaluation together with the patient to see if it was effective. The new knowledge built in that cycle can be used to the next decision. A useful method based on the idea of theory and action is the Plan–Do–Study–Act (PDSA) cycle (Fig. 7) (13,14). How the PDSA model can help us to work on improvement in health care in our own setting is further explored in the second part of this chapter.

An illustration of how the different knowledge systems need to be put together for improvement is the following equation suggested by Batalden and Davidoff (9):

Generalizable scientific evidence + Particular context → Measured performance improvement

The context is in this case is the adolescent rheumatology clinic.

The "+" in the equation represents the variety of methods available for connecting evidence to the particular context, degree of agreement, and priorities for implementing the scientific evidence, while the arrow symbolizes your strategy and execution plan for making improvements in the particular context (Fig. 8).

This equation provides a framework for the second part of this chapter, which provides practical advice on how to gain deeper knowledge of your particular context—the clinical microsystem of adolescent rheumatology. Suggestions on how to get started in your work to improve performance measures and outcomes with and for patients and families is illustrated.

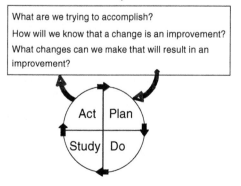

Model for improvement

What are we trying to accomplish?
How will we know that a change is an improvement?
What changes can we make that will result in an improvement?

Act | Plan
Study | Do

Figure 7 The improvement model: The Plan–Do–Study–Act (PDSA) cycle.

Science-based Improvement

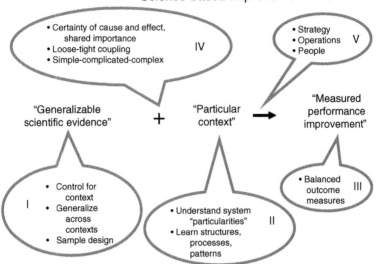

Figure 8 Evidence-based improvement equation. *Source*: Courtesy of Batalden PB, 2006.

THE ADOLESCENT RHEUMATOLOGY CLINICAL MICROSYSTEM

Microsystem Basics

A clinical microsystem is the "place" where patients, families, and health care teams meet. This place can be the rheumatology outpatient practice or an inpatient ward. Based on years of research and field testing, Nelson et al. (4) have promoted and advanced helpful concepts to guide gaining deeper knowledge into the microsystem, which results in improvements and improved measured results for patients, families and health care professionals. The clinical microsystem is defined as "a small group of people who work together on a regular basis to provide care to a discrete subpopulation of patients. It has clinical and business aims, linked processes, and a shared information environment, and it produces performance outcomes. Microsystems evolve over time and are often embedded in larger organizations. They are complex adaptive systems, and as such they must do the primary work associated with core aims, meet the needs of their members, and maintain themselves over time as clinical units" (4). This definition provides a clear understanding of the rheumatology microsystem in the population of adolescents with rheumatic diseases being cared for by an interdisciplinary team of health care professionals.

What do we need to know about our microsystem, the adolescent rheumatology clinic?

How can we help to provide the best possible evidence based care in our microsystem for every patient, every day and how do we know how our system is performing? How can we decrease unwanted variation, improve processes and start to learn from performance and outcome measurements in a "value compass."

To have deeper understanding of the rheumatology clinical microsystem, the anatomy and physiology should be explored.

The anatomy is the structure of the clinical microsystem and includes the following elements as shown in Figure 9 (4).

The 5 Ps: Purpose, Patients, Professionals, Processes, and Patterns

The *purpose* of the clinical microsystem is often stated as the desired outcomes for the patient population being cared for.

The patients (and families) are defined in categories of chronic, acute, preventive, and palliative care needs. Subpopulations of patients can be defined through specific diagnostic groups. Patient satisfaction, top diagnoses, patterns in volumes of patients seen by day, week, month, and season are all explored.

The *professionals* include all members of the care team providing care for the patients including administrative, clerical, support staff, physical and occupational therapists, social workers, nurses and physicians. Increasing knowledge of the professionals includes staff satisfaction data and information, understanding how professionals spend their time in the microsystems and gaining insight if the Professional roles are being optimized as defined by professional education, training and licensure.

The *processes* are the interactions between the patients and professionals intended to meet the needs of the patients. Often these processes of care are not well known or agreed upon by the professionals in the microsystem due to lack of discussions about "how" care is delivered.

The *patterns* are the results of the interactions within the clinical microsystem. What is the leadership like, who talks with whom, what are the measured clinical outcomes for patients, what makes the members of the microsystem proud and how often do they meet as an interdisciplinary team to discuss quality and safety.

A helpful collection of tools for gaining deeper knowledge of the 5Ps is the Clinical Microsystems' "A Path to Healthcare Excellence" (18) (www. clinicalmicrosystems.org) which provides an organized clear path forward to guide the process of deepening your knowledge of your rheumatology clinic or inpatient unit.

Once an interdisciplinary team together begins to learn about the microsystem they work in through the review of anatomy, they can then explore the physiology of their microsystem (Fig. 10) (4).

The physiology of the clinical microsystem includes a group of patients or subpopulation with a need, entering a health care setting with some

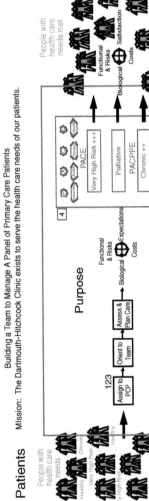
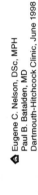
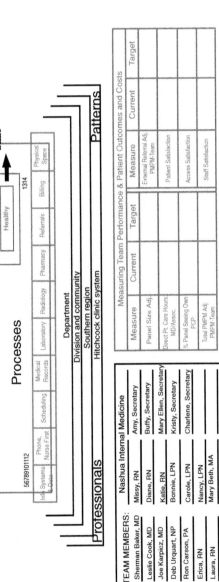

Figure 9 Clinical microsystem anatomy. *Source:* Adapted from Ref. 4.

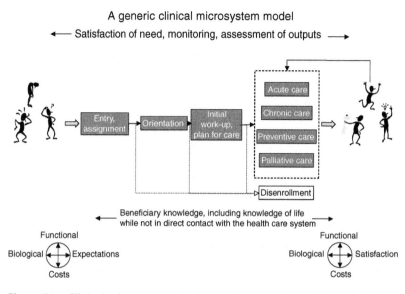

Figure 10 Clinical microsystem physiology. *Source*: Adapted from Ref. 18.

degree of orientation occurring, assessment, diagnosis and plan of care designed with and for the patient with measured result as the patient leaves the microsystem of care. An important note here is to notice in this diagram the balanced measures of the patient(s) that are assessed at the beginning of the physiology of the microsystem and then re-measured after progressing through the microsystem. The balanced measures are framed in the clinical value compass model (4).

The Clinical Value Compass is a framework to use to track measures over time for a single patient or a subpopulation of patients. The Clinical Value Compass informs us if our processes and system improvement is making a measurable improvement for patient outcomes (Fig. 6).

The use of the registry and associated technology in practice supports the clinician and the team in being able to review outcome and process data in real time during a patient encounter to immediately see and track if the plan of care is effective. The registry also provides safety features in the process of care to know medication types and doses.

HOW TO GET STARTED

"Assess, Diagnose, and Treat" Your Rheumatology Microsystem

Assessment

Helpful tools and methods are available including Clinical Micro-systems' "A Path to Health Care Excellence Toolkit: Quality by Design" (www.clinicalmicrosystem.org) to support busy clinical care teams to move forward to assess, diagnose and treat their clinical microsystem.

The path forward includes the following steps (4): "Create an interdisciplinary lead improvement team." This lead improvement team will guide the process of assess, diagnose and "treat" the rheumatology microsystem. The members of the lead improvement team are responsible for exploring the 5Ps of the microsystem using the microsystem workbook tools and worksheets. The members have primary responsibility to "bridge" the knowledge about the microsystem between the lead improvement team and the professional colleagues in the microsystem they are representing through regular multi-media communications. The lead improvement team should hold weekly one hour meetings to explore the data and information of the microsystem to make a diagnosis and design the path forward to make measurable improvements.

Once the 5P assessment is completed, the lead improvement team should identify a "theme" of improvement to focus improvement activities and follow the Dartmouth Microsystem Improvement Curriculum and ramp (4) to design improvements through rapid tests of change to result in measurable improvements.

The Improvement Model is based on the PDSA model popularized by Tom Nolan and his colleagues (Fig. 7) (13). The model for improvement provides a clear path forward for making small rapid tests of change using improvement science. The model poses three questions to be answered when making changes.

1. What are we trying to accomplish?
2. How will we know that a change is an improvement?
3. What changes can we make that will result in an improvement?

Testing good ideas using the PDSA model includes measuring results using run and control charts that track data over time.

The significance of this "path forward" to improve care for adolescents with rheumatic conditions is that the method promotes and encourages interdisciplinary professionals to work and learn together *differently* than they have in the past. Traditional health professional education promotes "silos" of professional practice whereas this method encourages focus on the patient and family and design of interdisciplinary processes of care and improvement. This path forward also invites interdisciplinary teams to engage in making changes that are small and manageable and to avoid the daunting feeling that there is too much to change and the sense of hopelessness. Instead the model gives clear direction and encouragement. Arthur Ashe, professional tennis player reminds us of this in his statement:

"Start where you are, use what you have, do what you can."

Diagnose

Once you have made your assessment of your rheumatology microsystem, you can begin to identify what you do well and what you could improve in your system of care. What is your diagnosis for your microsystem? You may have multiple diagnoses related to ensuring evidence based practice consistently, improving "hand offs" in the rheumatology care process to other microsystems to ensure consistent, reliable care, improved communication within your microsystem or between other microsystems, and improved documentation processes. If you review the improvement ramp (Fig. 11), you will see after identification of a diagnosis or "theme" for improvement based on assessments, you will move through a series of steps to narrow the focus from a broad theme to a specific process. For example, you may learn through your assessment process that rheumatology patients are not regularly evaluated following recommended guidelines for laboratory or uveitis check ups. You may wish to increase the number of communications and follow up with the adolescent. This will be a specific focus.

Treat

An important aspect of "treating" your microsystem diagnosis is to be mindful of "best practice" and review the literature for evidence based practice, best practices, and benchmark with other rheumatology clinics.

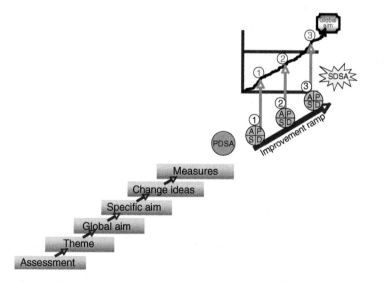

Figure 11 Dartmouth microsystem improvement ramp. *Source*: Adapted from Ref. 4.

Table 3   What Can You Do Tomorrow?

Arrange regular weekly meeting time for your interdisciplinary lead improvement
  team including patients and family members
Start to reflect on your 5Ps
Begin the Dartmouth Microsystem Improvement Curriculum (Quality by Design,
  pp. 119–229)
Review the outcomes of other rheumatology clinics to find the best
Draft a clinical value compass for your adolescent rheumatology patients and begin
  to collect data
Start development of a registry to track quality, outcomes, and to inform your
  practice and learning
Be transparent with your data with public displays of outcomes

Designing processes that eliminate waste and rework is essential in
improvement work. How can we improve outcomes and processes for
patients and families and at the same time improve the workplace for health
care professionals? The Institute for Healthcare Improvement (www.ihi.org)
and clinical microsystems (www.clinicalmicrosystem.org) provide rich
resources to aid the health care professional with current ideas and methods
to make improvements.

When you have identified a change idea to "treat" your microsystem
process, using scientific methodology to test improvements is key. The
Improvement Model, PDSA provides the methodology to test ideas in rapid
fashion in the clinical setting to make improvements and measure results.
The model encourages answering the question "How will we know if change
is an improvement?"

Follow Through

The improvement process done through an interdisciplinary team is a
continuous process. The professionals in the rheumatology microsystem
should commit to long term efforts to improve and sustain processes of care.
Creating a strategic plan for improvement and displaying results and
progress via storyboards and data walls help to keep the microsystem alert
to improvement and progress being made (4). Inviting patients to
interdisciplinary improvement teams is resulting in more focused improvement that patients and families desire- not only what health care
professionals decide should be improved. Patient and family involvement
in clinical improvement remind us of the importance of being patient
centered (www.familycenteredcare.org) (Table 3).

SUMMARY

Through providing the current state of quality in health care including
current recommendations of the Institute of Medicine, we have painted the

picture of the "chasm" that exists in current health care delivery systems. Based on this we have created a path forward for busy health care professionals caring for adolescents with rheumatic conditions to be able to take charge of current practice by convening a group of interdisciplinary professionals to learn new improvement knowledge and skills to improve processes of care. The clinical value compass and the registry provide frameworks for tracking results over time and that improvements are truly seeing whether resulting in better outcomes. It is hoped that identifying the key resources and materials that can help professionals "work on the work" to begin improving both the care we provide and the outcomes desired by adolescents, families, and health care providers. After all, "every system is perfectly designed to get the results it gets." It is up to the members of the rheumatology microsystem to design the system to be the best it can be with the goal of achieving the best care for young people in adolescent rheumatology.

REFERENCES

1. Berwick DM. Escape Fire. Designs for the Future Healthcare. San Fransisco: Jossey-Bass, 2004: 209.
2. Batalden PB, Berwick, DM. Personal conversation, Boston, 1996.
3. Övretveit J. Integrated quality development in public health care. A comparison of six hospitals' quality programs and a practical theory for quality development. Oslo: Norweigan Medical Associations' Publication series, 1999.
4. Nelson EC, Batalden PB, Godfrey MM. Quality by Design. A Clinical Microsystems Approach. San Fransisco: Jossey-Bass, 2007.
5. Manning FJ, Barondess JA, eds. Changing health care systems and rheumatic disease. Institute of Medicine. Washington D.C.:National Academy Press, 1996
6. Institute of Medicine. To Err is Human: Building a Safer Health System. Washington D.C.: National Academy press, 2000.
7. Institute of Medicine. Crossing the quality chiasm: A new health system for the 21st century. Washington DC: National Academy press, 2001.
8. Berwick DM. 15th Annual National Forum on Quality Improvement in Health Care, "My Right Knee" Plenary, New Orleans, Louisiana, December 4, 2003.
9. Batalden PB, Davidoff F. What is "quality improvement" and how can it transform health care? Qual Safety Healthcare 2007; 16(2):2–3.
10. Batalden, PB, Godfrey MM. Personal conversation, Dartmouth, 2006
11. Neuhauser D, McEachern J, Headrick L. Clinical CQI. A Book of Readings. Oakbrook Terrace: Joint Commission, 1995.
12. Nelson EC, Batalden PB, Ryer JC. Clinical Improvement Action Guide. Oakbrook Terrace: Joint Commission, 1998.
13. Langley GI, Nolan KM, Nolan TW, et al. The Improvement Guide. A Practical Approach to Enhancing Organizational Performance. San Francisco: Jossey-Bass, 1996.

14. Batalden PB, Stoltz P. A framework for the continual improvement of health care: building and applying professional and improvement knowledge to test changes in daily work. Joint Commission J Qual Improv 1993; 19(10): 432–52.
15. Deming WE. The new economics—For industry, Government, Education. Cambridge, MA: MIT Press, 1994.
16. Wheeler, DJ. Understanding variation: The key to managing chaos. Knoxville, TN: SPC Press, 1993
17. Brunner HI, Taylor J, Britto MT, et al. Differences in disease outcomes between medicaid and privately insured children: possible health disparities in juvenile rheumatoid arthritis. Arthritis Rheum 2006; 55(3):378–84.
18. Godfrey MM, Nelson EC, Batalden PB. Clinical Microsytems: A Path to Healthcare Excellence. Chicago, IL: American Hospital Association, 2005.

APPENDIX: WEBSITES

www.IHI.org
www.clinicalmicrosystems.org
www.familycenteredcare.org

19

Young People Have the Last Word

Amy Abrams
Coventry, U.K.

David Lewis and Akikur Rahman
Birmingham, U.K.

Toni Neufille
London, U.K.

Heather Clarke
Department of Paediatric and Adolescent Rheumatology, Birmingham Children's Hospital, Birmingham, U.K.

INTRODUCTION

"Nothing about us, without us" is a phrase that is often heard during conversations with young people in today's world. Consultation with and the participation of young people is a vital component of adolescent health service, research, and development (1,2). Their rights "to be heard" are enshrined in Article 12 of the United Nations Convention on the Rights of the Child (3). It asserts that children and young people should be able to express their views on all matters of concern to them and to have those views taken seriously in accordance with their age and maturity (3).

Young people have had few opportunities to evaluate the health services that they receive (4–9). In a multicenter U.K. study, the perceived quality of health care for young people with juvenile idiopathic arthritis (JIA) was significantly lower than they would like (10). It is important that the views of young people are not inferred by either their parents or professionals, who often have discrepant agendas for their health care (6,7,11–13). Marginalizing young people's views may result in practices and policies that have little meaning for those they are intended to benefit. Cleary highlighted is that there are two primary ways patients exert influence over the quality of their health care—exit and voice (14). Children and young people are unlikely to use the power of the former. Health care providers should therefore continue to advocate opportunities and skills training (15) for young people to be able to "give opinions" that are listened to, respected, and, when necessary, acted upon (1).

This chapter has therefore been included to enable the voices of young people to be heard with respect to the adolescent rheumatology professionals and services they would like. Contributions to the chapter were invited via the authorship of this book in addition to previously unpublished anonymous quotes from a series of focus groups held in the United Kingdom to determine the unmet transitional care needs of adolescents with JIA (16).

WHAT DOCTORS AND HEALTH PROFESSIONALS SHOULD KNOW ABOUT YOUNG PEOPLE

> Kids have changed over the years. They don't sit back and listen anymore. If there is a chance for their point to be heard, they will say it. Teenagers like to have fun and be childish at times, but we do like to be treated as adults and given choices, and not have choices made for us.
>
> Katie, 15 years (U.K.)

> Doctors and health professionals should know that young people like people to talk to them. They should understand that it's not the parents who have the condition; it is the young person's and that who the doctors should be discussing it with.
>
> Laura, 17 years (U.K.)

> We do not want to be treated different to any other young person.
>
> Ryan, 12 years (U.K.)

> Doctors and health professionals should know that young people want to enjoy their teenage years as much as possible. We want independence, and we can make our own choices and have our own opinions. We are becoming adults and have the opportunities to make something of our future lives.
>
> Amy, 15 years (U.K.)

> Many doctors and health care professionals just cannot see the difference between a ten-year-old and a sixteen-year-old.

However, they should know that young people of all ages have different needs and therefore require helpful support and advice from their rheumatology team. Healthcare professionals should appreciate that ten-year-olds, may not require the same support and advice as fifteen-year-olds who are going through a difficult stage in their lives because of several reasons, not just their illness.

Doctors and other health care professionals should know that, a sixteen-year-old for who has juvenile arthritis, life can sometimes be hell. Not always, but there are times when I am immobile, housebound and restricted to the same people, day in day out. As well as affecting my general well-being, it also affects my social life, which is not good.

Akikur, 16 years (U.K.)

Other doctors must understand that rheumatology doctors are well qualified and equipped for their job of looking after care of teenagers with lupus. Teenagers with lupus need a doctor who can explain clearly what is happening and going to happen. Young people with lupus need a doctor as well as a friend.

Samiyya, 16 years (U.K.)

Doctors and health professionals should know what it's like to be a kid. It would help them get better in the best way without trying to take away things we like.

Hannah, 14 years (U.K.)

The main aspect that they need to be aware of is that the coping with a disease such as juvenile arthritis is only half of the battle. Like all other young people of a similar age, arthritis or rheumatic sufferers have to deal with the growing up issues that face everyone. Doctors and health professionals should be experienced or be able to deal with aspects of growing up, education, social relationships, being independent and getting jobs. This, in turn, will help and benefit the young person if the health professionals have prior knowledge and are able to communicate effectively with the patient.

David, 23 years (U.K.)

I really don't like being treated as my "parents' child." I find people who respect me for who I am so much easier to get on with.

Matthew, 16 years (U.K.)

WHAT DOCTORS AND HEALTH PROFESSIONALS SHOULD KNOW ABOUT WHAT IT IS LIKE TO BE A YOUNG PERSON LIVING WITH A CHRONIC RHEUMATIC CONDITION

You can never really know what it's like. You can describe the pain you go through, but they don't know how bad it is until they have the illness themselves. It makes you sad and angry inside. I became frustrated and very angry. When I'm out with friends and they are running about having fun, I know that I can't join them physically because I'm just too tired. Some days can be worse than others. I can wake up full of energy, but lose it just as easily, and just can't be bothered to even move on other days. You get annoyed with people always saying you're putting it on—all the tiredness and people treating you differently because of your illness—when all you want is to be treated like everyone else. Having this illness makes doing things I love like swimming, running or being out with friends harder, so you have to do your best and hope it's good enough. We are the ones stuck with the illness—we had no choice, but we just struggle on and enjoy each day as it comes.

Katie, 15 years (U.K.)

Arthritis does not restrict the freedom of the young person's mind. We young people don't want to be treated any differently to those young people who are more fortunate. Living with juvenile arthritis is not easy. I try to get involved with as many things as possible so not to get left out of things. Being at school with arthritis is quite daunting but you have to go on as normal. Arthritis does not get in the way of a good education. Having arthritis means I have restricted movements and find it hard to get around school, especially with lots of students pushing and shoving trying to get out of one door. Having friends around, you feel more safe, friends also help to take your mind off things. I would like to be more independent and sometimes friends can be a little too overprotective of you, but it's nice to know they care and will always be there for you when you need them. Living with arthritis is hard but you just have to get on with it.

Amy, 15 years (U.K.)

Physicians and other health professionals should know that suffering from JIA not only involves joints but the whole person: pain, hopelessness and anxiety. Frequently I am the centre of attention—at home, with my parents, as well as at school. However, I feel like a dark horse at the same time. Take, for instance, dancing, inline, basketball or sports at school, where I've got to sit at the side-line because of my illness. This hurts! Swimming and cycling are the remaining choices—but they aren't cool any more are they? My first boyfriend, my first love, left me because of JIA, too. He wouldn't accept that I have to be an inpatient at a special clinic for several weeks each year.

Anxiety is always a big point. Fears concerning my personal future. Will I get a healthy baby even though I took all that medicine for years, for instance? Or will I end up sitting in a wheelchair? Numerous treatment options have been started and stopped. But nobody has answered my question—what will the final outcome be?

When I feel like a roller coaster, I am glad about the constant support from my parents as well as from my girlfriends. That there is somebody to lean on and to be comforted. Hopefully, other young people with peers will experience this in the same way. Health professionals should not only be able to listen. Apart from medical expertise it is important to maintain a holistic review. This is nicely put in a verse: "What could be more important than knowledge? asked the brain. "Feelings and intuition" answered the heart.

Katherina, 15 years (Germany)

I think the doctors should know that not everyone knows the long medical words. I also think doctors shouldn't be afraid to tell kids exactly what's wrong. I think doctors should know that we are still normal people.

Emma, 10 years (U.S.A.)

Doctors and health professionals should know that you don't like jokes about your height *every time* you see them! They should know that in their examinations if they say "move your leg" and "does this hurt?" it definitely will if you have arthritis.

Ellen, 14 years (U.K.)

Doctors should know that it is difficult being a teenager and then having an illness just tops it up. People (most) always degrade teenagers, which I feel they should not do. Teenagers are not children and they know what is what. I do feel that the majority of teenagers do take things to extremes, meaning they make mountains out of molehills, though, when it comes down to treatment, patients try to work with doctors to decide a suitable way.

Most doctors may know that first year of being diagnosed is the hardest, it is difficult for everything to sink in, the hospital visits, etc. Talking and having a close bonding relationship should be achieved by both the doctor and patient. Talking things over is always best.

Samiyya, 16 years (U.K.)

Doctors should know that it's hard to have the disease in everyday life because you are different from other children. So if you get supported enough you can get through it and feel normal again.

Hannah, 14 years (U.S.A.)

They should know our feelings: frustrated, angry, sad, tired, aching, fed-up, upset.

Ryan, 12 years (U.K.)

The main factor is the opinion of "being different." Although everyone is different in some way, in my opinion this is the major factor that results from suffering with arthritis during the growing up years. It can come as a shock to someone to be diagnosed with arthritis in these years, especially if they have previously been fit and active. The unpredictable nature of arthritis is somewhat difficult to overcome and, indeed, explain to others. This means tasks that are easy on some days, become mammoth tasks the next and is an important aspect that needs to be understood by all people, especially health professionals.

David, 23 years (U.K.)

I like a doctor who shows understanding and patience for the trial a young arthritic has to endure, appreciating the intense pain and disruption of life that comes with the disease.

Matthew, 16 years (U.K.)

I think health professionals should know what illness the young person has had and listen to what the patient has to say and how they feel, besides just talking to the patient. The best way to cope and help yourself on a daily basis and try not to get too down hearted and feeling that medication is not helping you.

Jodie, 12 years (U.K.)

My parents prolonged my recovery time. Every time I have a flare I now try not to tell them because they do my head in! When they do eventually find out, I either get treated like a four-year-old or an elderly person—they wrap me up in cotton wool.

Doctors could improve this situation by talking directly to us and involving us in our treatment and by allowing us to make decisions for ourselves.

Akikur, 16 years (U.K.)

I am 16 years old and have had arthritis since I was 14. The pain of my arthritis sometimes restricts me from doing things. My joints swell and I have difficulty in moving. The pain hurts so much that sometimes I have to be carried upstairs.

As a 16-year-old my parents do help me sometimes, but at times parents get very over protective and don't really know they are doing it. When I have flare-ups I sometimes tell them and sometimes not because they tell me to stay in the house, and I really don't want to. Just because I have arthritis, it does not stop me from having a social life.

Doctors sometimes treat you as a child—like the way doctors talk to your parents and not you—but I feel we need to be treated as adults. Since the age of 15, I have been going to clinic on my own so doctors have no choice but to speak to me.

Lesley-Anne, 16 years (U.K.)

Living with juvenile arthritis is very hard because some people don't understand that you're still the same person as you were, it's just that sometimes you struggle to get around. You also get people saying that they totally understand because they have it too, but what they do not understand is that it's not the same as they are a lot older than you are and it's a different type of arthritis to theirs.

Laura, 17 years (U.K.)

Growing Up ... and Going Out

I'd just like to be a normal teenager again ... just getting out with the girls. You can't go to parties.

You can't get anywhere on your own when you're a teenager.

It's very difficult having a social life and to stay with all your mates, to do what they want to do and do what you want to do at the same time. There's, like, clubs I can't go to, or go and talk to boys or do anything stupid. I can't even dance with my mates because I'm in agony. It's really depressing to deal with, as well as difficult.

It's about confidence, going out with other people, and there are things that you think you can't do, but you can do. But you just don't have the information or mobility to do them.

Growing Up ... as Seen by Other People

I just feel like people are always looking at us—if I'm in a wheelchair and if I'm wearing my neck brace. I mean I should use the wheelchair more than I do really, but I'll not use it because I'm afraid that I look different. People look at us differently and I think that's hard, especially for teenagers.

Older people see it as an old person's disease. They don't believe that young people can suffer with it, and that we can have problems or pain like they can.

People don't like to sit next to you because they think they're going to catch it and stuff.

If you haven't got like a big bandage on or something like that, they don't realize the pain.

People think now that I've got quite an attitude problem because I'm so used to having to fight for stuff.

They sort of wrapped me in cotton wool. I always remember I wasn't allowed to go on the school trip, because my physiotherapist and doctor said I was too delicate.

The trouble is ... the thing is when they say you can't do something, it's wrong. They should let you go, because we have probably all found our limitations anyway. It's better finding them for ourselves. Everybody finds their own limitations, so why not let the kids do the same thing.

Growing Up ... Looking After Yourself

It does get very embarrassing, especially if you're stuck in the bath and you can't get out. You just get embarrassed, especially if your parents are there, and you don't want your parents to pick you up out of the bath. You don't want your parents taking you to the toilet. It's embarrassing.

Because I've got problems with my shoulder as well, so I have to choose tops which I can get on easily, and they're not always the ones I like, but I find the others hard to get on.

I couldn't do simple things like put my socks on and things like that, and it was only when I came into hospital that I realized—this occupational therapist came round, and she said you can get gadgets that do this and that. They don't tell you that either, so you have to rely on, like, your mom, dad or a friend to do things. Like your shoelace comes undone, and you can't do it up, so you have to ask your friend to do it.

I find it hard to buy shoes because one of my feet is bigger than the other, so it's really hard to buy a pair of shoes that fit both feet.

Well, I mean, the most dreaded thing is of course starting periods, how do you go on with that when you can't even pull your own knickers down? How can you manage to put your pad on or use a tampon? Would you want your mom doing that?

It would be very useful if somebody sat there saying you can drive.

Growing Up ... At School

I just think teachers need to know more about it. They don't really know.

They [teachers] just sort of think it's alright just give you some painkillers or something or just send you home, but they don't actually talk to you about it or anything you know.

My PE teacher makes me do things I don't want to do, because it hurts, and she hasn't listened to me and let me do what I want. She makes me do things that ache my leg.

I was at was a fairly big school and they'd got no downstairs classrooms.... Downstairs were all the gyms, the swimming pool, offices, assembly halls, that sort of thing and the most they could do was clear out a storeroom for me. That was no good, so I had a bit of tuition at home and then I was sent to a unit, right across town. It was like for naughty boys and girls. It was where all the waggers and expelled kids got sent to. I was chucked in with them.

Well my school's quite big, so it's hard to get about it, but you've got to go from one room to another, which are always quite far apart, a lot of stairs and things—it's hard to get up and downstairs all the time.

It was always like the big thing you came to exams because you're writing slow. I constantly had to write in capitals. I couldn't write joined up. It was awkward.

I got bullied very badly which led me to have quite bad mental problems. I had a nervous breakdown and so I was moved to a school for disabled children.

I was moved to a school for disabled children and so it was just a natural course that when you came to the end of your schooling years you were advised as to disabled colleges for disabled people, ... They seem to go more on the negative side of things rather than positive ... . You've got to go to a college for disabled people because the mainstream cannot cope with you—not that you can't cope with mainstream, mainstream cannot cope with you. So I went to a residential college for disabled children and lived there for 2 years in the college... . I couldn't cope with them, and they couldn't cope with me because they were used to people with cerebral palsy and spina bifida and all those sorts of things which have a set course. And so they couldn't cope with a fluctuating disability, and because it caused so many problems and I'd been told for so many years that mainstream couldn't cope with me— then a disabled college couldn't cope with me—I was thinking "Well nobody can cope with me then. What do I do?"

Growing Up ... into the World of Work

You've got to have the confidence. I mean ... I went to see the careers officer, and the careers officer sat there and said "What do you want to do?" I said "I want to be a singer ... ," "Oh be realistic and grow up. All you can do is work in an office. You can be an office clerk and that's it," and so that's what I trained for, but last year I actually had my first professional booking and I got paid £60.00 for three minutes work you know.

I wanted to be a teacher. I was told I couldn't be a teacher because I couldn't stand up all day in front of a class. Then I talked about being a receptionist, things like that. I couldn't do that because of typing on the keypads all day would make my fingers flare up. Everything you came up with, basically, an obstacle was put in front of you.

Yes. I always put "in remission," I always put I haven't had any problems for years. If I'd put I was in a wheelchair, they wouldn't have given me the interview.

I mean I was basically looking at jobs, and I was talking to my parents about it, and they were thinking, you can't do this because you can't stand up too long, you can't stand up too long because your back'll start hurting or your legs'll start flaring up, and in the end I just totally defied it. I mean I went to hairdressing college. I'm a fully qualified hairdresser now.

Growing Up ... Meeting Someone Special!

It's hard, especially, like, as you get older and you start getting into relationships. That's always hard because you're like "shall I tell the person straightaway" because what happens?—I'm good now, but what happens in a few months, I might have a little bit of a bang, I might fall over—will it come back?—and then having to try and explain that.

When you are at the hospital, the boyfriend does get shoved out the way. But it's like now. I want him here. He's in my life. He looks after me. He needs to know, so it was really difficult the first couple of times he came with me, they weren't going to tell him what was wrong with me.

When I was 12 they were going to put me on a drug that would make me sterile. They didn't tell me about it. They took my mom into the office and said, "We want to give him this." She said "Does it make him sterile? Go and ask him."

One big issue that comes up with people—but they don't talk about it, and it's never dealt with, and people are too embarrassed to ask doctors about it—is the problem with sex, and either they don't want to ask because they're embarrassed or they think that they're too young and they shouldn't be—and it's all different issues to do with that. I mean, not only just the problems of the arthritis itself, the pain and things like that, I've never been spoken to at all about, and I didn't realize that there would be a problem, I hadn't even thought about it because I'm on such high doses of steroids and I'm on them all the time. I'm constantly suffering with thrush. Nobody ever, ever discusses that. Nobody says "well you could do this to help or you could do that." I mean what do you do when it's just too painful or you start passing it on to your partner, because you've got it so bad that ... .

All I've been told is if and when I get pregnant, there's a good chance that my hips and my leg joints would flare up because of the extra weight to carry. That's it, that's all I've been told. When I think about the tablets I'm on, whether you can actually still take them when you're pregnant, and stuff like that, I don't know.

WHAT WOULD YOUNG PEOPLE HAVE LIKED THEIR RHEUMATOLOGIST (OR A RHEUMATOLOGY TEAM MEMBER) TO HAVE TOLD THEM WHEN THEY WERE FIRST DIAGNOSED?

The total truth.

Ryan, 12 years (U.K.)

Oh, I'm dreadfully sorry, we've made a mistake, you don't have arthritis. Oh well, you can go home.

Ellen, 14 years (U.K.)

To be honest, the first thing that I would have liked a rheumatologist to say to me when I was first diagnosed in, "I'm only kidding. There's nothing the matter, take these tablets, and the tiredness, lack of eating, hair loss, rash and other symptoms will go and you will be normal again.

Katie, 15 years (U.K.)

I would have liked my rheumatologist to tell me that there are other kids that have the disease that are just like me.

Hannah, 14 years (U.K.)

I would have liked my doctor to have known that I am shy and sometimes afraid to ask questions.

Emma, 10 years (U.S.A.)

Since I was diagnosed at a very young age I cannot remember what my specialist told me and my parents. If I had been diagnosed with juvenile arthritis at an older age, I would have liked to have been told exactly what my disease was about and how would it affect me and my family and my future. And what could I do to make my life a little more comfortable.

Amy, 15 years (U.K.)

I would have liked him or her to be 100% straight with me. Why hide anything from me? It'll only hurt me more later.

Matthew, 16 years (U.K.)

When I was first diagnosed, I was very young, so it is hard for me to say what they should have told me because I probably would not have understood. However, when I was at an age where I did understand, it might be that they assumed I already knew.

Laura, 17 years (U.K.)

They need to explain it, right from the moment it's diagnosed. This is what it is, this is what can happen, and they need to do it in simpler terms.

We really need an informed medical team, because when I first got diagnosed, I was told that I was going to grow out of it when I was 18. So I hung on to the hope of growing out of it when I was 18.

There was no explanations as to why you should be doing that. It's all very well being told you should be doing this, you should be doing that, but why? They don't tell us enough about why we should be doing it.

I would have liked to have talked to someone who'd had arthritis, tried to get a job, and knew how to work round it.

I was just concerned that I couldn't hold a pint with one hand and I had to use two. Solution? Just stick to bottles.

You need encouragement, but sometimes people can be negative, saying "well I don't think you'll be able to do this." But until you actually try it, you're not going to know.

WHAT DO YOUNG PEOPLE THINK IS DIFFERENT ABOUT THE WAY HEALTH PROFESSIONALS LOOK AFTER A YOUNG PERSON WITH A CHRONIC RHEUMATIC CONDITION COMPARED TO A YOUNGER CHILD OR AN ADULT?

Doctors [who look after young people] ask "How have you been?" and if you aren't confident talking to doctors and say, "Alright," they still ask you if your joints are aching, have you any headaches lately? But if you go to an adult doctor, and they ask "How have you been lately?" and you say "Alright," they don't ask you all those questions. They say "Ok then, see you in 6 months," and you go. I think the adult doctors are probably much stricter and not as kind compared to the other doctors, who probably have a better sense of humor.

Katie, 15 years (U.K.)

I think my family is a little too over-protective of me sometimes, which has its advantages and disadvantages. I do need a little more looking after than a young person without a chronic condition, and having a family around me makes me feel more secure and happy. Although, when you are approaching adult age, you need more independence, and sometimes it's hard for my family to see this. Health professionals treat me with care and respect. I need to feel secure around them, like with my family. Doctors see that I am becoming an adult and give me help and advice to make my future as easy as possible.

Amy, 15 years (U.K.)

It is different because they treat you in a different manner. They are nice to you and make you special because of how you are, but they don't patronize you like they would if you were younger.

Hannah, 14 years (U.K.)

I think younger kids really might not understand what is happening very well and might be really afraid. Older kids can understand more and are able to know more.

Emma, 10 years (U.S.A.)

They treat us more like adults and explain options and choices to us.

Ryan, 12 years (U.K.)

When you are younger—aged 10–19 years—these in my opinion are the "learning years." Clinic consultations are conducted, with many members of the medical team and your parents and asking the questions making the decisions for you, and this, as you can imagine, can seem overwhelming to the patient at this stage. However, you do learn from this, and then as you grow older you can make the decisions and ask the questions for yourself. Then, when you are feeling able, you are encouraged to attend the clinic on your own, which enables you to build a trusting relationship with the health professionals and creates a more informal atmosphere, which in turn helps the patient to relax and trust the professionals.

David, 23 years (U.K.)

I think it is important to remember that the teenage years are the worst possible time for someone to obtain arthritis, so patience and understanding are crucial.

Matthew, 16 years (U.K.)

A doctor can listen to a 10- to 19-year-old, what they have to say and how they feel towards the treatment. They are the ones who can write down and ask questions.

Jodie, 12 years (U.K.)

WHAT MAKES FOR A GOOD RHEUMATOLOGY CLINIC FOR YOUNG PEOPLE AGED 10 TO 19 YEARS—FROM THEIR PERSPECTIVE

Clinics need to be a places where you can learn about your condition and how you can make living with your condition as easily and comfortably as possible. The people in the clinic need to treat young people with respect and with good manners. When you leave a clinic you should feel you have learned something new about your condition. I also feel that clinics should give information on work for young people with a chronic condition.

Amy, 15 years (U.K.)

Lot's of fun, games, fast service, magazines, more teen books—and a water cooler wouldn't be bad either!"

Ellen, 14 years (U.K.)

A good rheumatology clinic would have people who would make you feel welcome and make you laugh so you're not so stressed.

Hannah, 14 years (U.K.)

A good clinic has friendly people, light colors, cool magazines and nice doctors.

Emma, 10 years (U.S.A.)

All the people that help us—care for us. They try to treat us like adults even when we want to cry or shout.

Ryan, 12 years (U.K.)

The essential ingredient in any clinic is to meet others who are similar to you that you can talk to. This in turn results in a more confident approach to going to clinic as supposed to fear. Also, the waiting areas need to be more adult or young person orientated as supposed to being geared to children and people of an older generation. Also, a multidisciplinary team that can provide the close interaction and support young people need is crucial. Probably the most important of all though is that clinic consultation times need to be longer so that the patient doesn't feel rushed. If this is achieved, then a much more relaxed informal, organized and well-structured clinic will benefit all young people.

David, 23 years (U.K.)

I would enjoy a clinic that involved meeting fellow arthritics, a social and accommodating clinic, yet efficient.

Matthew, 16 years (U.K.)

The doctors looking after me are very different from the ones looking after older people with rheumatic conditions. They sit down at the beginning of the appointment and ask how you are. They have a general chat with you, which makes me feel more at ease whereas in an adult clinic they go straight into what seems to be the problem at the moment, then what they ask can do to help or make me feel better. I think the Rheumatology clinic is good for young people because it makes them feel more of an adult because it's not called a children's clinic, but also as they get older it helps them to prepare for when they move to an adult clinic.

Laura, 17 years (U.K.)

Since the introduction of the adolescent clinic, life in general has improved for me. I have met other young people who are in the same situation as I am, which has provided me with a network of people other than my parents I can depend on for support and advice.

In the past three years I have been attending the adolescent clinic here. I see more sympathetic doctors and other health care professionals who understand the difference between a ten-year-old and a fifteen-year-old.

I believe that the Adolescent Clinic could develop its services in the following ways:

- Offer careers advice
- Offer counselling to the parents of patients
- Provide teaching of medical student doctors and other health care professionals
- Have appointments with a group of young people that I am familiar with and then rotate them around. This provides the opportunity to improve young people's social life.

Akikur, 16 years (U.K.)

In the adolescent clinic, I have met some other people with the same problem. Also, throughout the hospital there are various projects taking place where you can meet other adolescents with different problems. I believe that these projects are fantastic way to get to know people, and this makes my social life better so I don't have to stay in the house. Adolescent clinics should take place in every hospital and in every department where there are adolescents.

Lesley-Anne, 16 years (U.K.)

The whole team has to be able to work together, and the patients have to work with the doctors by telling them what's wrong or else the doctors can't help. The doctors should listen to the patients' ideas, and the patients should listen to the doctors' because the doctors' ideas normally help make people feel better. The patients have to feel able to trust the doctors with the private stuff they tell them, and the patients have to trust the medical advice. Everyone has to have respect for each other. The doctors all need to have a good sense of humor, and not be strict and boring.

Katie, 15 years (U.K.)

It's all for babies and kids, it's all like teddies all over the wall, and when you get to your teens, you don't want to see the teddies and rattles and dolls.

Just really simple things like, you know, because ... if we had magazines, we could actually read them. That makes you feel a bit more at ease.

COMMUNICATION WITH HEALTH PROFESSIONALS— THE YOUNG PERSON'S PERSPECTIVE

You want to say all these things, but then you stop yourself and you think you're just a teenager.

They think that ... you won't understand what it means or how it'll work, but you do really; you just need a little more information sometimes.

Some of the medical terms, like these quite big long posh words .... I didn't know what they meant. I didn't understand. I didn't want to ask.

They do talk way over your head.

They talk at you.

He talks down to you, well with me anyway. He never seemed to realize that I had grown up. He thought I was still a child.

Your options should be discussed as well in front of you with your parents... not while you're getting dressed in the treatment room.

You get really fed up with other people making the decisions because it is your body, and you want a say in it.

Somewhere, the parents can't butt in. How many people just sit there and their parents just like go off, and it's like about them, excuse me, this is about me thank you very much.

I don't know why they ask parents, it isn't parents that have got the arthritis.

Sometimes it's better when I'm by myself. I just speak up more.

You'd feel a little bit more independent, this is good because it is my body and my arthritis, and I'm talking about it and you haven't got your parents there all the time.

My parents are quite cool. They ask "Do you want us to come in?" and I say no I'd rather go in by myself, because I feel that I achieve more by going in and talking to him, if they're there, he (the doctor) just ignores me and talks to them, and I just come out and don't feel any thing has been achieved.

If you've been with the same person, a long time, you get a little bit of attention, and you do ask more questions. But... when you're jumping from pillar to post—like I was seen by 6 doctors in one year—then I just didn't want to talk to them, but if you stay at the same doctor you tend to get a bit closer, to open up.

LAST YEAR I GOT ARTHRITIS

Last year I got Arthritis
Some people in my school
They thought it was contagious
I told them it wasn't
They took it quite cool

I was scared they wouldn't
But to think that
I was a fool
Because they're my friends
They should understand
That the doctors didn't tell me
I would get swelling in my hands
I would've liked my mum to be
As helped as children, just like me
But the health professionals
They help children more than adults
My mum is very poorly as well as me
But, of course I got more help
Than my mum

When I was first diagnosed
I had to stay in hospital
I was disappointed
Not only because I had Arthritis
But, they didn't have any good toys
They just had them for younger girls and boys.

Jennifer, 10 years (U.K.)

GROWING UP AND MOVING ON

Growing up and moving on
All the kids' things will be gone
You get annoyed with people who joke
And wish that they will choke

When you have an illness that lasts for long
You don't feel like singing a happy song

All your friends can do what hobbies they want
And you sit inside your house and don't

Hospitals have lots of memories
Like going to a special shoe sole place
And they say "try these on"

Or when you've been in an operation
Sometimes you get a lot of frustration

Afterwards mum would give me plenty of treats
Like coke, chocolate and fruity sweets

The staff are always very nice
But they have to be as quiet as mice

The things that make a clinic good
Are pink rooms that put girls
In a better mood

Noora, 11 years (U.K.)

ARTHRITIS IS MEAN

Arthritis is mean
Arthritis is cruel
I didn't like it
But I got to miss school

How long you are in for you do not know
You need to drink and eat to keep you on the go
You may not want to but you have to
The doctors and nurses will help you.

They ask questions, it's really boring
Soon they'll have you snoring and snoring
When they take blood it seems mean
But doctors are really keen.
When you feel better
And can take off your own sweater
Avoid the cannula, it's not nice
It busts your hopes by a real slice

After that it will feel nicer
When they've taken out the slicer
After that you can go home
And leave the hospital dome

James, 10 years (U.K.)

WE ARE YOUTHS WITH A DISABILITY NOT
A DISABLED YOUTH

Life can be hard *sometimes* for all the youth
But we have *always* to take the rough with the smooth

I was only three when I became ill
So mum and dad took the bitter pill

Speak *to* us so we know you care
Not *about* us as if we're not there

No building bricks, dolls or toys
Just things that matter to young girls or boys

Sophie, 16 years (U.K.)

SUMMARY

"Listening to" the written "voices" of the young contributors in this chapter makes it is clear that they want their voices and opinions to be heard and to be active participants in their care. In the clinical setting they want professionals who understand about their diagnosis and what it is like to be a young person living with a chronic condition. Professionals need to acknowledge the challenges involved in balancing life with a chronic condition with life as an adolescent in the 21st century. Young people want to be treated with respect, to take a lead their consultations and be fully informed. Their words echo research findings in which their peers (adolescents with JIA) considered knowledgeable and honest staff as best practice in transitional care provision (10). The wealth of expertise of these young people should also be recognized in future service development and multidisciplinary medical education. A model of good practice in this area is the Youth Health Talk Project developed by the University of Oxford (www.youthhealthtalk.org). As one young participant in an adolescent rheumatology research project stated: "It's not about arthritis is it? It's about living with it." (16).

REFERENCES

1. Royal College of Paediatrics and Child health. Coming out of the shadows. A strategy to promote participation of children and young people in RCPCH activity (June 2005) www.rcpch.ac.uk
2. Department of Health. You're welcome quality criteria. Making health services young people friendly. October, 2005 (www.dh.gov.uk).
3. United Nations. Convention on the rights of the child. Geneva: United Nations; 1989.
4. Aasland A, Flato B, Vandvik IH. Patient and parent experiences with health care services in pediatric rheumatology. Scand J Rheumatol 1998; 27:265–72.

5. Chesney M, Lindeke L, Johnson L, Jukkala A, Lynch S. Comparison of child and parents satisfaction ratings of ambulatory pediatric subspecialty care. J Pediatr Health Care 2005; 19:221–9.

6. Jacobson LD, Wilkinson CE, Pill RM, Hackett PMW. Communication between teenagers and British general practitioners: a preliminary study of the teenage perspective. Ambulatory Child Health 1996; 1:291–301.

7. Litt IF. Satisfaction with health care. The adolescent perspective. J Adolesc Health 1998; 23:59–60.

8. Margaret ND, Clark TA, Warden CR, Magnusson AR, Hedges JR. Patient satisfaction in the emergency department–a survey of pediatric patients and their parents. Acad Emerg Med 2002; 9:1379–88.

9. Vandvik IH, Hoyeraal HM, Fagertun H. The first stay in a pediatric rheumatology Ward. Associations between parent satisfaction and disease and psychosocial factors. Scand J Rheum 1990; 19:216–22.

10. Shaw KL, Southwood TR, McDonagh JE. Young People's satisfaction of transitional care in adolescent rheumatology in the UK. Child Care Health Dev 2007; 33:368–79.

11. Waters E, Stewart-Brown S, Fitzpatrick R. Agreement between adolescent self-report and parent reports of health and well-being: results of an epidemiological study. Child Care Health Dev 2003; 29:501–9.

12. Ennett ST, DeVellis BM, Earp JA, Kredich D, Warren RW, Wilhelm CL. Disease experience and psychosocial adjustment in children with juvenile rheumatoid arthritis: children's versus mothers' reports. J Pediatr Psychol 1991; 16:557–68.

13. Shaw KL, Southwood TR, McDonagh JE. Growing up and moving on in Rheumatology: parents as proxies of adolescents with Juvenile Idiopathic Arthritis. Arthritis Care Res 2006; 55(2):189–98.

14. Cleary PD. The increasing importance of patient surveys. Now that sound methods exist, patient surveys can facilitate improvement. Br Med J 1999; 319: 720–1.

15. Beresford B, Sloper P. Chronically ill adolescents' experiences of communicating with doctors: a qualitative study. J Adolesc Health 2003; 33:172–9.

16. Shaw KL, Southwood TR, McDonagh JE. Users' perspectives of transitional care for adolescents with juvenile idiopathic arthritis. Rheumatology 2004; 43:770–8.

Index

t = location of tables.
f = location of figures.